Rates of autoimmune diagnosis have been rising dramatically and so too has interest in the Autoimmune Protocol (AIP), a science-backed dietary and lifestyle program. Feedback from thousands of practitioners and millions of patients, as well as new research, has indicated that AIP needs an update: Many patients see results before extensive dietary eliminations. In *The New Autoimmune Protocol,* leading AIP authority Mickey Trescott not only explains the basics of autoimmune disease and new medical research but also provides a new addition to the protocol: Modified AIP Elimination, which makes relief achievable by many more autoimmune sufferers.

The New Autoimmune Protocol includes detailed meal plans and more than seventy AIP-friendly recipes, divided into two essential sections:

- Core AIP Recipes & Meal Plans: the standard AIP elimination protocol (excluding all grains, gluten, dairy, legumes, nightshades, processed vegetable oils, nuts and nut oils, seeds and seed oils, alcohol, and processed food chemicals)
- Modified AIP Recipes & Meal Plans: the new AIP elimination protocol, which is less restricted and now includes ghee, rice, pseudo-grains, legumes (except soy), and seeds

This book arms you with flexible meal plans, delicious recipes, and the knowledge you need to regain your vitality, whether you decide on Core or Modified AIP.

The New Autoimmune Protocol

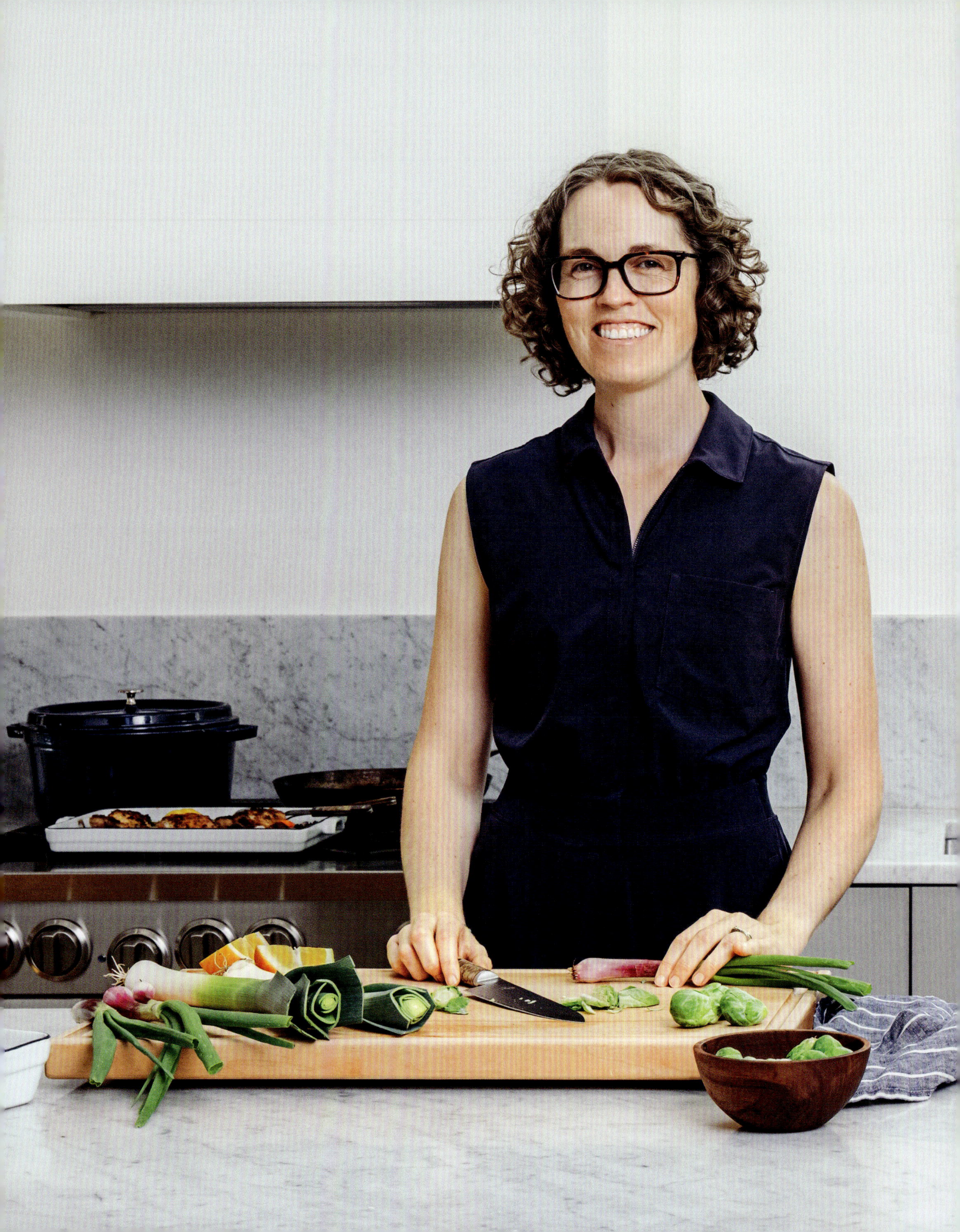

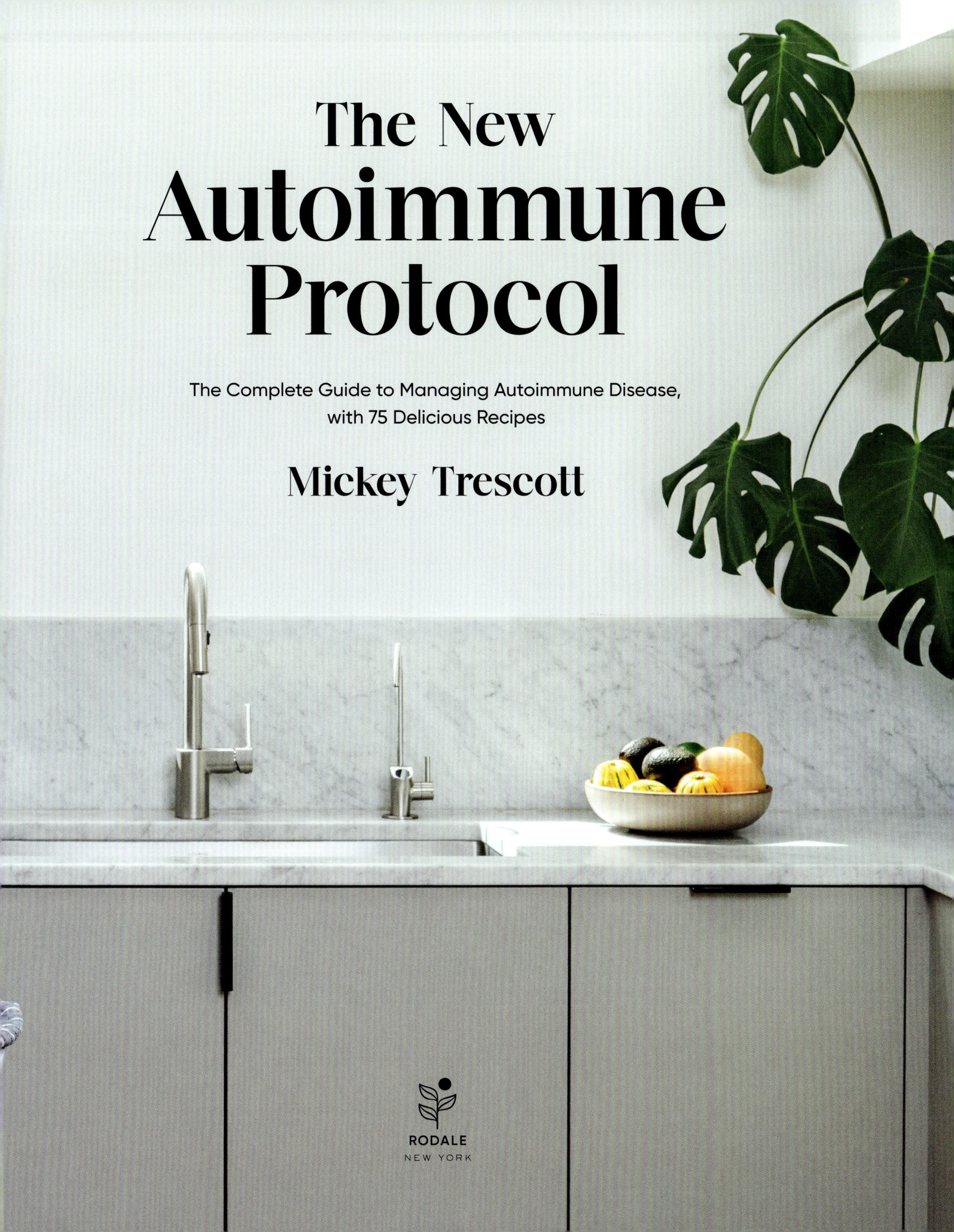

The New Autoimmune Protocol

The Complete Guide to Managing Autoimmune Disease, with 75 Delicious Recipes

Mickey Trescott

RODALE
NEW YORK

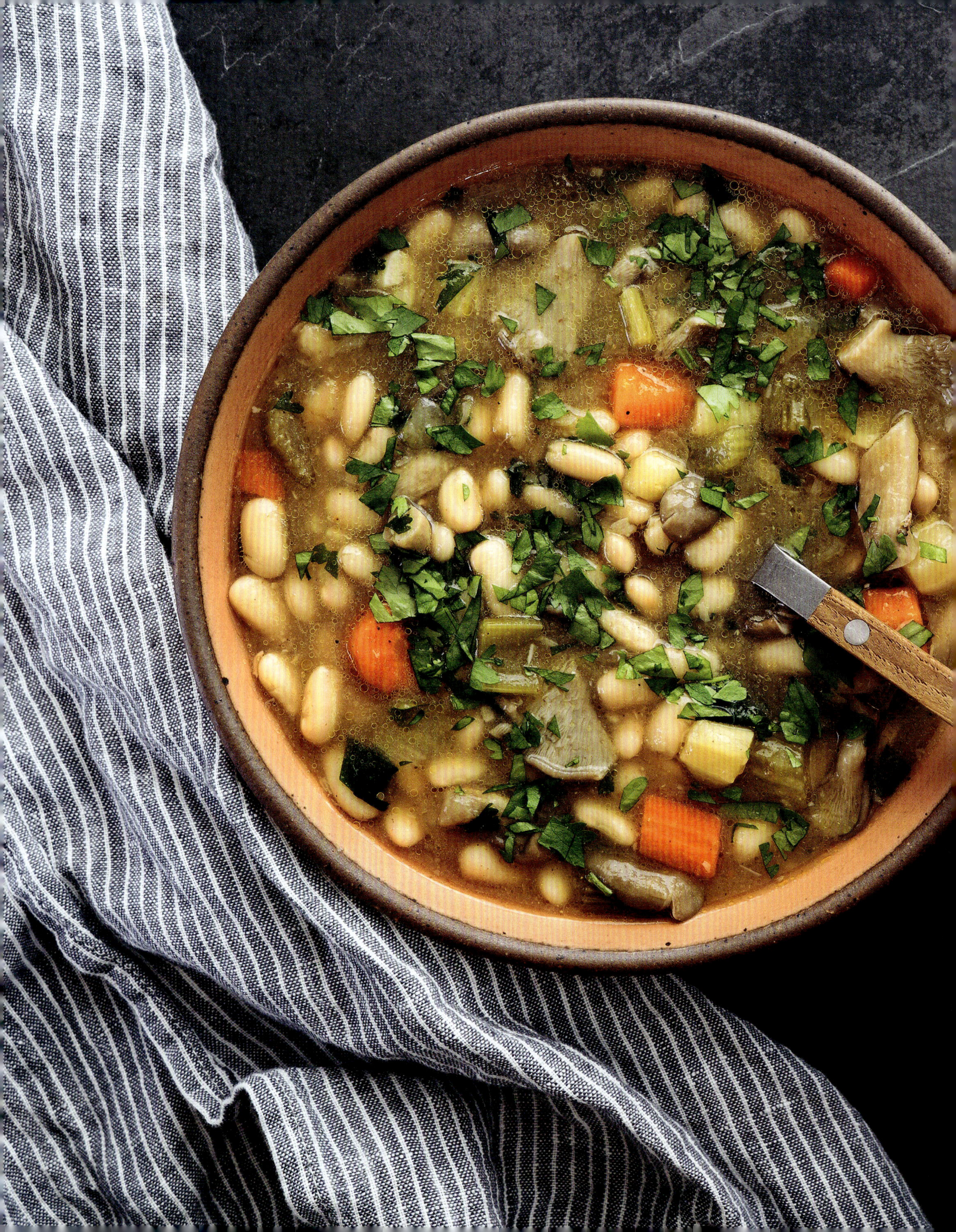

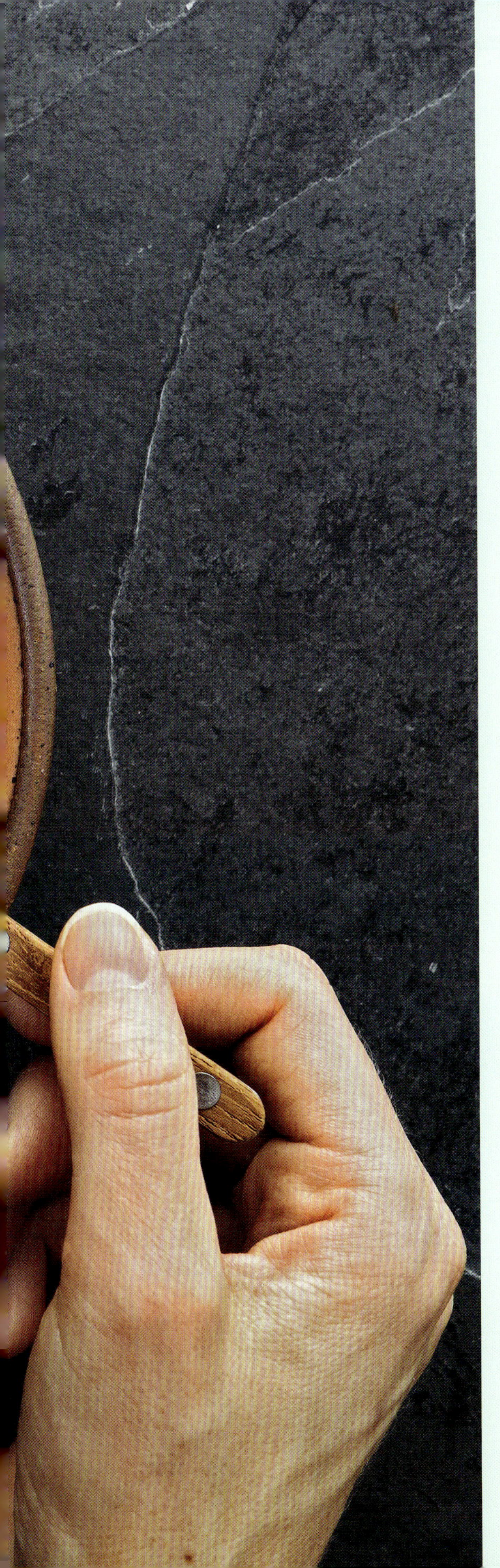

For Stacy—who is always
planting seeds.
This is the tree that grew.

Contents

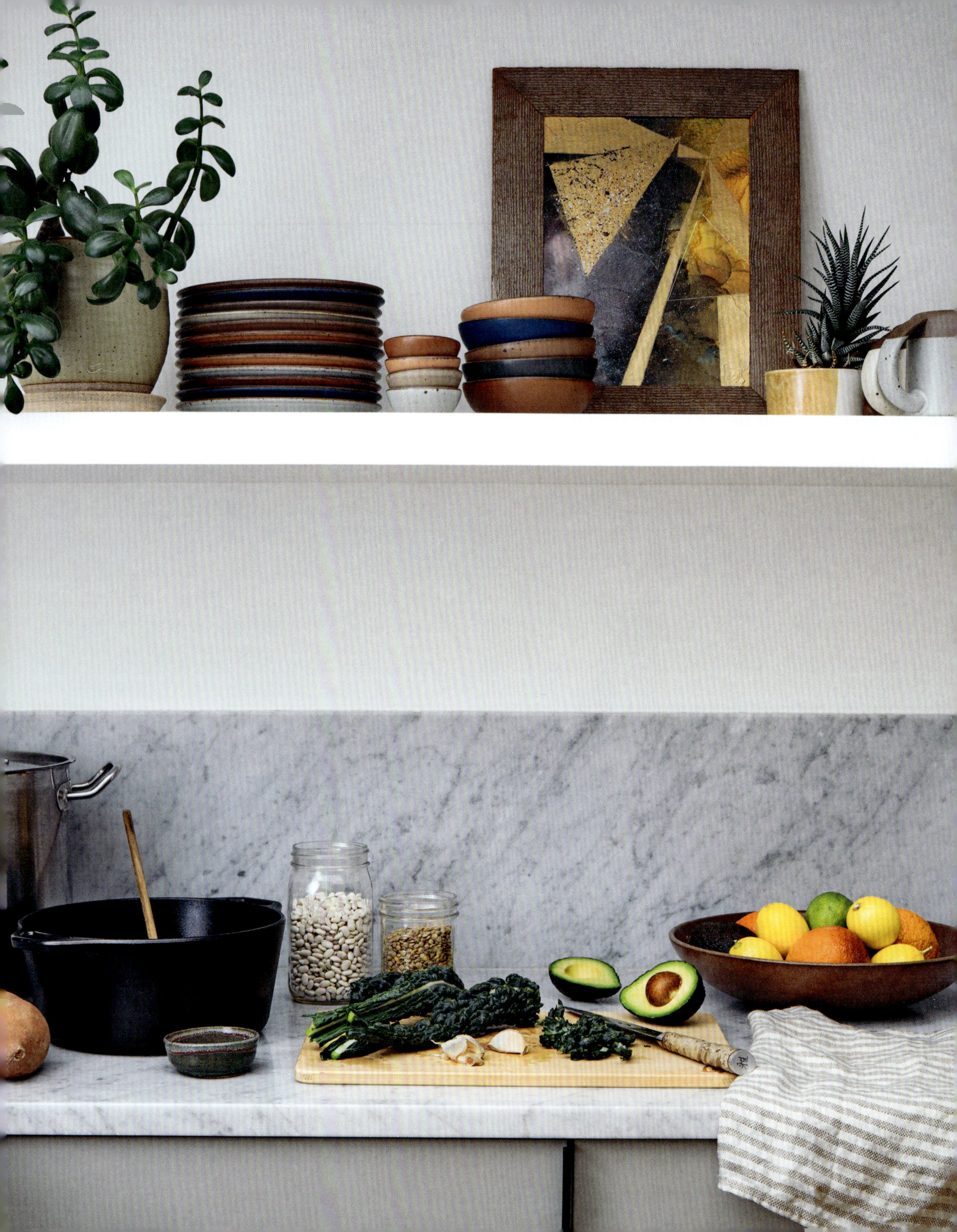

Preface

Some of life's discoveries come just when you need them. I remember feeling overcome with a mix of relief and hope as I stumbled across the Autoimmune Protocol for the first time—I was in my twenties and in the depths of my first autoimmune health crisis: completely overwhelmed by debilitating symptoms, exhausted from searching for answers, and plagued by the fear that I'd be sick for the rest of my life. I had recently lost my job due to unrelenting symptoms, and I'd been through countless unproductive medical appointments. Despite my persistent symptoms, doctors had little to offer besides diagnosing me with two autoimmune conditions, wishing me good luck, and sending me on my way. Anyone who has struggled with an autoimmune diagnosis knows this feeling well—the crushing mix of frustration, fear, and the hope that if you just keep looking or asking, there might be a path forward.

On the "tolerable days," which seemed to be few and far between, I continued combing online to see if there was a complementary approach that I was missing, since I had run out of options with my healthcare providers. I eventually came across the Autoimmune Protocol (otherwise known as AIP)—a structured dietary and lifestyle program that immediately stood out as a potential path to progress. The moment I read about it, something clicked, and I knew it could be the key to sustainably recovering my health.

This was in 2011, and the Autoimmune Protocol was just a vague idea beginning to take form. There was no "official" guidance or instructions—just a list of seven broad food categories to avoid and some theorizing about why it might work. In my research online and in support forums, I learned that other autoimmune patients were reporting that they experienced food sensitivities and chronic nutrient deficiencies, and that they found lifestyle factors (like high stress or lack of sleep) to be significant triggers of symptoms. So much of this rang true for me, too.

After everything I had been through and what was at stake, it wasn't hard to convince myself to start the elimination diet and make some lifestyle changes to see if my health would improve. And it did—week by week, my symptoms reduced, and in six months, I was able to return to a baseline of health that enabled me to live well, despite autoimmune disease. I wasn't alone in this transformation—other autoimmune patients were also discovering AIP, sharing their experiences online, and forming the foundation of a growing community. Grateful for the tools that helped us heal, many felt a deep responsibility to spread the word, hoping to offer guidance and encouragement to those still searching for answers.

THE AUTOIMMUNE PROTOCOL

Let's back up a bit—what is AIP, exactly? AIP is a systematic and evidence-based approach to determining which foods and lifestyle components are supportive of your best health, even if you experience chronic illness like autoimmune disease. This is done through implementing a specific dietary and lifestyle protocol with three consecutive phases—transition, elimination, and reintroduction—usually over a period of three to six months.

How does it work? The AIP dietary approach removes food-driven sources of inflammation and increases nutrient density, while the lifestyle approach includes prioritizing practices that are important for managing health, like improving sleep, stress management, and finding balance with exercise. Through carefully working through each phase of AIP, you learn how these dietary and lifestyle strategies impede or support your best health and arrive at a personalized, sustainable structure to confidently manage your health going forward.

GROWTH OF THE AIP MOVEMENT

In the early days of the AIP movement, the biggest challenge in adopting the protocol was simply finding recipes. What do you eat if you are avoiding grains, legumes, eggs, dairy, nuts, seeds, and nightshade-family vegetables? Before my own illness I had worked as a personal chef, prepping and batch-cooking healthy meals from scratch for busy families with complex dietary needs. While navigating the protocol myself, I decided to put my skills to use creating and sharing AIP recipes online; I also went back to school to study nutrition. It turns out, a lot of autoimmune patients had heard about AIP and were searching for resources, so this led to self-publishing the very first recipe book devoted to AIP, *The Autoimmune Paleo Cookbook*, in 2013. I had a simple goal for this passion project: to make it easier for the next person looking to begin AIP, hopefully making their path to success a little smoother by sharing everything I'd learned on my own.

I knew the AIP community would grow—hundreds and eventually thousands of others were sharing their stories online. What I didn't know was how fast these stories would spread. In a few short years, *The Autoimmune Paleo Cookbook* had become a viral best-seller and my website, Autoimmune Wellness, was serving AIP recipes, food lists, and resources to millions of people per year, facts that still amaze me. Seeing the impact firsthand, I realized that AIP wasn't just a personal experiment, it was becoming a revolution in how people approached wellness with autoimmune disease.

This explosive growth led to another phase in the history of AIP—one that I never saw coming, not even in my wildest dreams. Starting in 2015, medical research teams took interest in the Autoimmune Protocol and began conducting studies into its usefulness for managing specific autoimmune conditions. Since then, formal medical studies have been performed using AIP for conditions including Hashimoto's thyroiditis, Crohn's disease, ulcerative colitis, psoriasis, and rheumatoid arthritis, validating anecdotal evidence of the usefulness of AIP for these common autoimmune conditions. While many of us who adopted AIP in the early days were told that there was no research on AIP and that it couldn't possibly be helpful, we now have a growing body of evidence showing efficacy of the protocol, which is incredible! In addition to validation, this research also paved the way for greater awareness and accessibility in the medical community.

Around the same time the AIP medical research began, many forward-thinking healthcare providers became interested in using AIP with their patients. In 2017, this led me to collaborate with my AIP nutrition colleagues to create AIP Certified Coach, a program training healthcare providers in best practices in implementing AIP with their patients and clients. Since then, more than a thousand providers from both the conventional and natural healthcare worlds, including physicians, naturopaths, researchers, nurses, dietitians, physical therapists, holistic nutritionists, and health coaches, have completed the program and incorporated AIP in their work. Watching AIP become an integral part of so many healthcare practices is a powerful reminder of how far we've come—and how much potential there is to continue making a difference.

Today, AIP stands on a foundation that didn't exist fourteen years ago—a thriving patient community of millions, a growing body of medical research validating its effectiveness, and a network of experienced healthcare providers trained in its implementation and customization. This collective knowledge has given me an invaluable opportunity to analyze what works, refine the approach, and improve it for the next wave of people seeking personal healing. The insights gained from countless patient experiences, clinical research studies, and healthcare provider feedback have all led to the first major update to AIP since its inception, and the driving force behind the approach in this book.

All this to say—you are learning about AIP at the perfect time in its history. My goal in writing *The New Autoimmune Protocol* is to present a fully updated and refined protocol for you to benefit from all this knowledge and experience that has come since the early days of AIP.

THE NEW AUTOIMMUNE PROTOCOL

I'm excited to present the new and improved Autoimmune Protocol, with comprehensive changes to the transition, elimination, and reintroduction phases, which work together to make the protocol easier to implement and sustain.

If you're already familiar with the Autoimmune Protocol, the first major change you'll notice is that I've completely reworked the transition phase. Previously, transition had no structured approach—it was simply assumed that each person would figure out how to bridge the gap between their current diet and lifestyle and full AIP implementation on their own (which understandably was challenging and led many people to give up altogether). Through my experience coaching people through this process, I've seen firsthand the value of specific, strategic steps to complete for making a smooth and sustainable shift in dietary approach. The new transition phase integrates this knowledge into a clear, guided process that helps you accurately assess your baseline, define your goals, evaluate your readiness, and pinpoint the key actions needed to transition smoothly and effectively into the elimination phase.

The New Autoimmune Protocol also introduces the first major update to the elimination phase since AIP was first developed. This phase is what most people associate with AIP—focusing on which foods are removed, and for how long. In 2023, I embarked on an in-depth exploration of the elimination phase with my partner and co-teacher at AIP Certified Coach, Jaime Hartman. Our goal was to determine what was working and what could be improved to better support the next wave of people trying the protocol.

Through interviews with AIP researchers, reviews of medical studies, and surveys of the AIP Certified Coach provider community, Jaime and I found that while the original protocol remained valuable, there was also a need for a more accessible option. The result was a shift to two distinct elimination phase approaches: Core AIP, which follows the traditional elimination and reintroduction framework, and Modified AIP, a more flexible, expansive option designed to improve affordability and accessibility while still delivering consistent results.

Last, *The New Autoimmune Protocol* includes updated guidance for completing the protocol—the reintroduction phase. In the past, there was minimal direction for navigating food reintroductions, as the focus was primarily on maintaining the elimination phase. That led many to experience trouble determining which foods were causing symptoms or staying in the elimination phase for so long that other problems would crop up. With new insights and a deeper understanding of how to successfully structure and approach reintroductions, guidance has been refined and updated to make the process smoother, more effective, and predictable.

These updates bring the Autoimmune Protocol into the present, making it more relevant and practical than ever. *The New Autoimmune Protocol* is designed to set you up for success with ease. It's adaptable to your unique needs, and it's now more affordable, accessible, sustainable, and achievable than ever before.

HOW TO USE THIS BOOK

Your journey with the Autoimmune Protocol is unique, but you don't have to navigate it alone. *The New Autoimmune Protocol* is your guide to embracing each phase of AIP with confidence and clarity. Think of this as a complete resource you can turn to at every stage—from learning the foundational science and strategies, to finding support through practical tips, discovering delicious recipes, and even troubleshooting when things don't go according to plan.

Wherever you are in your story, this book is designed to meet you there. Whether you're easing into AIP gradually or diving in all at once, you'll find the resources, guidance, and encouragement you need to create a protocol that works for your life. Start where you feel ready—take in the science, jump straight into the recipes, or follow along step by step. You're in the right place, and this book is here to help you succeed.

ABOUT THE RECIPES

In addition to being your complete guide to the Autoimmune Protocol, this book contains two collections of recipes, one for each option for the elimination phase—Core AIP and Modified AIP. You'll find that the recipes and materials specific to Core AIP are coded in red, and the recipes and materials specific to Modified AIP are in blue. No matter which option you end up embarking on, all the recipes in this book will be relevant to your journey, as all Core AIP recipes are compliant with Modified AIP, and Modified AIP recipes can be enjoyed after reintroductions following Core AIP (this might seem confusing now, but you'll learn all these details in Chapter 3!).

There are a few key things you should know about my process and how I approach developing recipes for AIP. I've been at this for more than fourteen years, and I've learned some very valuable tips and tricks for making AIP not only achievable, but also enjoyable. Here is a list of factors I consider when developing recipes for the elimination phase:

- **Simple ingredient sourcing.** I prioritize ingredients that can be found at most regular grocery stores, year-round. Successfully implementing AIP does not require that you shop at specialty grocers, online, or at farmers' markets (although those options can be helpful, if they are accessible to you!).
- **Nutrient density.** In addition to the foods eliminated on Core or Modified AIP, nutrient density is an essential part of the protocol, and I try to include key nutrient-dense ingredients in every recipe, if possible, to maximize healing potential.
- **Classic flavors.** Instead of trying combinations that take some getting used to or are a less-than-yummy re-creation of something that is not included in the elimination phase, I like to focus on flavors that are truly delicious to anyone, whether they are following AIP or are a family member or friend along for the ride.
- **One-pot meals and minimal cleanup.** I emphasize recipes that create complete meals and use the least amount of kitchen equipment to minimize cleanup.
- **Batch-cooking potential.** Cooking for AIP means you'll be making just about all your meals from scratch, so I write recipes that make additional portions for leftovers to reduce the amount of time you'll need to dedicate to food preparation.
- **Simple techniques and accessible tools.** For those with minimal cooking experience, I've developed these recipes to be simple and easy to follow, with no requirement for advanced or expensive cooking tools (like pressure cookers, stand mixers, air fryers, and more).

Each recipe draws inspiration from the vibrant flavors of global cuisine and the transformative power of real, whole foods. Whether you're preparing meals for yourself or your family, these dishes are crafted to bring joy and healing to your table. To make things even easier, I've included meal plans and additional resources to help you stay organized and inspired. My hope is that these recipes will show you just how fulfilling and enjoyable eating for your health can be.

Even though your goal isn't to stay in the elimination phase of AIP long-term (you'll learn more about this in Chapter 3!), I've designed these recipes to be so flavorful and versatile that you'll want to keep making them long after you've completed the reintroduction phase. So, flip through the pages, give them a try, and see for yourself how "normal" and nourishing eating on AIP can be. Let these meals support you through every stage of your healing journey. You've got this!

Mickey

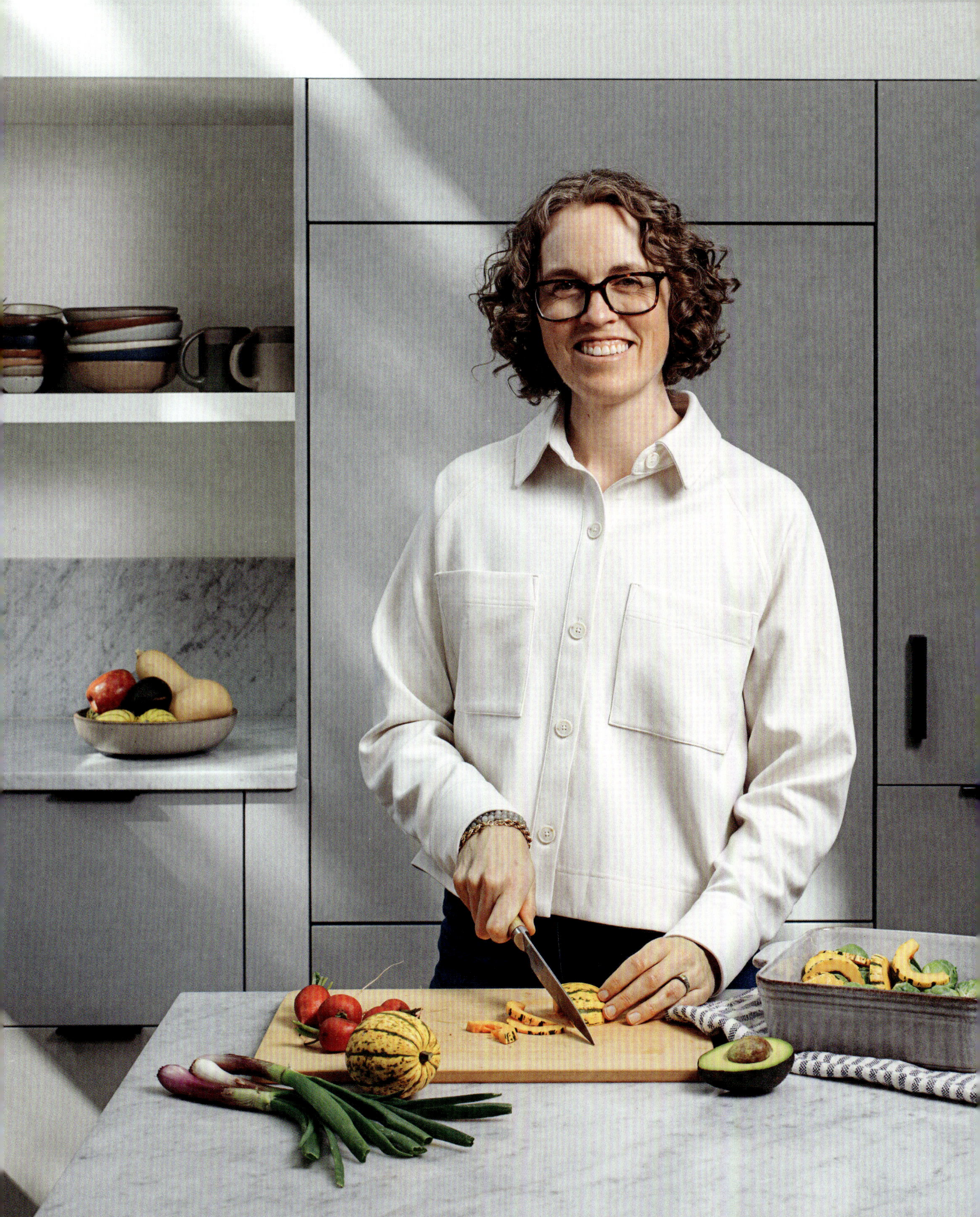

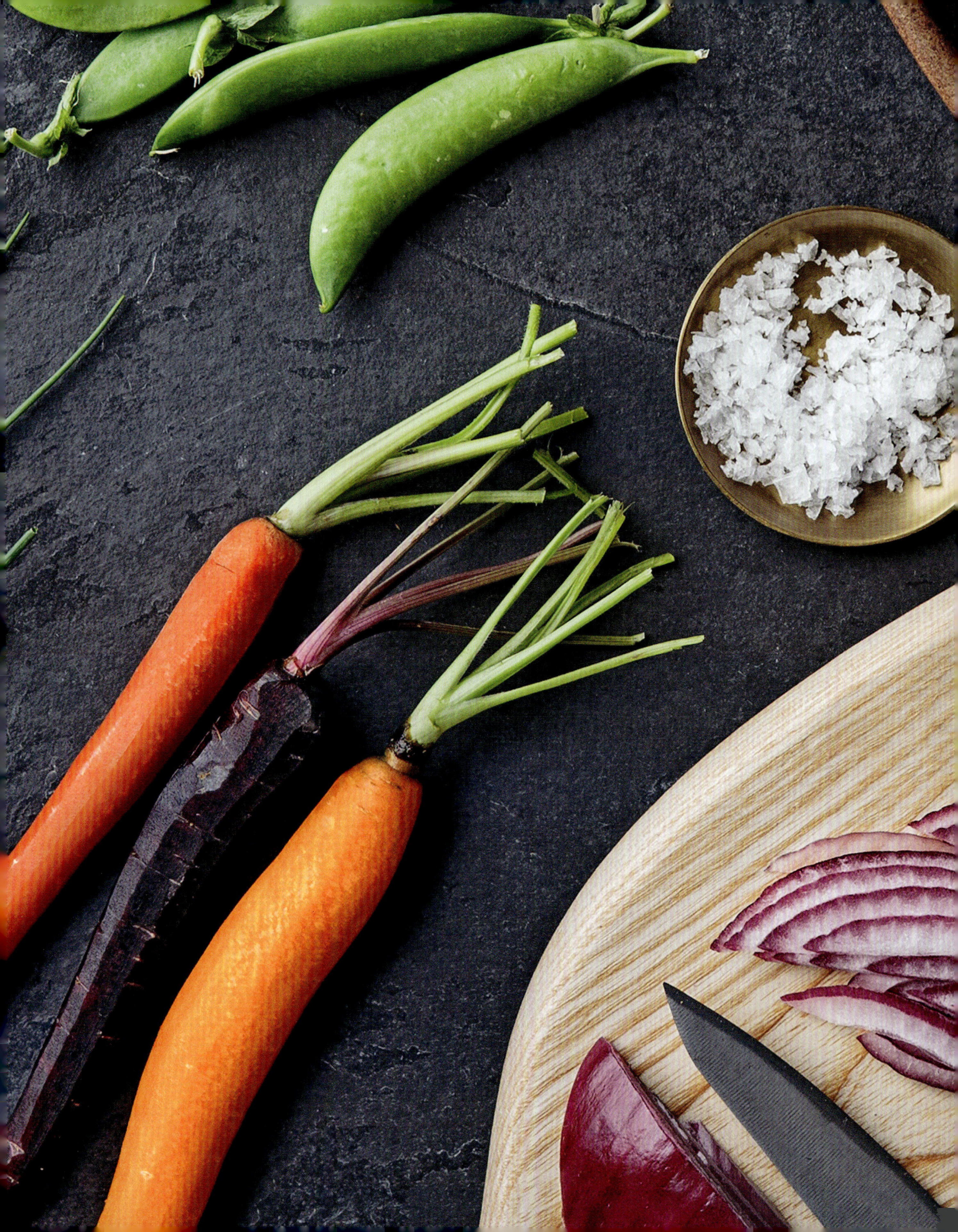

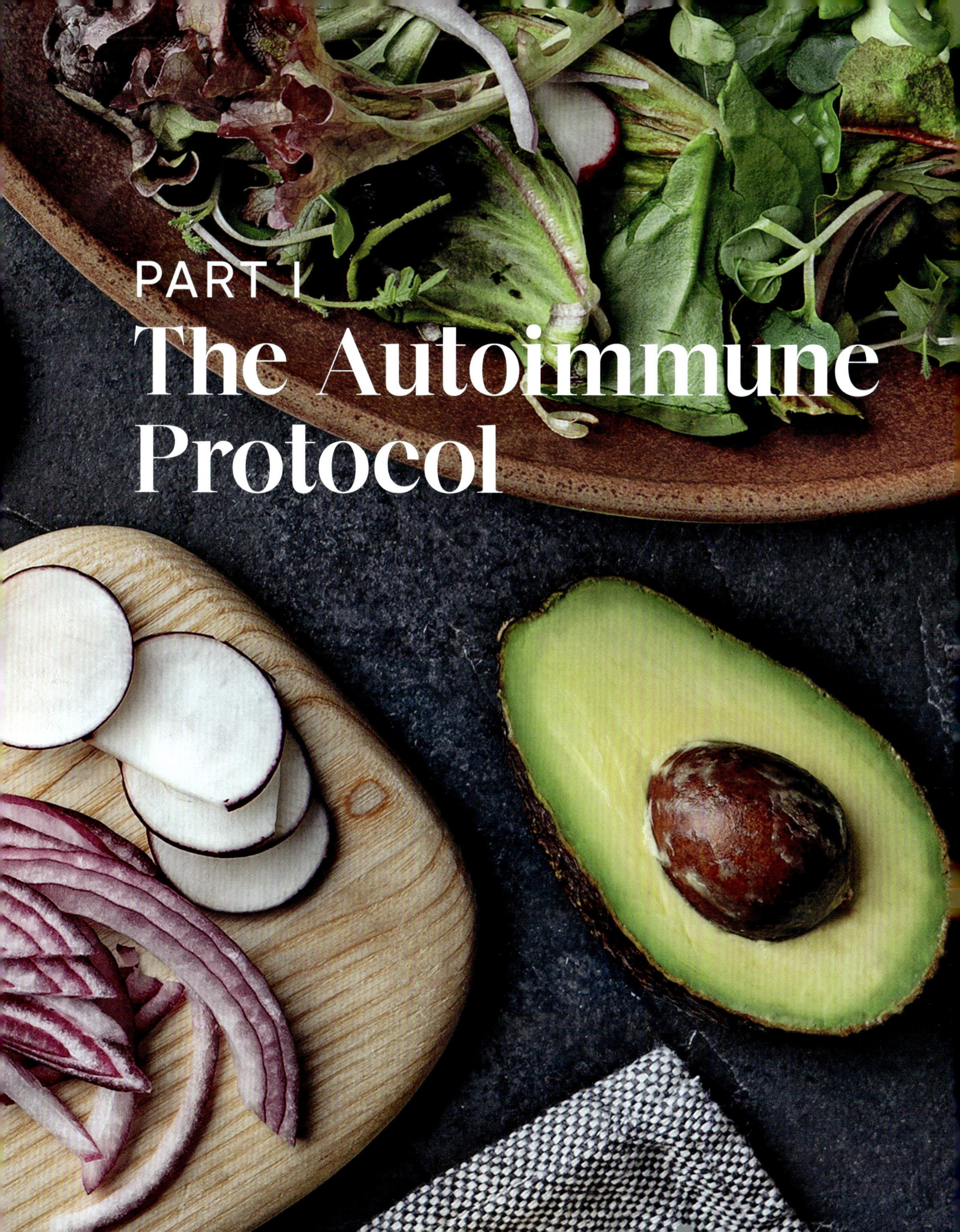

PART I

The Autoimmune Protocol

CHAPTER 1

Autoimmune and AIP Basics

In my twenties, while researching Hashimoto's thyroiditis—the condition I had just been diagnosed with—I came across a term that was entirely new to me: "autoimmune." I quickly discovered my condition was an autoimmune disease affecting the thyroid. Despite growing up in a family with multiple doctors, I knew little about autoimmune disease. This was likely due to the misconception that they are rare and the tendency for patients to keep their diagnoses private. This quest led me to not only learn about my autoimmune thyroid condition, but also the immune dysfunction at the root of autoimmune disease in general.

Simply put, autoimmune disease begins when your immune system starts targeting parts of your own body, resulting in symptoms related to loss of function or damage (in my case, the autoimmune attack on my thyroid led to hypothyroidism, or a lack of thyroid hormone). While these aspects of your immune system are finely tuned and calibrated to deal with infections and allergies (like viruses, bacteria, and other pathogens), once they start targeting your own cells, the pattern becomes difficult to reverse. Your immune system keeps a memory of every exposure, which heightens future responses. You can easily see how this is a problem when the trigger is a part of your own body!

It's no coincidence that so many people either have or know someone with an autoimmune disease—these conditions rank as the third most common cause of chronic illness, impacting an estimated 18 to 22 million Americans, with women making up 78 percent of those affected.[1] And if it seems like everyone has a *different* autoimmune disease, that's because there are more than one hundred distinct conditions with confirmed autoimmune processes. The most common autoimmune diseases include rheumatoid arthritis, which affects the joints; Crohn's disease, ulcerative colitis, and celiac disease, all of which affect the digestive tract; multiple sclerosis, which affects the myelin sheath in the brain; and psoriasis, which affects the skin. Because your immune system is present in every cell, organ, and system of the body, autoimmune diseases can affect those areas, too.

Despite how common they are, being diagnosed with an autoimmune disease is often a long, challenging process. Autoimmune Association surveys show that patients report diagnosis taking about three to four years after having seen four to six physicians, with most of them reporting multiple rounds of dismissal from doctors and specialists.[2] If you are currently navigating your diagnosis journey and struggling to feel heard, just know that I see you; I've been there, too.

Each autoimmune disease has its own hallmark symptoms based on which organs or systems of the body are affected, and these symptoms can range from a mild annoyance to life-threatening. Within specific autoimmune disease categories, symptoms can vary widely from patient to patient, with many falling far outside the spectrum of what is considered "classic" for a particular condition. To make it even more difficult, symptoms of many autoimmune conditions are nonspecific, like joint pain, fatigue, and brain fog. This makes them impossible to quantify and categorize and can lead to further dismissal from providers and loved ones alike ("Are you *really* that tired all the time?").

Autoimmune disease is challenging to treat, with the conventional approach primarily centered on symptom management. If you've got Hashimoto's thyroiditis or type 1 diabetes, you might be prescribed thyroid hormone or insulin to replace what your body doesn't make. If you've got rheumatoid arthritis, you might be prescribed an immunosuppressant to dampen your immune system's relentless attack on your joints. Or if you have Crohn's disease or psoriasis, you may be prescribed a round of steroids to help your body come out of a flare. While these treatments are important, you've probably already discovered that they come with additional challenges—including access, cost, and the high burden of side effects.

Even when autoimmune patients are "well managed" on medication, medical research shows that we often experience chronic symptoms and decreased quality of life.[3,4] I found myself here after my own diagnosis, when I was told by both conventional and naturopathic providers that my hormone levels did not require treatment, despite having symptoms that were debilitating enough that I could not hold a job. These kinds of experiences often lead autoimmune patients to seek out complementary therapies to manage our health, as well as make dietary and lifestyle changes to live well despite our chronic health challenges. In fact, I'm sure it is the primary reason why you've picked up this book—and precisely where the New Autoimmune Protocol comes into play.

WHERE DID THE AUTOIMMUNE PROTOCOL COME FROM?

The Autoimmune Protocol (otherwise known as AIP) originally took root in a tight-knit community of women who implemented it to help manage a collection of very different autoimmune diseases—multiple sclerosis, rheumatoid arthritis, psoriasis, Hashimoto's thyroiditis, and Crohn's disease, specifically. I was in this group who originally connected online through autoimmune support forums. Initially we got together to share our stories and offer each other support; later we started writing about our positive experiences using AIP on our personal blogs and social media. Even though each of us was trying to manage a different autoimmune disease, we all saw incredible improvements to our health that were even expanded from our primary disease symptoms. Out of this small group, the AIP community grew as anecdotes and stories about how effective it was for those seeking healing spread like wildfire across all corners of the internet.

The original idea for AIP as a protocol didn't have one defined source—it emerged around 2011 as a collaborative framework that was shaped by health researchers and an autoimmune community that was both dedicated to searching for answers and interested in self-experimentation. In all honesty, many of us who discovered AIP in these early days were looking for *anything* that would help us feel better. This earliest form of AIP was influenced by the functional medicine community, which had been advocating for the use of elimination protocols for chronic health issues for many years, and the ancestral health community, which was interested in research investigating how modern foods lead to chronic conditions like autoimmune disease. From there, health researchers like Dr. Sarah Ballantyne played a major role in consolidating and forming AIP into a defined protocol that was then implemented by greater numbers of the autoimmune community and later shared far and wide.

At the same time, forward-thinking complementary and functional medicine healthcare providers started using AIP in their practices as a tool to help their patients manage autoimmune disease. Anecdotal and clinical evidence about AIP's usefulness for both common and unusual autoimmune diseases continued to spread online. This resulted in an increased awareness and even more backing from healthcare providers to the point that AIP became the standard dietary recommendation for autoimmune patients. This led me to co-create AIP Certified Coach, an advanced training that teaches healthcare providers best practices in using AIP with their patients and clients, which has now trained more than one thousand practitioners of both conventional and natural medicine worldwide. You'll hear a lot about what this group of providers has learned in their many years' experience implementing AIP throughout this book.

In 2015, an autoimmune patient single-handedly changed the trajectory of the AIP movement. This patient with inflammatory bowel disease (IBD) asked their gastroenterology specialist at Scripps Research if they could try AIP for a month before resorting to a surgical bowel resection to manage their disease. The specialist wasn't familiar with AIP but gave them clearance to try AIP before resorting to the procedure. On follow-up, she found that AIP had been incredibly effective, as the patient's symptoms had resolved and they no longer needed surgery. Being a gastroenterology researcher, she asked them for more information about the protocol, which led her to my website and later collaboration on the first of what would eventually become four medical studies investigating the efficacy of AIP for IBD. The incredible results of this research were consistent with the patient's case report and inspired other research teams around the world to test AIP as an intervention for other autoimmune diseases, including Hashimoto's thyroiditis, rheumatoid arthritis, and more. If you can't wait to hear about the research results, don't worry—we'll take a deep dive later in this chapter!

This brings us to the New Autoimmune Protocol, which is the fully updated and refined protocol as it stands today. With more than a decade of self-directed use within the autoimmune patient community, practitioner-guided use within the AIP Certified Coach community, and recent results from the AIP medical research, the protocol has been updated to accommodate everything we've learned.

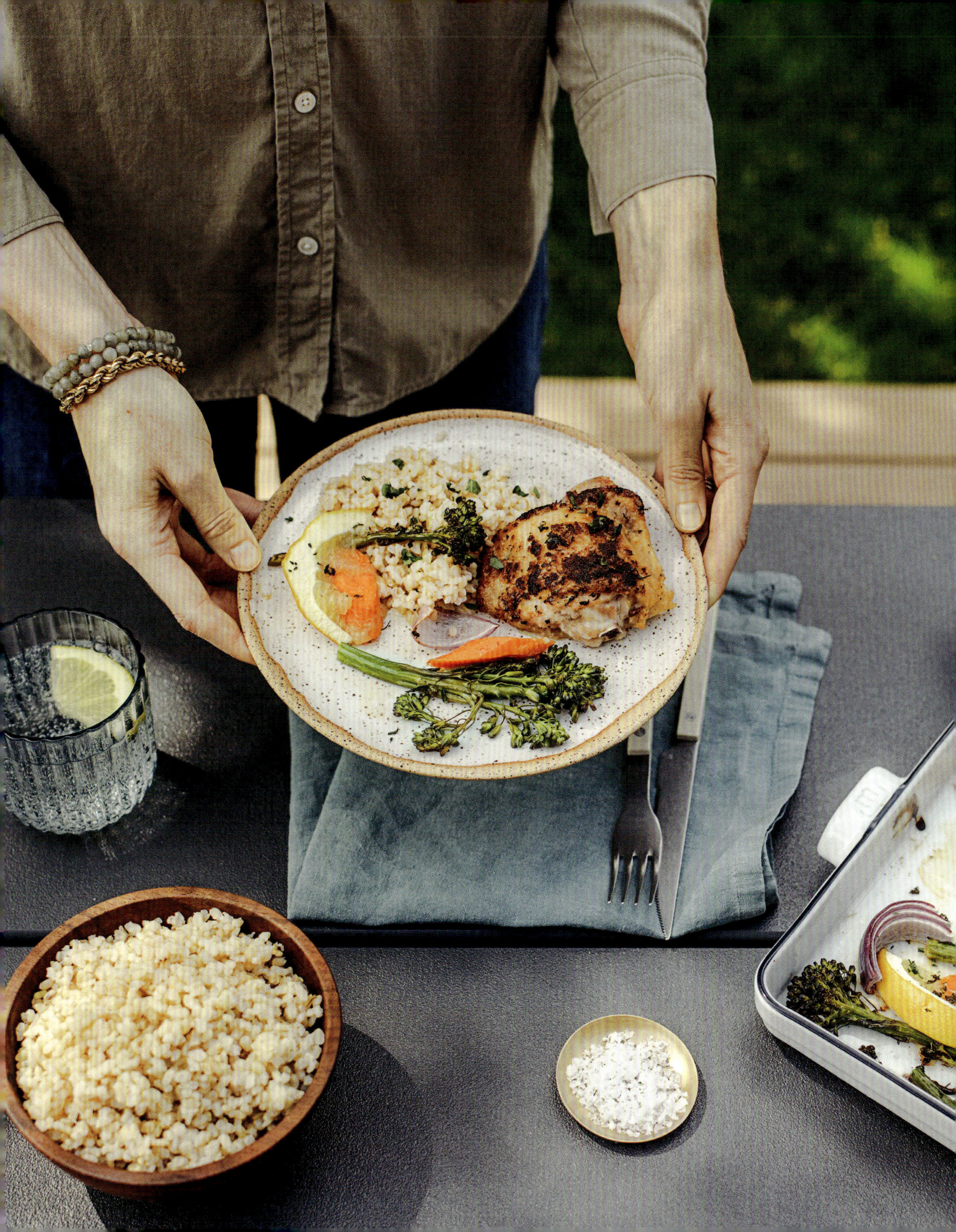

WHAT IS THE AUTOIMMUNE PROTOCOL?

But what is the Autoimmune Protocol, exactly? Here's the elevator pitch: AIP is an evidence-based elimination and reintroduction dietary and lifestyle protocol focused on repairing gut health, balancing hormones, and regulating the immune system. The dietary component includes removing food-driven sources of inflammation and restoring nutrient density, while the lifestyle component includes prioritizing quality sleep, stress management, and proper movement to promote balance and health for those with autoimmune disease. Through carefully working through the phases of AIP, you learn how these dietary and lifestyle strategies impede or support your best health and arrive at a personalized, sustainable structure to confidently manage your health going forward.

Since its inception in 2011, AIP has grown from a theoretical framework based on early medical research on the effects of *individual* food and lifestyle components to a tested, evidence-based protocol informed by medical studies using the *complete protocol* as an intervention in real people with specific autoimmune diseases (which is amazing, for having been around for barely more than a decade!). This shift is important, as AIP is the only comprehensive dietary and lifestyle protocol that has been tested for efficacy in multiple autoimmune conditions affecting different organs and systems of the body.

Now, the number one thing that people get wrong about AIP is that they think it is a diet meant to be implemented long term. You'll hear me repeat this throughout these pages, because this is an important point: AIP is not a *diet*! The difference is in the name—Autoimmune *Protocol*, which speaks to the dynamic process you work through over time, discovering which dietary and lifestyle components affect your health. The goal is not to maintain the eliminations of AIP forever (in fact—I specifically don't recommend this!), but to discover an expansive way of eating that yields your best individual health with autoimmune disease. Go ahead and take a deep breath as you let go of the idea that you'll have to maintain the most restricted phase of AIP forever—phew!

This is how it looks: You spend some time thoughtfully transitioning your diet to the elimination phase, a period where you strictly avoid specific foods for 30 to 90 days, while adding in certain nutrient-dense foods and prioritizing lifestyle factors that are known to influence symptoms and health for those with autoimmune disease. At this point, you are likely experiencing a positive shift in your symptoms and well-being. You then enter the reintroduction phase, where you systematically reintroduce foods, one by one, to determine which are tolerated and which cause symptoms. Each of these phases has its own guidelines and options for modifications, with the goal of being adaptable to your unique needs and yielding a completely customized and health-supporting diet after completion.

Think of yourself on a road trip, with your destination being an approach to diet and lifestyle that helps you most easily and sustainably manage life with autoimmune disease. The elimination phase of AIP is like a highway, where you can quickly cover a lot of ground on your way to that destination. The transition phase represents your on-ramp to the elimination phase, and the reintroduction phase represents your off-ramp. Just as with a road trip, you aren't sure exactly how long it will take you to get there, and you want to leave well-equipped to navigate any challenges that spring up along the way. Think of this book as the map, helping you plan and consider your options for a successful journey.

What can you expect to learn from navigating AIP? While the initial phases of the protocol may look similar from person to person, the dietary approach that you end with may look drastically different post-reintroduction, even if your friend, relative, or a health influencer you follow shares a similar health history or autoimmune condition. Instead of a one-size-fits-all approach, AIP is a completely flexible framework that allows you the joy of discovering what works for you and teaches you to sense your body's feedback to your routines so that you can make an informed decision about choices that affect your health going forward. How powerful is that?

If you have any experience with autoimmune disease or chronic illness, you already know how much can change over time. The beauty of navigating AIP is that it not only teaches you how to discover which foods and lifestyle factors influence your health and symptoms currently, but it also helps you plan for adjustment during periods of remission or flare. Even after experiencing healing, if your health shifts in the future, you have firsthand experience of which dietary and lifestyle factors are most effective at quickly relieving inflammation and symptoms in your own body from your experience working the phases of AIP.

HOW DO WE KNOW THE AUTOIMMUNE PROTOCOL WORKS?

In the early days of the AIP community, there were a small number of healing stories fueling a growing group of autoimmune patients ready to take healing into their own hands. Personally, I was motivated to begin AIP after watching Dr. Terry Wahls's healing testimony in her TED talk—what an inspiration! Today, if you go searching for individual accounts of healing using the Autoimmune Protocol, you'll find literally *thousands* of them, on every corner of the internet—in blog posts, podcast episodes, book reviews, autoimmune support groups, forums, social media, and more. Autoimmune patients who have used AIP successfully are talking about it, *everywhere*!

Early on, most of these healing anecdotes were from those who suffered from the most common autoimmune conditions—rheumatoid arthritis, Crohn's disease, ulcerative colitis, psoriasis, Hashimoto's thyroiditis, Graves' disease, and celiac disease. But over time, stories of those using AIP to successfully manage more unusual conditions, as well as multiple coexisting conditions, emerged—like myasthenia gravis, lupus nephritis, multiple sclerosis, alopecia, psoriatic arthritis, hidradenitis suppurativa, ankylosing spondylitis, scleroderma, lichen planus, and mixed connective tissue disease (this is in no way an exhaustive list—but I'm aware of many folks in the AIP community reporting success with those conditions). I've been compiling individual stories for more than ten years on my Autoimmune Wellness website, and some of the results autoimmune patients have shared with me are absolutely astounding. Here is a selection:

- Jolaine was diagnosed with ankylosing spondylitis after twenty-one years of searching for answers. After trying every type of dietary approach out there to help manage her chronic pain, she noticed a massive improvement just days into the elimination phase of AIP. While she was still needing crutches to grocery shop during the earliest days of transitioning to AIP, by the time she began reintroducing foods, she could walk without pain (and now enjoys her favorite sports like running and cycling once again!).
- Michelle was diagnosed with palmoplantar pustulosis, a rare autoimmune condition that caused painful skin flares on her hands and feet along with persistent digestive issues. The physical symptoms quickly began to affect her mental health, leading to panic attacks and emotional exhaustion. Within two weeks of implementing AIP, the inflammation in her hands noticeably subsided, and over time it helped her regain both physical health and emotional resilience.
- Jaime was diagnosed with Crohn's disease at age nineteen. Surgery and medication managed the bowel symptoms, but severe extra-intestinal complications including anemia and crippling enteropathic arthritis in her thirties led her to consider other factors, including diet and lifestyle. AIP has allowed her to return to an active life that includes running marathons, and she reports feeling better now in her early fifties than at any other point in her life.
- Nick's journey with autoimmune disease began in his teens with ankylosing spondylitis, later followed by psoriasis and psoriatic arthritis. After experimenting with dietary changes, he discovered AIP and began to experience significant improvements. Over time, his pain lessened, his energy returned, and he was able to reduce his medications. While he's faced setbacks along the way, Nick now enjoys long stretches of pain-free living and continues to use AIP as a cornerstone of his healing.

- Jennifer was diagnosed with relapsing-remitting multiple sclerosis at thirty-eight after sudden, unexplained numbness started in one arm and then spread throughout her body. A handful of treatments that either didn't work or had unpleasant side effects led her to try AIP. This slowly brought her body back to balance, helping her feel in control of her health and enjoying a dramatically improved quality of life.
- Jacqueline began experiencing strange and debilitating symptoms as a teenager, but it wasn't until college that her health declined so drastically she became bedridden. She was eventually diagnosed with mixed connective tissue disease—a complex autoimmune condition that includes features of lupus, scleroderma, and polymyositis, often affecting the joints, muscles, skin, and internal organs. Jacqueline turned to AIP with guidance from a healthcare provider. By following a personalized version of the protocol, she experienced steady and lasting improvements and is back to studying, creating art, and living a life she once feared might not be possible.

Amazing, right? If you are in search of more inspiration, be sure to check out the Stories of Recovery series on my Autoimmune Wellness website, where I've compiled more than seventy-five interviews with real autoimmune patients detailing their successes with AIP.[5] I've been passionate about sharing these stories because I know how it feels to be in the position of just getting by with chronic symptoms after all treatment options have fallen short—I know I'm not alone in this. Finding success with AIP literally helps autoimmune patients see a future where we can live our dreams, and nothing can stop us from sharing our experiences with the next person who might be suffering and in search of answers.

While these personal healing stories have fueled the exponential growth of the AIP community and highlight the potential of AIP to help manage complex autoimmune diseases, medical research has also begun to validate its effectiveness, providing scientific evidence to support these firsthand experiences. We'll discuss this next.

THE AUTOIMMUNE PROTOCOL IN MEDICAL RESEARCH

While healing stories are inspiring and offer valuable insights, they are not considered scientific evidence, as they lack the controlled conditions needed to draw definitive conclusions. Fortunately, there has been increasing interest in studying the Autoimmune Protocol, and we have an emerging body of research that can now inform how AIP is used in general as well as for specific conditions. If you've got a skeptical provider or relative, or just want to see the results, this section is for you!

This AIP medical research formally began in 2015, with results of the first pilot study published in 2017. Since then, studies have been conducted using AIP as an intervention for inflammatory bowel disease (IBD), Hashimoto's thyroiditis, rheumatoid arthritis, and psoriasis. This research is a key component of how AIP has moved from a theoretical framework based on individual dietary and lifestyle components into the realm of an evidence-based protocol that has been put to the test in real humans managing their conditions.

As you'll learn in the following research reviews, results have been overwhelmingly positive and indicate that AIP shows promise at improving quality of life and managing symptoms for those with autoimmune disease. A snapshot: For those with IBD, two studies report 73 percent of patients reaching clinical remission in as early as six weeks using AIP.[6,7] In those with Hashimoto's thyroiditis, AIP has been shown to decrease symptom burden in multiple studies, with one study showing a 29 percent decrease in hs-CRP, a marker of inflammation, and a second study showing an average weight loss of eight pounds over the course of twelve weeks despite eating the same amount of calories, as well as a reduction in thyroid swelling as seen on ultrasound.[8,9] While we still have a lot to learn, these results indicate that AIP can be a useful tool for managing the negative impacts of symptom burden and low quality of life for autoimmune patients.

While this book is more about implementation than science, taking a deeper look at the research can help you glean insights into how you might approach using AIP and build confidence in what you're trying to achieve in changing your habits. On the following pages, I've summarized each of the medical studies on AIP to date, detailing the key points about each intervention as well as the specific results that were observed.

While these results using the Autoimmune Protocol as an intervention for autoimmune disease are promising, it should be noted that research in this area is still in the infancy stage. Critics are quick to point out the small sample size of the pilot studies and the nature of self-reported data in the surveys. However, those who are familiar with the research process know that small steps must be taken before large ones—a pilot study provides a proof of concept, to show safety and that there is something there worth exploring further. These studies show that answer is a resounding yes! From here, interested research teams can build on what has been explored to date, and design larger, more controlled studies that can better add to what we know about how dietary and lifestyle interventions can help those with autoimmune disease live healthier lives.

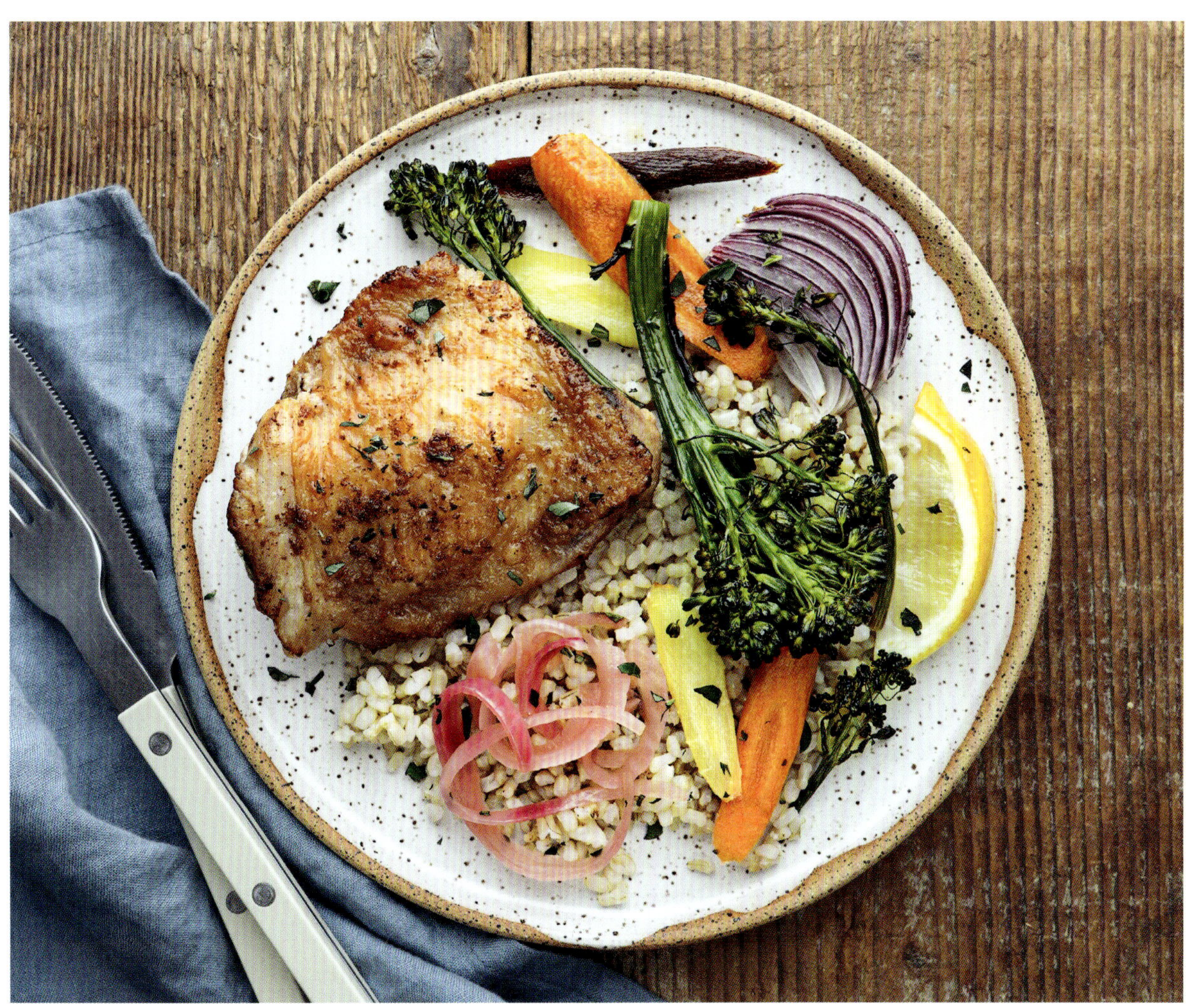

The Autoimmune Protocol for IBD (Crohn's Disease and Ulcerative Colitis)

1 / PILOT STUDY ON EFFICACY OF AIP FOR IBD

The first study into the efficacy of AIP was a prospective cohort study conducted by Dr. Gauree Konijeti and her team at Scripps San Diego: "Efficacy of the Autoimmune Protocol Diet for Inflammatory Bowel Disease." A group of 15 patients with active Crohn's disease or ulcerative colitis was guided in a 6-week transition and a 5-week elimination in accordance with Core AIP. Some notable statistics about the study participants were that the mean disease duration was 19 years and that about half of the patients (47%) were on biologic therapy going into the study. These were patients who had longstanding disease and had not achieved clinical remission even with the use of powerful medications according to the conventional standard of care. Surveys, labs, and physician assessments were conducted at baseline, week 6, and week 11, and endoscopy, radiology, or biomarker assessments to assess mucosal healing were conducted both at baseline and the end of the study.

INTERVENTION: Patients were guided through a 6-week transition phase, slowly removing two food groups per week and adding in foods to increase nutrient density. At 6 weeks, participants were in Core AIP elimination phase and maintained this for 5 weeks. For both phases, a group health coaching program was used as the model to guide patients in implementation and provide support in transitioning and maintaining the dietary and lifestyle intervention.

RESULTS: At week 6, 73% of the patients had achieved clinical remission, and all in this subset maintained this remission during the elimination phase. It should be noted that at week 6 participants were still in the transition phase and had yet to enter the elimination phase of Core AIP, indicating that the dietary changes were effective very quickly. There was no difference in the rates of remission between patients with Crohn's disease and patients with ulcerative colitis. Although patients were advised not to make any medication changes during the study, four patients discontinued or reduced their medications and all in this subset either achieved remission or measurable improvement in scores representing disease severity.[10]

2 / STUDY ON AIP AND QUALITY OF LIFE FOR IBD PATIENTS

A second study was published analyzing changes in quality of life using the data from the prospective cohort AIP IBD pilot study: "An Autoimmune Protocol Diet Improves Patient-Reported Quality of Life in Inflammatory Bowel Disease." Here, the Short Inflammatory Bowel Disease Questionnaire (SIBDQ) was used to assess IBD disease activity and quality of life at baseline and at weeks 3, 6, 9, and 11 of the study. SIBDQ scores of over 50 indicate good health-related quality of life.

RESULTS: For patients who completed all surveys in the AIP IBD pilot study, SIBDQ scores improved from 46.5 at baseline to 61.5 at the end of the study, showing a considerable improvement in health-related quality of life over the period that Core AIP was implemented as an intervention.[11]

3 / STUDY ON AIP AND INTESTINAL RNA EXPRESSION IN IBD PATIENTS

A third study was published using data from the prospective cohort AIP IBD study, this time analyzing genetic expression in stool samples of 4 patients with ulcerative colitis: "The Autoimmune Protocol Diet Modifies Intestinal RNA Expression in Inflammatory Bowel Disease." RNA expression was examined in tissue samples at baseline and end of the intervention and compared for patterns or changes. This type of analysis is experimental, but points to reasons why an intervention may be effective at producing the types of tissue-level changes seen in the AIP IBD pilot study.

RESULTS: 324 significant differentially regulated genes were identified following the AIP intervention, with 167 downregulated and 157 upregulated. Downregulated genes included those associated with inflammatory T-cell responses that lead to autoimmune inflammation. Upregulated genes included those associated with a T-regulatory cell response that lead to immune modulation and transcriptional pathways associated with mucosal healing and DNA repair. It is interesting to take these results together with the results of the AIP IBD pilot study to see how an intervention like Core AIP might be working in terms of altering genetic expression in the intestine, which is the site of inflammation and damage in the case of IBD.[12]

4 / SURVEY ON AIP DIETARY PATTERNS AND IBD

In addition to observing the effects of Core AIP as an intervention for IBD patients, Dr. Konijeti and her team at Scripps also wanted to survey those who had already successfully used Core AIP to help manage their IBD: "Clinical Course and Dietary Patterns Among Patients Incorporating the Autoimmune Protocol for Management of Inflammatory Bowel Disease." Patients were surveyed on how long they had a diagnosis of IBD, if they were on medications and which ones, how they went about implementing Core AIP, and which foods they reacted to as reintroductions.

RESULTS: 78 IBD patients submitted surveys, with a mean age of 39.4 years and mean disease duration of 13.4 years. 73% of respondents reported achieving clinical remission after implementing Core AIP, and 32% of them reported discontinuing steroids after implementing AIP. Most respondents reported reintroducing foods between 5 weeks and 1 year of implementing Core AIP, with only 12% reporting needing more than 1 year in the elimination phase. In terms of foods that respondents reported unable to reintroduce, gluten (58%), processed foods (52%), nightshades (46%), dairy (42%), and non-gluten grains (29%) were the worst offenders.[13]

The Autoimmune Protocol for Hashimoto's Thyroiditis

1 / FIRST STUDY ON THE EFFICACY OF AIP FOR HASHIMOTO'S THYROIDITIS

This prospective cohort study was modeled after the IBD study, except this time, the patients had Hashimoto's thyroiditis, the most common autoimmune disease: "Efficacy of the Autoimmune Protocol Diet as Part of a Multi-disciplinary, Supported Lifestyle Intervention for Hashimoto's Thyroiditis." Dr. Abbott and his team led a group of 17 women with Hashimoto's thyroiditis on a 6-week transition and 4-week elimination phase in accordance with Core AIP. Surveys quantifying symptom burden and lab tests assessing thyroid hormones, antibodies, and inflammatory markers were performed at the beginning and end of the study. Functional medicine lab tests such as urine organic acids and comprehensive stool analysis were performed at baseline.

INTERVENTION: The intervention was the same as the AIP IBD study that preceded it, using a group health coaching program. Patients went through a 6-week transition as they gradually eliminated foods and added in foods to increase nutrient density. At 6 weeks, participants were in the full elimination phase of Core AIP and maintained this for 4 weeks.

RESULTS: 16 participants finished the study, 1 dropped out due to pregnancy. Clinical symptom burden as indicated on a Medical Symptom Questionnaire (MSQ) decreased from an average of 92 (standard deviation 25) at baseline to 29 (SD 20). No changes in thyroid hormone levels or antibodies were seen, but 6 out of 13 participants lowered or discontinued their thyroid hormone medication dosage, and hs-CRP, a marker of inflammation, decreased by 29% from baseline to end of the study.[14]

2 / SECOND STUDY ON NUTRIENT DENSITY AND EFFICACY OF AIP FOR HASHIMOTO'S THYROIDITIS

Another prospective cohort study using AIP for Hashimoto's thyroiditis was conducted in Poland: "Effects of Autoimmune Protocol (AIP) diet on changes in thyroid parameters in Hashimoto's disease." The research team led 20 patients with Hashimoto's thyroiditis through a 12-week elimination phase in accordance with Core AIP, using personalized meal plans. Assessments included prior diet analysis, body composition, thyroid hormones, thyroid ultrasound, and symptom burden surveys.

INTERVENTION: Patients were assessed for prior diet intake and then prescribed individualized, 12-week Core AIP meal plans based on their anthropometrics. Prior diet was compared to prescribed AIP diet for nutrient density.

RESULTS: Blood test analysis showed thyroid-stimulating hormone (TSH) significantly decreased from a mean of 3.72 to 2.69 mU/L. Free T3 and T4 significantly decreased, although both stayed within reference ranges (3.31 to 2.88 pmol/L; 1.36 to 1.20 ng/dL, respectively). A comparison of thyroid ultrasounds showed the right lobe volume decreased by 5% and the left lobe volume decreased by 6%. Anthropometric measurements showed that mean weight decreased from 69 kg to 65.5 kg (152 pounds to 144 pounds). Mean body fat percentage decreased from 33% to 29.5%, indicating that twice as much weight was lost from fat than muscle. Analysis of questionnaires showed a broad improvement of symptoms reported by Hashimoto's thyroiditis patients.

NUTRITIONAL RESULTS: Analysis of nutrient intake via prescribed AIP diet showed there was a broad increase in nutrient density during the intervention. Specific nutrient intake increases included beta-carotene (550%), fiber (162%), folates (198%), long-chain fatty acids (262%), potassium (196%), vitamin A (341%), and vitamin C (886%), with other nutrients like B vitamins, iron, zinc, and magnesium demonstrating considerable increases.[15]

The Autoimmune Protocol for Rheumatoid Arthritis (RA)

1 / QUALITATIVE RESEARCH ON THE EFFICACY OF AIP FOR RHEUMATOID ARTHRITIS

Julianne McNeill, a nutritionist and PhD candidate based in New Zealand, performed graduate research involving interviews with 10 people who had been successful using AIP to manage their rheumatoid arthritis. These 90-minute interviews investigated how they implemented Core AIP, how they decided what to eat and what to avoid, and the foods they perceived as problematic or safe to eat. The group included 1 man and 9 women, mean age 41.7 (28 to 60 years), and mean reported time on AIP was 2.9 years (6 months to 5 years).

RESULTS: A few themes were reported in the interviews. First, most patients had been introduced to Core AIP through a holistic practitioner. The most significant barrier to implementation was changing to a restrictive diet, and most participants reported planning ahead with a specific start date and making a rapid transition. The most significant barrier to maintaining the diet was the attitudes of others, and having the support of at least one person was instrumental in success in maintenance. The primary motivation was lack of pain, and all participants reported the effects were worth the effort required.[16]

2 / PILOT INTERVENTION STUDY ON THE EFFICACY OF AIP FOR RHEUMATOID ARTHRITIS

Another study by Julianne McNeill was performed in patients with rheumatoid arthritis in New Zealand: "What Is the Efficacy of the Autoimmune Protocol (AIP) Diet in People with Rheumatoid Arthritis? A Mixed-Methods Pilot Intervention Study." The preliminary results were presented at the Nutrition Society Conference in 2022. Initial analysis shows potential for Core AIP to improve fatigue, pain, and sleep in patients with RA.[17]

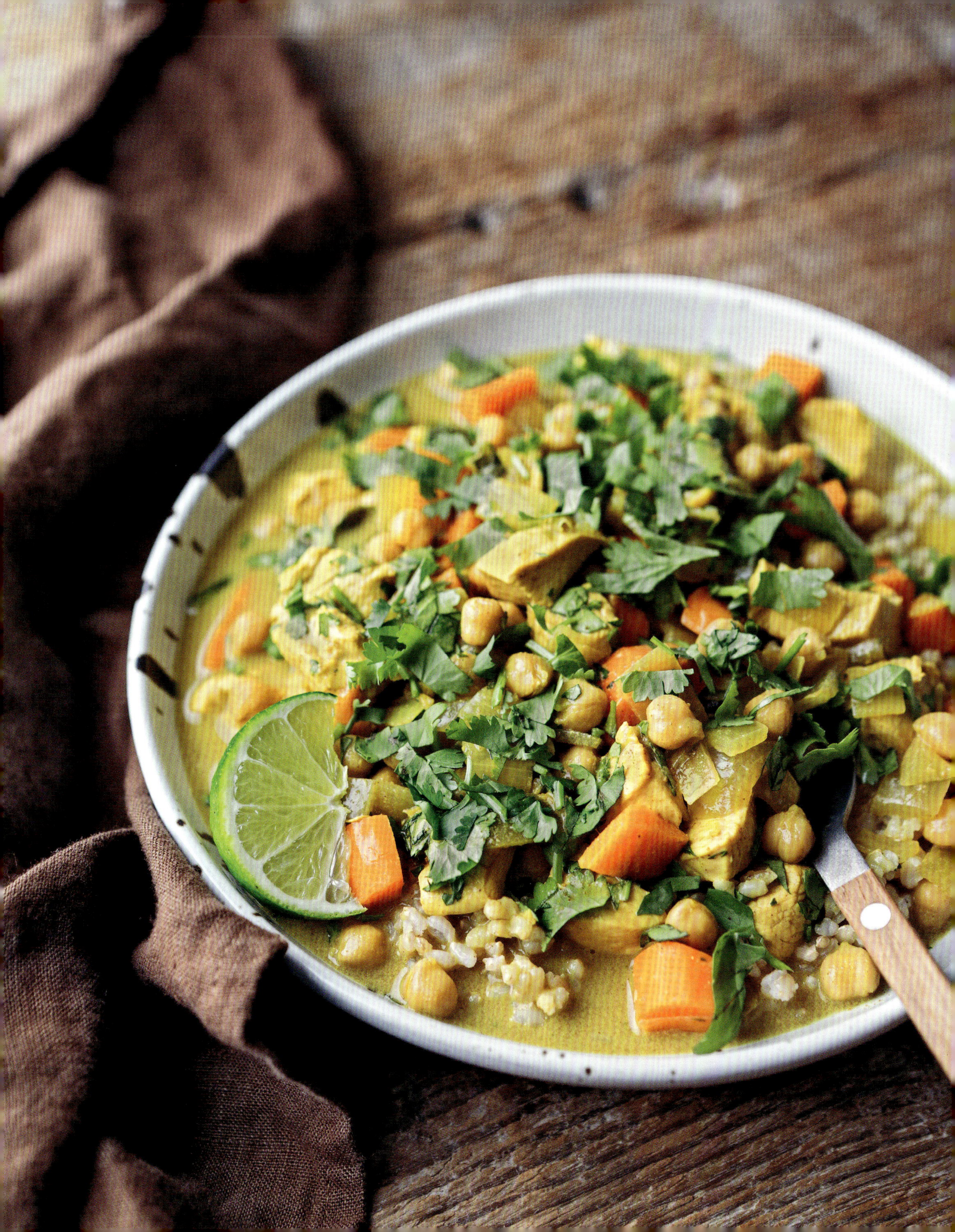

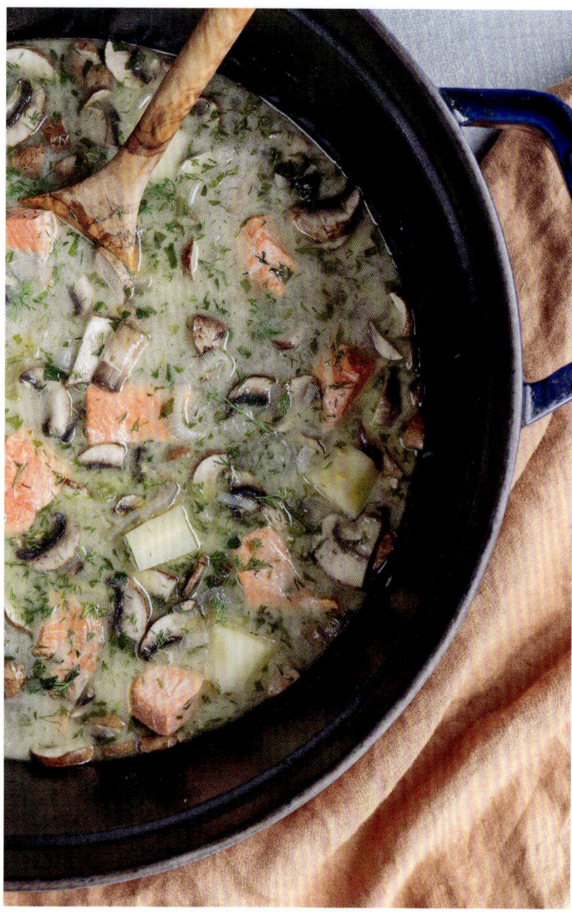

HOW DOES THE AUTOIMMUNE PROTOCOL WORK?

These anecdotes and medical research results show us how powerful the Autoimmune Protocol can be for people with autoimmune disease—but how, exactly, is it working to improve our health? The short answer is that AIP combines specific dietary and lifestyle interventions that produce effects in key areas of concern for autoimmune patients. Because AIP involves making changes in areas that have each individually been shown to produce benefits for autoimmune patients, it is likely that these effects are synergistic—meaning they are more powerful when used in combination. A breakdown of each of these key areas follows.

Identifying Food Allergies and Sensitivities

AIP helps you discover any food allergies or sensitivities you might have through a thorough elimination and reintroduction protocol. Food allergies differ from food sensitivities due to the specific type of immune response involved. Allergies involve immunoglobulin E (IgE) antibodies and usually elicit an immediate, strong response, which can often be life-threatening. Food sensitivities, in contrast, do not involve IgE antibodies but can elicit a different type of immune response, or be due to non-immune mechanisms. They typically come on more slowly, sometimes appearing days after exposure, and can have a range of effects from mild discomfort to severely debilitating.

There is a lot of misconception out there surrounding food allergy and sensitivity, the largest being that if you have a food allergy or sensitivity to something you are eating, you'd already know. While you are likely to know if you have an extreme food allergy (especially if it is life-threatening), there are more subtle allergy responses that can go undetected until you take some time off from eating the specific food. Among the thousands of people I've observed implementing elimination diets, just about *everyone* finds, after diligent elimination and reintroduction, some surprising, often-consumed foods were majorly contributing to their autoimmune symptoms (for me it was bell peppers and tomatoes—darn!).

Elimination and reintroduction protocols are still the gold standard for accurately identifying food allergies or sensitivities and continue to outperform every type of food allergy or sensitivity testing in comparison studies.[18,19] This is why popular food allergy blood tests are not a good replacement for a thorough elimination and reintroduction protocol.

Research shows that it is important for elimination protocols to last at least 2 weeks, with some recommending up to 4 weeks, especially to allow the immune system time to recover from more subtle food sensitivities—this is why AIP requires at least 30 days in the elimination phase (more on that later!). During the time spent avoiding potential dietary triggers, your immune system gets the opportunity to calm down and be less reactive. Once your immune system has found balance and you are feeling an improvement overall, you then proceed to the reintroduction phase, where you test each food, one by one, to see what reaction you get. Because you've done the hard work of avoiding potential triggers, it is more likely that those subtle reactions now elicit a larger response. While this can be uncomfortable, it is an important part of being able to identify which foods are supporting your health and which ones might be causing a reaction.

While food allergies and sensitivities can happen to anyone, studies show they are more common in autoimmune patients.[20,21] Autoimmune patients also tend to have specific food sensitivities that are not as common in the healthy population, like sensitivities to nightshade-family vegetables.[22] The Autoimmune Protocol is ideal for autoimmune patients, as it has been designed to avoid foods that have the highest likelihood of being food allergies or sensitivities in this group.

Correcting Nutrient Deficiencies and Promoting Nutrient Density

Next, AIP includes nutrient-dense foods that correct deficiencies and promote overall dietary nutrient density. Certain nutrient deficiencies are common with specific autoimmune diseases, such as iron deficiency and Hashimoto's thyroiditis, vitamin D deficiency and multiple sclerosis and rheumatoid arthritis, and zinc deficiency and psoriasis. Beyond these specific connections, everyone's immune system needs sufficiency in many key micronutrients for proper functioning, including vitamins A, D, C, E, and B, and minerals like zinc, iron, copper, and selenium.[23] In a standard Western diet, intakes of these nutrients are commonly below recommended minimums, with up to 45% of people failing to meet the requirements for vitamin A, 46% for vitamin C, 95% for vitamin D, and 15% for zinc.[24] This presents a major problem for those with autoimmune disease, as many may not be getting even the bare minimum of nutrients for their immune systems to function properly (much less heal and repair from the tissue damage and other effects resulting from autoimmune processes!).

AIP is designed to not only meet these minimum nutrient requirements for good health but go above and beyond in terms of nutrients that help support immune function, lower inflammation, and promote deep healing. This is done by adding in "nutrient-dense foods," or those with high levels of nutrients relative to the calories they contain. As a part of the Polish AIP study discussed earlier, researchers compared diets of the participants before and after transitioning to AIP. Unsurprisingly, they found a massive increase in nutrient density during the intervention. Specific increases included beta-carotene (550%), fiber (162%), folates (198%), long-chain fatty acids (262%), potassium (196%), vitamin A (341%), and vitamin C (886%), with other nutrients like B vitamins, iron, zinc, and magnesium demonstrating considerable increases.[25]

AIP is not only an elimination protocol, but one that adds in specific foods to increase nutrient density, and these additions are one more potential reason why it might help in managing your autoimmune disease. We'll be talking more about this in Chapter 5.

Lowering Chronic Inflammation

Inflammation is the body's natural immune response to infection or injury and, when appropriate, allows healing and repair. Unfortunately, autoimmune disease is often a source of *chronic* inflammation, which does not resolve and is often the cause of symptoms like joint pain and swelling. A leading theory on why AIP may be effective for managing symptoms for those with autoimmune disease is that it may be helping to bring down these high levels of chronic inflammation.

AIP can help manage inflammation in a variety of ways. First, food allergies and sensitivities are a major source of inflammation for those who experience them. You already know how effective AIP is at identifying these allergies and sensitivities, and eliminating potential triggers is going to help you feel better quickly. In terms of those nutrient-dense additions you'll be consuming on AIP, it is important to understand that inflammation is a process that is also nutrient-dependent, and there are specific foods included during AIP that are anti-inflammatory and promote

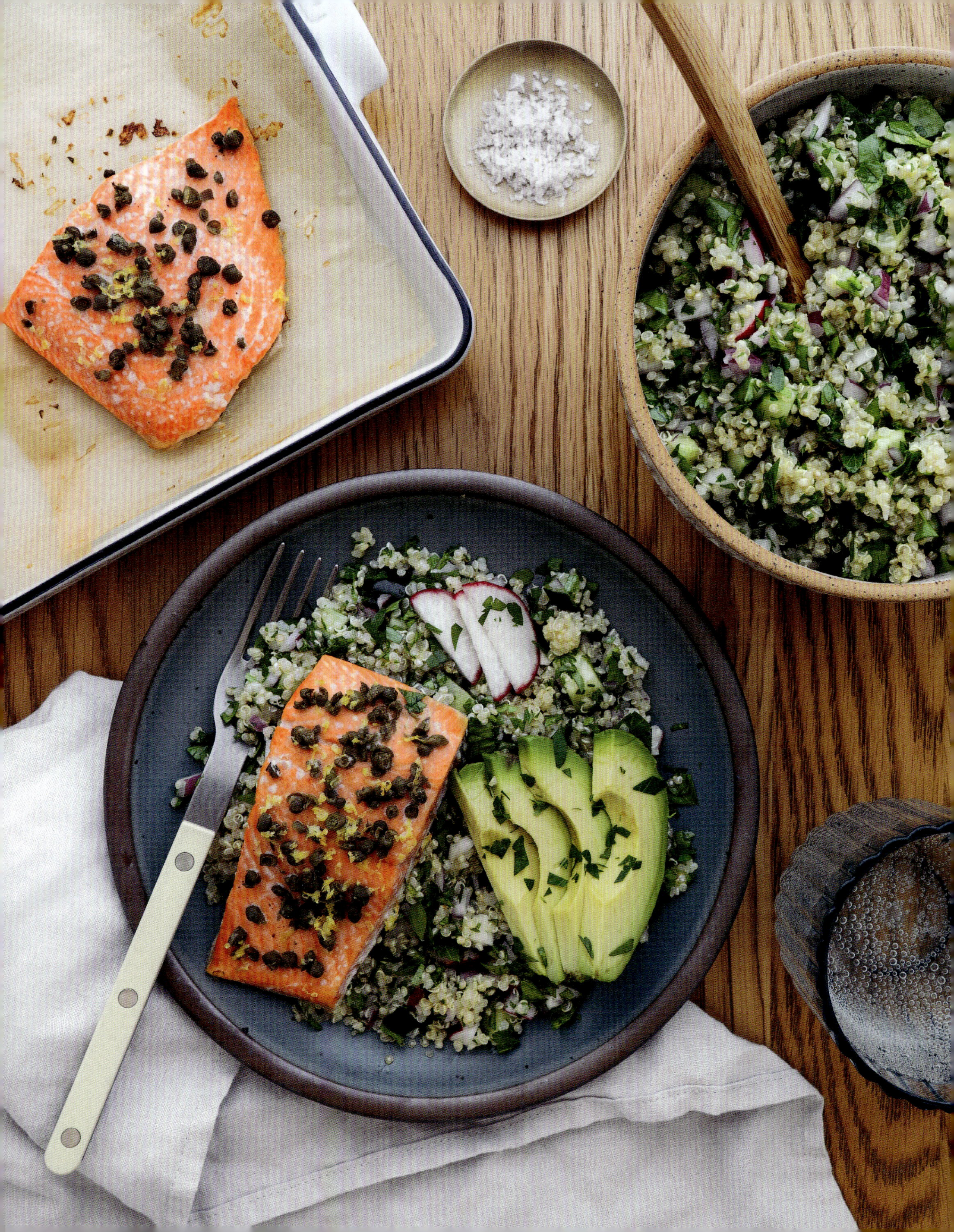

the resolution of inflammation (like lots of vegetables and omega-3 fats). What you're not eating (potential dietary triggers), and what you are eating (nutrient-dense, anti-inflammatory foods), are both responsible for the effect here.

How do we know AIP is effective at lowering inflammation? The biomarker high-sensitivity C-reactive protein (hs-CRP) is a blood test that helps identify levels of chronic inflammation and can be useful for tracking it over time. In one of the Hashimoto's medical studies, hs-CRP was measured before and after ten weeks of AIP and significantly decreased by 29%.[26] Similarly, in the AIP IBD study, fecal calprotectin, a measure of intestinal inflammation in patients with gastrointestinal conditions, improved from a mean of 471 µg/g (SD of 562) to 112 µg/g (SD of 104) after AIP.[27] Last, an analysis of intestinal RNA expression in the same group identified that after AIP, their tissue showed downregulated genes that were commonly associated with autoimmune inflammation.[28] While these studies weren't designed to measure the effects of AIP on inflammation specifically, they do show us that a part of the overall effect may be due to resolving or managing chronic inflammation.

Now that you understand the various potential mechanisms, it should be obvious that the effects of AIP are not likely due to the individual components of the protocol but the synergy of how all these interventions work together to help you feel better.

UPDATES TO THE AUTOIMMUNE PROTOCOL

Today, we have three things we didn't have fourteen years ago when the Autoimmune Protocol first took shape: a patient community in the millions, formal scientific studies, and the benefit of feedback from hundreds of AIP Certified Coaches using AIP in their healthcare practices. In 2024, Jaime Hartman (my partner at AIP Certified Coach) and I completed a high-quality analysis to see what is working and what could be made better for the next wave of individuals looking to embark on AIP. The result was the first major update to AIP, informed by medical research and patient experiences.

To gather information to update AIP, Jaime and I started by interviewing researchers who performed the AIP medical studies as well as those who had completed research in similar but relevant areas. We also consulted experts and writers in autoimmune health and functional medicine. Next, we surveyed and interviewed key members of the AIP Certified Coach practitioner community who run busy practices working with predominantly autoimmune patients or clients. Collectively, these providers have worked with thousands of autoimmune patients since they started using AIP in their work. Last, we considered recent scientific evidence for elimination diets, food allergies/sensitivities, and reintroduction protocols in consideration of this updated approach.

As a result of our search, we identified four key reasons why AIP needed to be updated:

1. Many patients in AIP medical studies saw results before reaching the full elimination phase, indicating that partial elimination might be just as effective for some people.
2. AIP Certified Coaches reported often customizing the existing protocol to suit their clients' and patients' specific needs. Despite this, they also reported high levels of efficacy using these less-restricted, customized protocols.
3. Other elimination diet medical research indicates stricter is not always better—recent studies using minimal food eliminations have also reported good results in patients with specific autoimmune conditions.
4. Increasing accessibility, affordability, and sustainability has the potential to widen the reach of AIP, removing some barriers caused by food access, cost, or implementation.

We noticed two contrasting themes from this exploration. First, that the original protocol still had high value and efficacy in both research and practice. And second, that many researchers and AIP Certified Coaches were confident that some patients would be

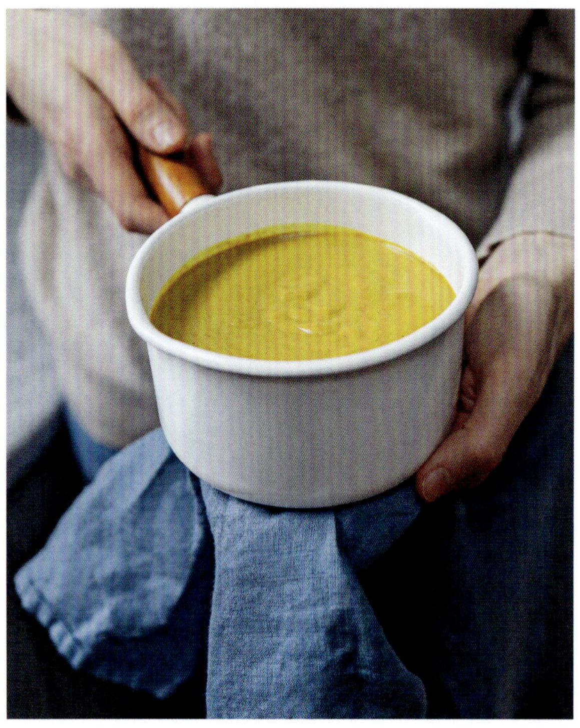

best served by a less-restrictive option. This led us to move forward in a way that honored both discoveries—to preserve the original protocol, while adding an additional option for the elimination phase.

The big update to AIP is this: The original elimination protocol, as used in the AIP medical studies and original AIP literature, remains unchanged and is now known as Core AIP Elimination. The intention is to preserve the original protocol for research comparison and to use with patients or clients who need a more comprehensive approach or can implement it easily (due to support, finances, or time). The new protocol, containing fewer eliminations, is known as Modified AIP Elimination. This new protocol incorporates what we've learned about foods that are well tolerated in the autoimmune community, and is simplified for ease of implementation, budget, and accessibility.

In addition to including Modified AIP as an elimination option, we also updated the official guidance and procedures for the transition and reintroduction phases of AIP based on feedback from coaches and current food sensitivity research. All of this is great news for anyone who has struggled to start or stick to AIP in the past!

IS THE AUTOIMMUNE PROTOCOL RIGHT FOR YOU?

At this point, you know where the Autoimmune Protocol came from, the stories that fueled the growth of the AIP community, and all the current medical evidence supporting its use for people with autoimmune disease. You *still* might have questions before deciding if it is right for you—which is completely natural, as embarking on AIP is a big commitment!

What if you have an autoimmune condition that hasn't been studied yet? While AIP has been studied for some of the most common autoimmune conditions, the fact that it hasn't been studied for all of them shouldn't discourage you from trying it (with the blessing of your medical providers, of course!). If you suffer from an unusual autoimmune disease, or one that is not currently confirmed but may be suspected to be an autoimmune disease, you might seek out disease-specific communities to see what other patients are reporting anecdotally and to seek inspiration. Over my years of traveling worldwide teaching about AIP, I have heard countless stories of recovery from people of all ages with autoimmune diseases both rare and common, and I guarantee you will find some personal stories to guide you!

Remember, there are more than one hundred autoimmune diseases, and the key factor that all autoimmune diseases have in common is an immune system that's gone awry. Even though each of these autoimmune diseases has its own specific patterns and symptoms, this shared foundation of immune imbalance is a key reason why AIP can work for a variety of conditions. AIP helps identify food and lifestyle-driven triggers of symptoms and has a balancing effect on the immune system, giving you a personalized foundation to manage your health.

Next, you might be wondering if you can combine AIP with conventional or natural medical treatment. Absolutely! The choice is not to use AIP as an alternative to conventional or natural medical care, but in conjunction with it. In fact, this is exactly how AIP has been used by many members of the AIP community, as well as in the medical studies discussed earlier. Autoimmune disease is often serious, and the smartest and most effective approach often involves using all options available to manage your health—including medication, surgery, alternative treatments, *and* things you can do on your own, like dietary and lifestyle modifications. While some of the patients in the IBD and Hashimoto's AIP medical studies showed a reduction in amount of medication necessary, conventional treatments like medication are often a key component of managing autoimmune disease and should not be avoided. Personally, I manage my autoimmune conditions with appropriate medical care (including thyroid hormone medication) *and* eating and living in a way that is supportive of my best health. You don't need to choose one or the other!

Last, there are some people for whom an elimination protocol like AIP is not appropriate—this includes you if your medical providers have concerns based on your specific medical history or needs, or if you have a history of an eating disorder. Others may need to bring in specialized support, like a dietitian or mental health counselor, to ensure that the protocol is implemented safely. While Modified AIP provides a less-restricted option that may better serve those for whom Core AIP is not appropriate, always follow the advice of your healthcare team before getting started. If you are looking for evaluation and support of a provider who understands AIP, be sure to check out the international AIP Certified Coach Directory at DIRECTORY.AIPCERTIFIED.COM.

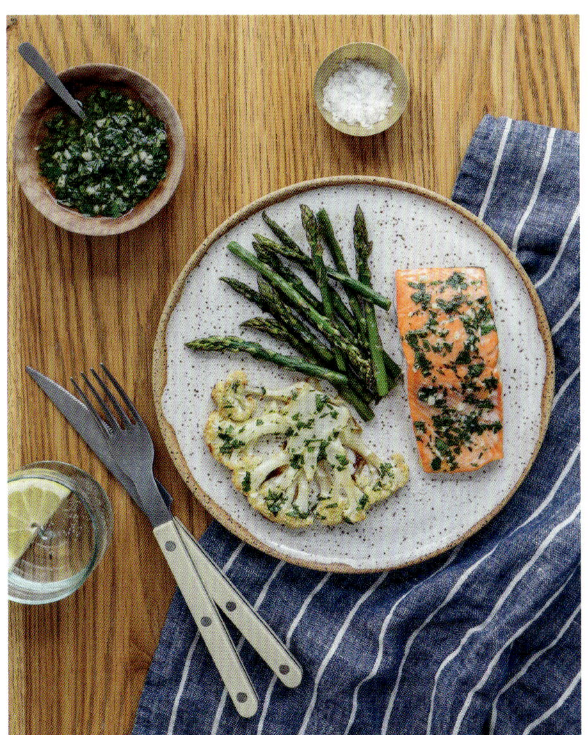

Discussing your plans to embark on AIP with your healthcare team can also get them on board for running any testing or tracking as you navigate the protocol. And who knows—reporting to them that you are trying AIP might inspire some curiosity about the protocol and interest in learning about it to implement with their other autoimmune patients, broadening the reach of the AIP movement!

***

You now understand that the Autoimmune Protocol is widely recognized and utilized as a powerful, evidence-based tool for managing autoimmune disease through dietary and lifestyle changes. Throughout the years it has evolved from a theoretical framework used by a few self-experimenting autoimmune patients to a defined and fully updated protocol, now used by millions of wellness-seekers. The new updates to AIP make it more affordable, accessible, and easier to implement, widening the reach of those who can use it to live their healthiest lives, despite autoimmune disease.

The New Autoimmune Protocol is followed in three consecutive phases: transition, elimination, and reintroduction. Each phase has its own guidelines and options for modifications, with the goal of being adaptable to your unique needs and yielding a completely customized and health-supporting diet after completion. In addition to the specific guidelines of the three phases, there are areas of diet and lifestyle where attention is paid throughout the entirety of the process. The following chapters will walk you through each of these phases of AIP. Now that you've got a great foundation of knowledge, let's get started digging in to the details!

CHAPTER 2

Transition Phase

The Autoimmune Protocol formally begins with the transition phase—the period during which you complete a series of specific action steps to best prepare you for success in the elimination and reintroduction phases that follow. Using our road trip analogy, the transition phase is the on-ramp to AIP, allowing you to gradually pick up speed and confidently merge onto the highway that is going to take you to your destination. You might be best served by a quick on-ramp, with a small list of tasks to complete before making your transition. Or you might do better with a longer on-ramp, one that gives you lots of time for preparation and practice, especially if you are new to some of the practices necessary for this big life change. What matters most is not the length of your transition phase, but how well it prepares you to confidently implement and stay compliant with the elimination phase.

You've already learned that navigating AIP is a deeply personal process with many options, and much of its strength comes from its adaptability to individual circumstances and preferences. This is especially true during the transition phase. Factors like your family influences, cultural background, geographic location, budget, lifestyle, and more impact how you might implement AIP successfully, or which obstacles you are likely to experience.

The original AIP did not include a transition phase—it was just simply assumed that each person would start the elimination phase when they "felt ready." You can see how that might have been difficult for those facing common barriers to implementation, and where AIP originally got the reputation for being incredibly challenging. When AIP medical research began and the AIP Certified Coach practitioner training was developed, a transition phase was created to help identify if a person was suited to making a quick transition (usually over a weekend), or a slow transition (usually over six weeks), and then various guidance was given to help them implement either one of those two options. The downside to these approaches to transition were that they only focused on dietary eliminations, without taking into consideration any of the other common barriers to implementing AIP (like mindset, support, finances, time, or commitment).

The New Autoimmune Protocol transition phase has been completely reworked to include five steps to produce the most successful transition to elimination. This expanded approach embraces personalization, recognizing that factors like your family influence, cultural background, geographic location, budget, lifestyle, and personal preferences profoundly shape your ability to implement AIP. Instead of focusing only on gradual eliminations, transition now includes self-exploration, goal setting, and the development of practices that will make your transition to AIP more adaptable and empowering for long-term success. I'm excited that you are discovering AIP at a time when you can benefit from all this knowledge and new and improved guidance!

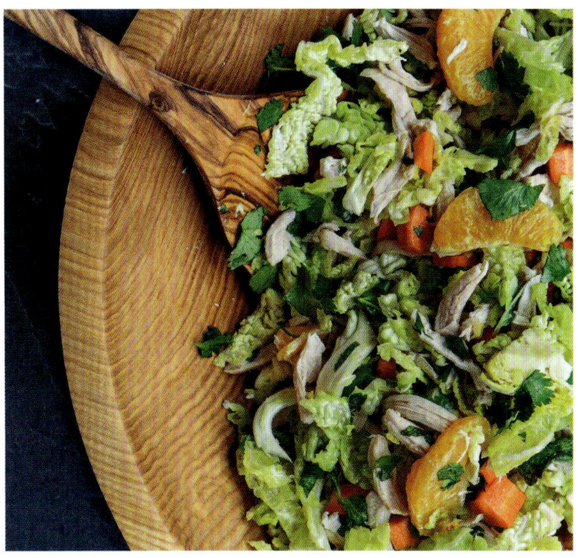

STEPS TO THE TRANSITION PHASE

During the transition phase, you'll complete these five steps, in order, which will lead you to a sustainable transition to the elimination phase. They are as follows:

1. **Track your baseline symptoms:** An accurate accounting of your current symptom burden will provide a foundation for measuring progress as you navigate both the elimination and reintroduction phases of AIP. Once you begin to make changes, it can be difficult to rely on memory to accurately determine what you used to experience; capture this initial record carefully.
2. **Develop your personal health vision:** Before making any changes, it is important to define what health truly means to you and to clarify what you hope to achieve with AIP. During this step you will identify what really matters in your life to help gain perspective and build motivation for your healing journey.

3. **Perform a confidence assessment:** This step involves taking an account of beliefs in your own ability to implement AIP. After completing this step, you'll have a detailed list of action items to complete before you implement the elimination phase as well as a better idea of how long your transition phase should last.
4. **Select your elimination phase start date:** Once you have developed your health vision and understand the specific action steps you'll need to follow to be most successful with AIP, you are ready to pick a date to start that allows you ample time to mentally and logistically commit to the transition to the elimination phase.
5. **Act on your preparation tasks:** The final step is to complete your list of preparation tasks that were generated in your confidence assessment. This might look like scheduling appointments with your medical providers, investing in some new cooking tools, asking friends or family for support, or practicing new recipes.

By following these five steps, the transition phase becomes a thoughtful, empowering process that sets you up to easily and sustainably transition to the elimination phase. Next, we'll discuss how to complete each step in detail, and which tools and assessments you'll use for this exploratory process.

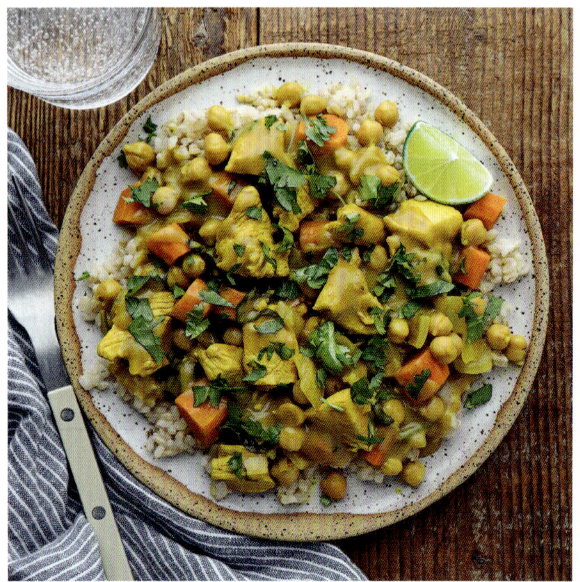

STEP 1: Track Your Baseline Symptoms

The first step in the transition phase is capturing your baseline symptoms, which you'll do by keeping a symptom journal. This step comes first, as it is something you can start immediately and provides the data you'll need to gauge progress made throughout the subsequent phases of AIP. Ideally, you'll complete one week of baseline symptom tracking before making any changes, even if those changes slowly move you toward the elimination phase. If you have a condition for which symptoms fluctuate from week to week, you'll want to try to track when symptoms are at their worst so you can capture your highest level of symptom burden.

Symptom tracking is a practice that you'll use in all three phases of AIP. During transition, your goal is simply to capture one week of baseline data. During elimination, you'll track consistently throughout the phase to gauge your progress. During reintroductions, you'll shift your tracking to help you make connections between eating foods and your symptoms. You'll learn more about symptom tracking as it applies to the elimination and reintroduction phases in Chapters 3 and 4, but for now, just understand that your goal in tracking for the transition phase is to capture your baseline symptoms for later comparison. It is recommended to complete this tracking right away, and once you've done this, you don't need to begin tracking again until you formally begin the elimination phase (more on that in Chapter 3).

On the following pages, you'll find sample weekly symptom journal pages for capturing your baseline data. (If you'd like a printable version of these pages, visit THEAUTOIMMUNEPROTOCOL.COM/PRINTABLES.) We'll discuss symptom tracking in greater detail in Chapter 3—just know you are free to use another method for your baseline symptom tracking if you are confident that is what you'll be using once you are in the elimination phase.

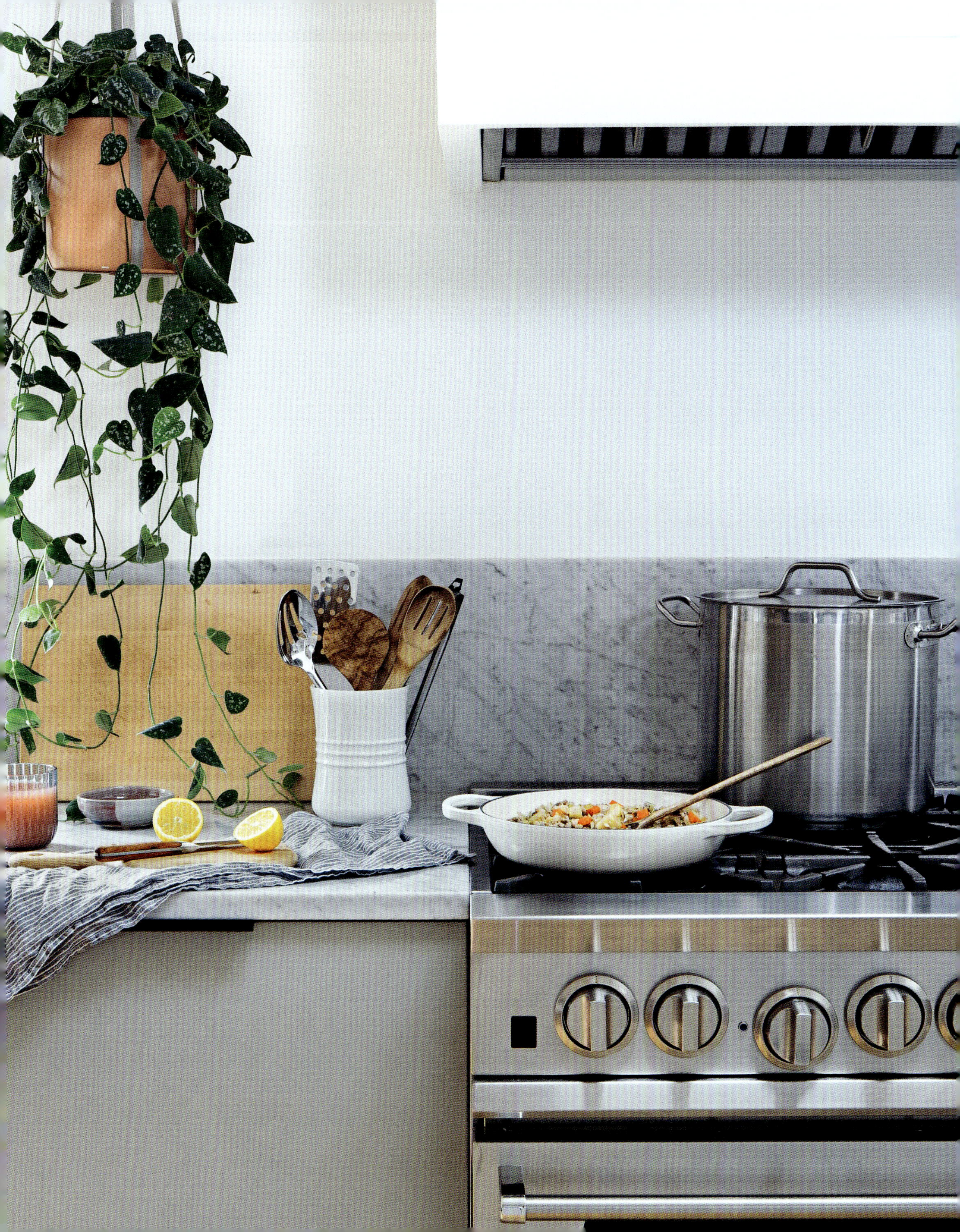

SYMPTOM JOURNAL PAGES

In each of the first four rows, record a number between 1 and 10 representing how you felt in that area on that day. Next, circle any digestive symptoms experienced on that day, note bowel movement scores per the Bristol Stool Chart (reference online), and add any notable symptoms using the list below to help you. Use a new form each week.

DATES: ____________________

	MON	TUE	WED	THU	FRI	SAT	SUN
ENERGY 1 = very low 10 = very high							
PAIN 1 = very low 10 = very high							
STRESS LEVEL 1 = very low 10 = very high							
MOOD 1 = very low 10 = very high							
DIGESTION (circle those that apply)	Belching Bloating Cramping Flatulence Heartburn Nausea	Belching Bloating Cramping Flatulence Heartburn Nausea	Belching Bloating Cramping Flatulence Heartburn Nausea	Belching Bloating Cramping Flatulence Heartburn Nausea	Belching Bloating Cramping Flatulence Heartburn Nausea	Belching Bloating Cramping Flatulence Heartburn Nausea	Belching Bloating Cramping Flatulence Heartburn Nausea
BOWEL MOVEMENTS	BM 1: BM 2: BM 3:	BM 1: BM 2: BM 3:	BM 1: BM 2: BM 3:	BM 1: BM 2: BM 3:	BM 1: BM 2: BM 3:	BM 1: BM 2: BM 3:	BM 1: BM 2: BM 3:
OTHER/ NOTABLE SYMPTOMS							

LIST OF NOTABLE SYMPTOMS

☐ Acne	☐ Dry hair, skin, or nails	☐ Neck aches or pains
☐ Anxiety	☐ Fatigue (from mild to unable to stay awake)	☐ Need for caffeine
☐ Backache or pain	☐ Headache (from mild to migraine)	☐ Phlegm, runny nose, or postnasal drip
☐ Breast tenderness	☐ Hives	☐ Pink bumps or spots
☐ Cough or need to clear throat	☐ Insomnia	☐ Rash
☐ Cravings (fatty)	☐ Itchy eyes, mouth, ears, or skin	☐ Sinus pressure
☐ Cravings (salty)	☐ Joint aches or pains	☐ Sneezing
☐ Cravings for non-food items (like chalk, dirt, or clay)	☐ Ligament aches or pains	☐ Stomach aches or pains
☐ Depression	☐ Low stress tolerance	☐ Tendon aches or pains
☐ Dizzy or lightheaded	☐ Muscle aches or pains	☐ Unrested after sleep

Were there any notable symptoms or those that need more explanation this week? If so, describe below:

STEP 2: Develop Your Personal Health Vision

The second step in the transition phase is developing your personal health vision—a powerful exercise that will serve as a foundation for your healing journey. Jaime Hartman, my partner and collaborator at AIP Certified Coach, introduced me to this model for identifying a person's unique vision of health and using it to create realistic and actionable goals for progressing through the phases of AIP. Even after you complete the protocol, you can refer to your work in this area to inform which practices you will continue to engage in.

The idea of a personal health vision is born out of the concept that there is more than one way to measure health. Some may view it through a conventional medical model and define health as the absence of disease or symptoms, or the ability to perform daily activities without physical or mental limitations. Those who subscribe to this model often focus on measurable physical outcomes, such as lab results like antibodies or other diagnostic testing that might indicate disease progression. Others may take on a more holistic model of health, which includes markers that go beyond the physical body, including mental, emotional, social, and spiritual well-being. Those who hold this view of health might feel that deficits in any of these areas are equally important or challenging as those that are physical. Finally, you may recognize that health is not a stable constant over time and may be open to even the most subtle shifts. If so, you are viewing health through a wellness model that includes an understanding that health is a dynamic state of equilibrium in many areas that can shift and adapt due to life circumstances. Within this model, subtle shifts in health are expected and resilience and adaptation celebrated.

Whether you primarily view your health through a medical, holistic, or wellness model—or some combination of the three—it is important to understand only *you* can determine your personal health vision (not your partner, your friends, or your healthcare providers). When you are ready to start the process, set aside an hour or two to complete the Personal Health Vision Questions (for a printable version, visit THEAUTOIMMUNEPROTOCOL.COM/PRINTABLES). Try to set aside a time that is quiet and during which you will be undisturbed. You might want to light a candle and play some soft music or perform this exercise outside in nature—pick a time and place in which you feel focused and grounded. Give yourself ample time to consider each question and journal your answers in detail.

Your process working through this exercise may be one journaling session, if your answers come easily and your personal health vision emerges from your writing. It is also possible that this exercise can inspire deeper thought and exploration, perhaps spurring you to discuss with a close friend or family member or research other books or resources on the topic. Feel free to stay in this process as long as you need to, emerging when you feel you accurately understand and have articulated your personal health vision.

PERSONAL HEALTH VISION QUESTIONS

Spend some time reflecting on the following questions before journaling your answers.

1. What does "health" mean to you, considering physical, mental, emotional, and spiritual aspects?

   For example: *Is health about having the endurance to climb stairs, go hiking, or play with your kids? Feeling at ease within your body? Being able to pursue your passions and goals? Engaging in activities that give your life meaning? Contributing to your community to find fulfillment?*

2. What are your top three health goals, and why are they important to you?

   For example: *Do you want to decrease joint pain so you can start a consistent exercise routine? Increase energy levels so you can participate in a* *favorite activity? Reduce anxiety to improve your quality of life?*

3. What activities or practices make you feel alive, balanced, and energized?

   For example: *Do you feel best after spending time in nature, taking a yoga class, or having a meaningful conversation with a friend? Playing with your children?*

4. How do you measure success when it comes to your physical, mental, and emotional health?

   For example: *Is it when your lab results show improvement, when you experience a symptom less often, when you wake up feeling energized, or when you feel resilient in the face of stress?*

5. How do you envision your life when you have realized your personal health vision?

   Try to be as specific as possible as you describe your life in this future time. What are some of the activities you will be doing? Who will you do them with? What will you be seeing and hearing? What will you be feeling?

STEP 3: Perform a Confidence Assessment

Now that you've tracked your baseline symptoms and developed your personal health vision, it is time to perform a confidence assessment. This exercise will help you determine which action steps are necessary and how long it will take you to complete the rest of the transition phase. You've noticed I haven't given a timeframe for completing the transition phase, which is because this is the step where you'll learn exactly how long it will take for you to be ready to start the elimination phase. As with many aspects of AIP, this is going to vary from person to person!

In this exercise, you'll use the Confidence Assessment Questionnaire (for a printable version, visit THEAUTOIMMUNEPROTOCOL.COM/PRINTABLES). For each question, you'll answer on a scale of 1 to 10 for confidence in specific key areas important to implementing AIP, with an answer of 1 representing your lowest level of confidence and 10 representing your highest level of confidence. Next, for any questions you scored below a 7, you'll list the exact reasons for your answer, as well as list any action steps that would bring that level up to above a 7. Last, you'll indicate how long it will take you to complete those steps (it could be days, weeks, or months). Be thoughtful and honest about your responses here, as they will dictate the rest of your approach to the transition phase.

The goal of the confidence assessment is not to get to the point where your answer is a 10 for every question once you've taken the steps indicated. Instead, the goal is to spend some time acting in the areas that are likely to present the largest barriers when you implement the elimination phase, so that you can be successful in your attempt. Essentially, you are prioritizing your time to raise your level of confidence in the areas that you identify will present the largest challenge for you in implementing AIP. These barriers won't go away, but many of them can be improved before beginning, which will lead to a much smoother and successful transition.

For example, in question 4, "How confident are you in your ability to handle basic cooking tasks?" you answer 4. Your reasons for answering a 4 are that your cooking skill only includes boiling water and heating convenience foods, and maybe rough chopping fruits and vegetables. The action steps you could indicate to bring this area up to a 7 might be taking an in-person cooking class, watching some instructional cooking videos online, and spending some time practicing basic cooking techniques at home. These action items might take you two to three weeks, if not a month, to complete thoughtfully. If you were to retake the confidence assessment after completing these action items, you would be ready to transition to the elimination phase if your answer is now a 7. If you need ideas about how to improve your score in each area, we'll be discussing each of them further in the following sections.

CONFIDENCE ASSESSMENT QUESTIONNAIRE

Answer each question on a scale of 1 (not confident at all) to 10 (extremely confident) to provide a clear picture of readiness and highlight areas needing more focus or support.

1. UNDERSTANDING OF AIP PRINCIPLES

How confident are you in your understanding of AIP, including the foods to include, foods to avoid, compliance, and the reintroduction process? 1 2 3 4 5 6 7 8 9 10

If below a 7, list the reasons for your answer:

____

What action steps would bring your confidence level to 7 or above?

____

How long will they take to complete? ______________________________

2. COMMITMENT LEVEL

How confident are you that you can remain committed to the process of AIP from transition, elimination, and reintroductions? 1 2 3 4 5 6 7 8 9 10

If below a 7, list the reasons for your answer:

____

What action steps would bring your confidence level to 7 or above?

____

How long will they take to complete? ______________________________

3. SUPPORT SYSTEM

How confident are you that supportive friends, family members, or community members will encourage you or help you implement AIP? 1 2 3 4 5 6 7 8 9 10

If below a 7, list the reasons for your answer:

____

What action steps would bring your confidence level to 7 or above?

____

How long will they take to complete? ______________________________

4. COOKING SKILL

How confident are you in your ability to handle basic cooking tasks like chopping, measuring, peeling, sautéing, roasting, boiling, and simmering, as well as following simple recipe instructions? 1 2 3 4 5 6 7 8 9 10

If below a 7, list the reasons for your answer:

What action steps would bring your confidence level to 7 or above?

How long will they take to complete?

5. KITCHEN AND EQUIPMENT ACCESS

How confident are you that you will have consistent access to a kitchen equipped with the necessary basic tools for preparing AIP meals? 1 2 3 4 5 6 7 8 9 10

If below a 7, list the reasons for your answer:

What action steps would bring your confidence level to 7 or above?

How long will they take to complete?

6. TIME MANAGEMENT

How confident are you that you have enough time each week for meal planning, grocery shopping, food preparation, and cleanup? 1 2 3 4 5 6 7 8 9 10

If below a 7, list the reasons for your answer:

What action steps would bring your confidence level to 7 or above?

How long will they take to complete?

7. GROCERY STORE ACCESS AND FAMILIARITY

How confident are you in your ability to access physical or online stores that sell AIP-compliant ingredients and find those items? 1 2 3 4 5 6 7 8 9 10

If below a 7, list the reasons for your answer:

What action steps would bring your confidence level to 7 or above?

How long will they take to complete?

8. FINANCIAL RESOURCES

How confident are you in your ability to afford AIP-compliant ingredients and any additional needs like basic cooking tools? 1 2 3 4 5 6 7 8 9 10

If below a 7, list the reasons for your answer:

____

What action steps would bring your confidence level to 7 or above?

____

How long will they take to complete? _______________

9. SOCIAL SITUATIONS

How confident are you in your ability to navigate social events, dining out, or family gatherings while staying compliant with AIP and explaining your dietary needs? 1 2 3 4 5 6 7 8 9 10

If below a 7, list the reasons for your answer:

____

What action steps would bring your confidence level to 7 or above?

____

How long will they take to complete? _______________

10. ADAPTABILITY AND WILLINGNESS TO EXPERIMENT

How confident are you in your ability to navigate challenges like adjusting recipes or your openness to trying new foods, recipes, and cooking techniques? 1 2 3 4 5 6 7 8 9 10

If below a 7, list the reasons for your answer:

____

What action steps would bring your confidence level to 7 or above?

____

How long will they take to complete? _______________

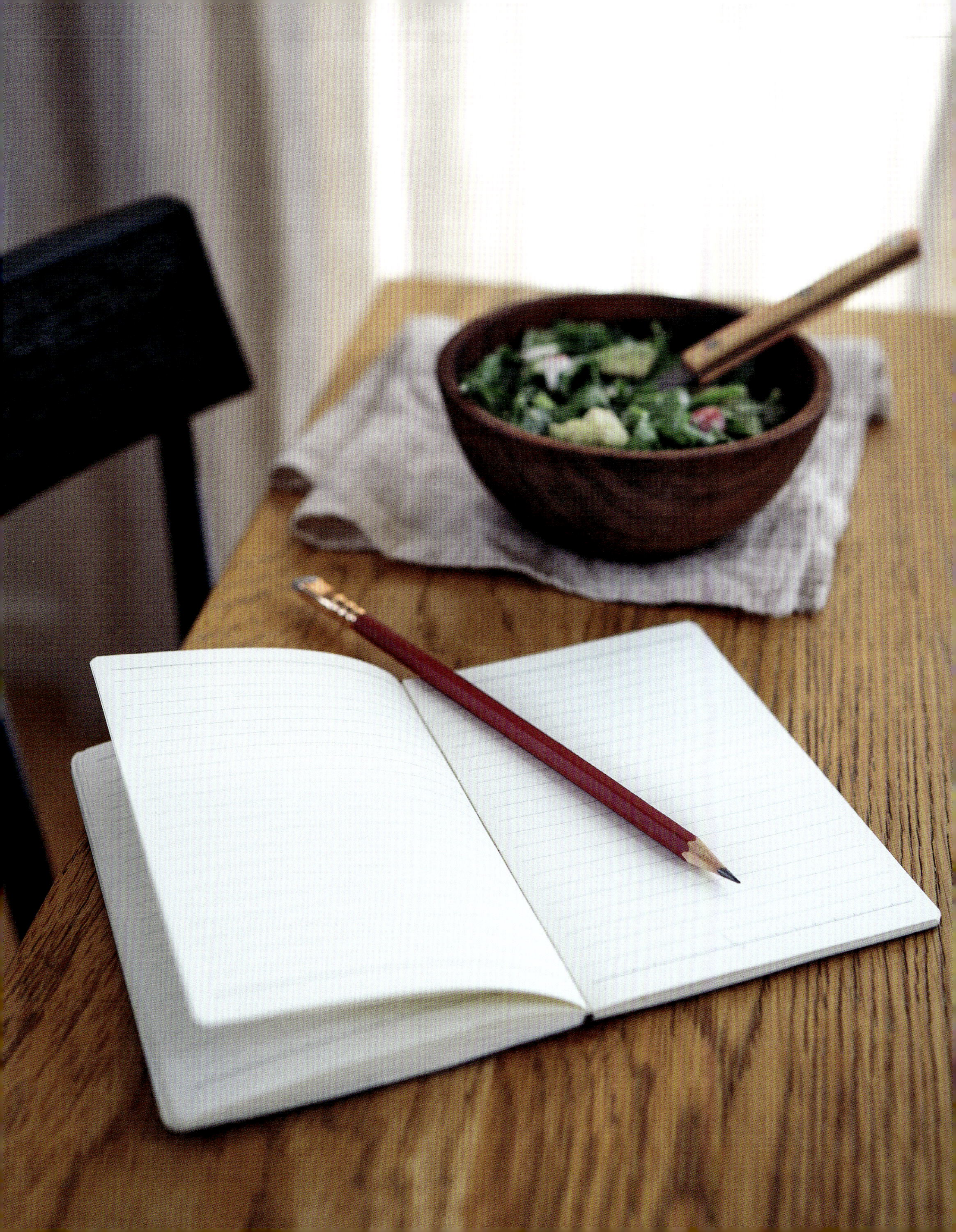

STEP 4: Select Your Elimination Phase Start Date

Now that you have completed the confidence assessment, you have a clearer picture of what needs to be done to make a sustainable transition to the elimination phase. You should have generated a list of action items—now you are ready to pick a start date! Sit down with this list and your calendar and come up with an option that gives you ample room to work through everything, as well as a little buffer for unexpected challenges or roadblocks.

What is a reasonable amount of time to dedicate to this process? If your assessment indicates you are confident and prepared to start the elimination phase (at least a 7 in all the questions on the assessment), your transition might be as short as a couple of weeks. Most people who have a couple of answers in the 5 or 6 range will do well with about a month to work through their action items. And if you noted many barriers to implementing AIP or need more time to act on your list, don't be afraid to spend a couple of months in transition!

In addition to how long it will take you to work through your action items in preparation for the elimination phase, you also need to consider the overall timing of implementing AIP as it relates to other commitments or challenges in your life. Events or activities like moving cross-country, a change in job, major travel, caretaking for children or sick family members, or planning major events like weddings are often very difficult to navigate alongside implementing AIP. While sometimes challenges are unexpected and you may need to adapt in the moment, if you have advance knowledge of a big event or change happening in your life, you may want to plan around it, if possible. It is unlikely you will have a perfect window to devote to navigating AIP, but waiting to begin until your life can best accommodate it will set you up for success in completing the protocol with ease.

STEP 5: Act on Your Preparation Tasks

Now that you've got your start date picked out, your final task is to act in all the areas you identified because of the confidence assessment. In the following section, you'll find some ideas for action items you can take in the areas where your confidence assessment indicated you need work. You also may have your own, more specific, action items to add to your list!

Understanding of AIP Principles

To successfully navigate AIP, you'll need an excellent working understanding of the protocol as you'll be implementing the elimination phase to 100 percent compliance and following the reintroduction procedure carefully. If you indicated a low confidence level in this area, simply reading Part I of this book (or perhaps rereading it, if necessary) will help you understand the finer points. You can also print the lists of foods to include, foods to avoid, and other materials for your chosen elimination protocol and post them on your refrigerator or keep them handy for reference (printable versions are available at THEAUTOIMMUNEPROTOCOL.COM/PRINTABLES).

You can also practice your understanding of what is allowed during the elimination phase of AIP before committing to your start date to avoid mistakes when the stakes are higher. This might look like taking the food lists to the grocery store and practicing reading ingredient labels, identifying which foods are suitable for your elimination. If there are any ingredients you aren't sure about, you can note them to research later. By doing this, you'll essentially be practicing the steps for determining if a food is compliant during the elimination phase, something that will become incredibly important to your success.

If you still feel confused or challenged by the details of AIP, especially if you intend to personalize or modify the protocol to your circumstances, consider hiring an AIP Certified Coach to help answer any questions or concerns you have about navigating AIP.

Commitment Level

Implementing AIP requires a high level of commitment to both begin the elimination phase and also to stay the course to complete the protocol. Fully evaluating your commitment level involves not only identifying how committed you are to beginning, but also honestly evaluating your confidence in remaining committed through the process of elimination and reintroduction. It is smart to anticipate the possibility that your commitment could flag at some point, and in case that happens, you should have some corrective plans in place so you can reach your goals.

If you've determined you have a low level of commitment to beginning AIP, you'll want to engage in some practices to build that up so that you can gain starting motivation. This might look like spending time reflecting on your personal health vision, your reasons for starting AIP, and what you hope to achieve through navigating the protocol. Additionally, you might have some other issues that need to be addressed before you are fully committed. For example, if time is a major barrier for you, consider when you could schedule your transition to AIP so that you have more attention to see the process through from start to finish. If you are lacking commitment due to being unsure if the protocol will help you and you are motivated by research, spend time reading the full-text articles of the AIP medical studies. Or, if you find personal stories inspiring, dig deeper with the Stories of Recovery series on the Autoimmune Wellness website or seek out AIP success stories in disease-specific support groups.

It is also possible that you identify as committed to beginning AIP now, but you have a history of starting and stopping lots of dietary or lifestyle changes in the past. This is a key indicator that even though you might not be presently struggling with commitment, some anticipatory work might help you avoid stopping due to encountering the same barriers you've struggled with in the past. Consider some of your past experiences to come up with an actionable plan for success should you find yourself lacking commitment to seeing the process of AIP through from start to finish.

Support System

It is important to identify your support network before implementing AIP so that you can engage them for different ways as you implement the protocol. If your assessment showed that you need improvement in this area, you'll want to take action to identify or strengthen your support network during the transition phase.

The first step here can be simply identifying who in your life is able to offer you support, and in what ways. You might create separate lists of people, those who can help with physical tasks like grocery shopping, cooking, or cleanup, and those who are able to offer emotional support like regular check-ins or vent sessions. They might be your partner or spouse, family members, and/or close friends—or they could even be members of disease or AIP-specific support groups. It is important not to rely on only one person to support you in all areas as you navigate AIP—this is a recipe for burnout on their end. Instead, try to think of delegating various support tasks throughout your network, and trying to match the right type of support with an ideal supporter. For example, your partner might not have experience with chronic illness, so asking for emotional support from a friend who also has autoimmune disease might be more helpful for support in this area (shoutout to Mary, who has been my Hashimoto's bestie since my earliest days on AIP!).

Next, you might set aside time to speak with these potential supporters and explain that you'll be implementing AIP and ask them for their support in specific areas. Many people find it awkward to ask for support or help, but our loved ones often jump at the opportunity to help us succeed in our goals. Informing your supporters ahead of time can also increase the chance that they will help you stay accountable, and help you stay positive in challenging situations. This might look like a friend who backs you up at a gathering where a host is giving you a hard time about not eating provided food, or who suggests your friend group gather for a walk together in the park instead of drinks out at a bar to socialize.

If you experience a lack of support within your immediate family or friend group, you might seek out additional community with people who understand. This can come in the form of local or online support groups focused on your specific autoimmune condition or AIP in general.

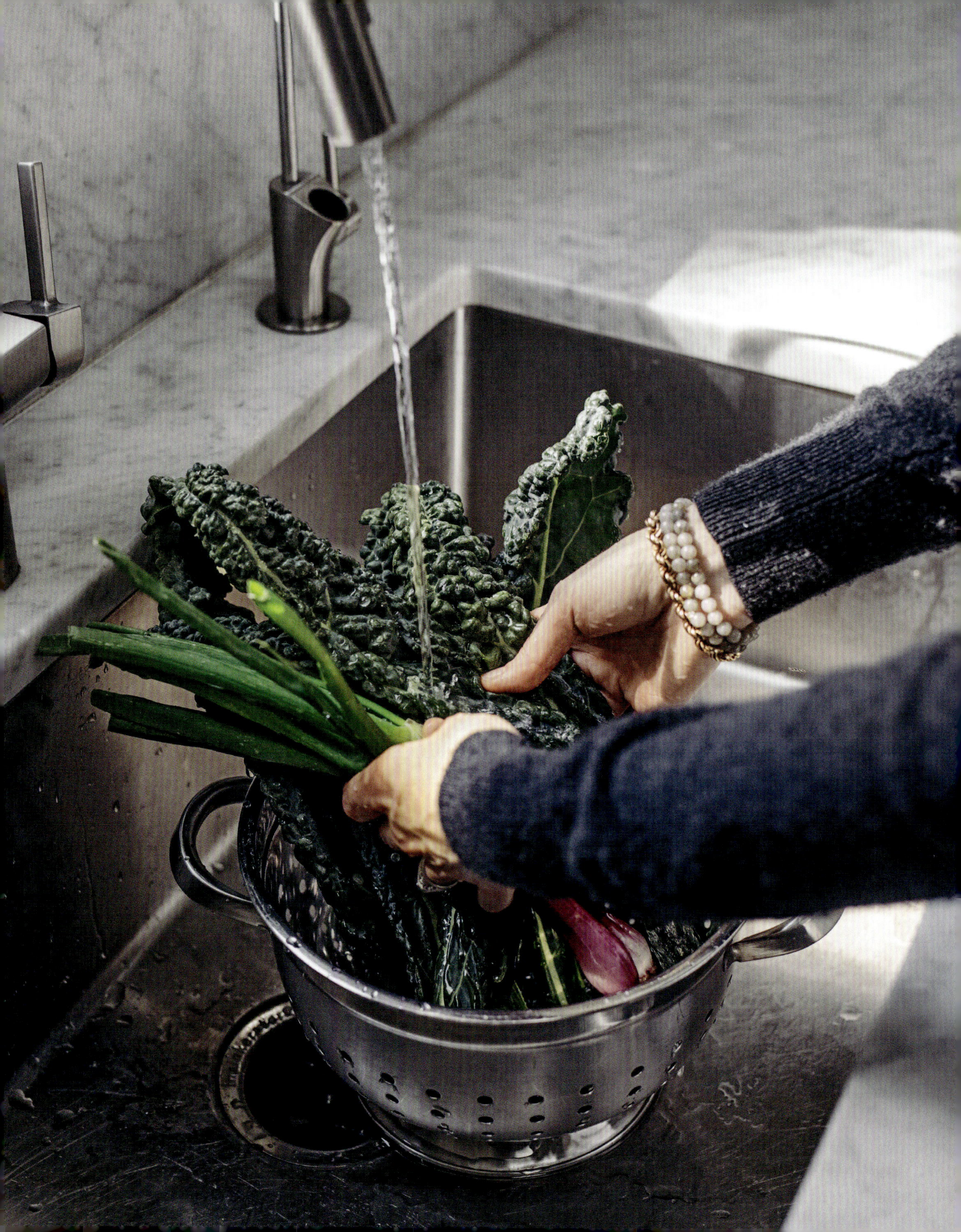

Cooking Skill

While you certainly don't need to be a gourmet chef to successfully implement AIP, you do need to perform basic cooking tasks to prepare your meals and be successful in the elimination phase. If you are unable to cook for yourself, this applies to your helper or supporter. If your confidence assessment indicated that you need to improve your cooking skill, there are a few ways you can achieve that during your transition phase.

First, you can take an in-person cooking class. This does not need to be an AIP-focused class, as you'll be completing this before you start the elimination phase. Look for a class that covers the essentials of basic cooking, like chopping, peeling, sautéing, roasting, boiling, and simmering. Steer clear of any advanced classes or those that focus on difficult or specific techniques—those won't be required to perform the basic cooking needed for AIP or any of the recipes in this book. If an in-person cooking class isn't accessible to you, there are a wealth of resources, both free and paid, for cooking instruction online. I recommend starting with YouTube, looking up each basic cooking task, and watching a detailed instructional video on the topic.

Once you've gained basic cooking knowledge in the form of in-person or online instruction, it is time to practice cooking at home. This might look like selecting some simple AIP recipes from this book and scheduling a couple of sessions per week to practice your skills and prepare some meals. You might feel like a few cooking sessions raises your confidence to the point that you feel you can implement AIP, or you might need a month to practice your new skills and spend some time until it feels routine.

Kitchen and Equipment Access

To prepare and cook your meals while on AIP, you'll also need access to a kitchen with basic tools available for cooking. If you answered with low confidence in this area, there are a few ways you can improve this.

Those who are in community living situations (like college dorms) sometimes have trouble accessing or using a kitchen regularly or are concerned with cross-contamination (especially if they have known food allergies, like gluten or dairy). Your action items for troubleshooting these situations are likely to be unique to your situation but might look like waiting to implement AIP until kitchen access is not a concern (such as a summer break) or doing some research on how to access a shared kitchen and planning for either cleaning shared tools and equipment or storing a separate set for your own use.

You might have access to a kitchen but lack the right tools or organization. It is a misconception that you need expensive or specific tools to implement AIP—if you have a kitchen that has been outfitted for basic cooking, you likely have what you need already. One action item could be to spend a weekend organizing your kitchen to provide easy access to items you'll be using most often and perform some cleaning and/or maintenance on items that you haven't used in a while. This organization might include storing those items and using that space for something you will be using every day or just creating more counter space. See the Kitchen Setup Guide on page 284 for a listing of tools you'll need as well as additional organization tips.

Another action item could be to inventory your kitchen tools to determine if there are any gaps in your setup. From there, you can research options to invest in that will help you fill those gaps and make cooking for AIP easier. Many people assume that they need large or expensive tools to implement AIP successfully (pressure cookers, high-speed blenders, air fryers, etc.) when a basic set of tools like sizable cutting boards, sharp knives, soup pots, a skillet or two, and some roasting dishes will set you up just fine to make most of the recipes in this book.

Time Management

Implementing AIP means that you will likely need to devote more time to things like meal planning, grocery shopping, food preparation, and cleanup compared to your usual routine. If your confidence assessment pinpointed trouble in this area, there are a few action items that could be on your list as you transition to the elimination phase.

First, you might create a time budget identifying how much time it will take you to complete each implementation-related task on a weekly basis. This time budget can then be used to create a realistic schedule of when you plan to execute each task so that you can budget the right amount of time accordingly. In addition, you might consider how you might save time. Practices like meal planning and batch-cooking can save an incredible amount of time when implementing AIP, and taking another look at those practices with an eye for how you can use them to save time is a great idea. You also might invest in tools that can help save time (such as a pressure cooker that can cook soups and stews in a fraction of the time). Last, you might consider other solutions to save time, such as fresh or frozen grocery or meal delivery services that cater to AIP, if these are accessible to you (see Resources on page 288 for more information).

Grocery Store Access and Familiarity

To transition to the elimination phase, you'll be shifting what you buy at the grocery store, often quite substantially. If your assessment indicated that grocery store access or familiarity is an area of low confidence for you, there are some ways you can improve.

First, print out the lists of foods to include and avoid for the elimination phase and take an exploratory tour of the grocery stores you already shop at. It is a misconception that ingredients for AIP need to be purchased at organic or specialty grocers. In fact, the recipes in this book include ingredients found year-round in most regular and big-box grocers for ease of access. Circle all the ingredients you can find regularly at the shops you already frequent. If there are still some items that you can't source at your usual stores, try visiting some other markets that you don't usually shop at to see if they offer anything extra. Again, make a note of which AIP ingredients you are likely to find there, so that can inform your grocery shop planning in the future.

Last, it is becoming increasingly affordable to shop for ingredients online, especially pantry items. If there are some items you just can't find at your local markets, be sure to check online retailers and compare prices to see if that is a good option for you (see Resources on page 288 for some recommended options, as well as the Core and Modified AIP Pantry Guides on page 286 for a list of ingredients to keep on hand).

Financial Resources

Shifting your diet to include fresh fruits and vegetables along with ample meat and seafood is likely to increase your grocery bill. If your assessment pinpointed that staying within your food budget is a primary concern for you in transitioning to AIP, use some of these tips to help keep your costs down.

First, you might make a list of AIP-compliant ingredients that are within your budget to prioritize in your meal planning. This might take referencing the food lists with prices at your local supermarkets, as well as online, to come up with the meats, seafood, fruits, vegetables, and other pantry staples that are affordable in your area. Next, you can explore deals at big-box stores or through buying in bulk. While some budgets don't allow for bulk upfront purchases, if you have some flexibility, you might be able to save some money on food expenses using this practice.

You can also consider if there are adjustments in other areas of your budget that could be temporarily reallocated to your food budget. This could include categories like eating out, coffee shops, or alcohol purchased at bars, which you won't be needing during your time on AIP. You can also consider other areas of your budget that may be less essential, like travel or shopping, if that works for you. Last, consider investing in only necessary tools to implement AIP. You don't need any fancy or expensive equipment to implement the protocol, and instead you can prioritize your finances to accommodate your grocery purchases.

Social Situations

To stay compliant with the elimination phase of AIP, you'll likely need to navigate ordering at restaurants, social events, and family gatherings, which can be challenging. If you find yourself with low confidence in this area, there are some things you can practice to increase your confidence in being able to navigate these social situations.

First, you might do some research into restaurants that might be able to provide AIP-friendly meals to you.

I usually start a restaurant search by looking for those that already cater to eliminations like gluten and dairy, as these places are usually less bothered by asking about ingredients or making additional modifications to their meals. If their website doesn't provide enough information, you can call or email to inquire more about their ability to provide for you. While it is unlikely you'll find a long list of establishments in your area that can serve you, it is possible that you might find one or two safe places to eat for special occasions while you are in the elimination phase. Identifying this ahead of time also gives you a location to suggest if someone asks you to eat out during this time.

Next, regarding social events, there are a couple of strategies you can use to increase your confidence here. First, you can arrive at social gatherings having already eaten and perhaps bringing an AIP-compliant beverage or snack to enjoy instead of what is provided. Another option is to arrange ahead of time to bring a full meal, if part of the gathering includes a sit-down dinner. (I used this approach to attending weddings multiple times during my original elimination, and found all caterers were happy to plate my provided meal in the back and serve it to me at the same time as the rest of the party.) Last, you can prioritize socializing in ways that don't require eating or consuming alcohol while you are in the elimination phase, to resist temptation.

Often discussing your dietary needs with others can be difficult. If you think this is an area you are worried about, you can practice what you'll say in specific situations. Often, a simple statement with a clear boundary is the way to go, versus overexplaining and trying to justify why you are eating a certain way. "I would love to attend your wedding, but I am eating a special diet. Do you mind if I bring my own meal to make things easy for both of us?" "Can we catch up over a cup of tea instead of a glass of wine this time? I'm working on my health and not drinking right now." Continue building a library of scripts to use when the need arises.

Adaptability and Willingness to Experiment

Those who are most successful on AIP tend to be able to adapt quickly to unforeseen circumstances as well as those who take an experimental approach to their time on the protocol. If you don't feel confident in this area, here are some action items to increase your ability to adapt and shift gears while implementing the elimination phase.

First, if you identify yourself as someone who lacks adaptability, make sure your on-ramp to the elimination phase includes small, incremental changes. This might look like taking some extended time in transition to practice cooking and eating AIP meals, gradually excluding food groups or increasing intake of foods that are new to you. By transitioning slowly, you give yourself more time to practice and adapt to the skills necessary for implementing AIP successfully.

Additionally, you might want to designate a time (perhaps once a week) to experiment with making some of the recipes in this book, especially those that include ingredients you have not prepared or eaten before. Acknowledge and celebrate each successful experiment, even if it is as simple as trying a new vegetable or cooking method. As your experiments yield positive results, make notes of your favorites to fall back on as you plan to implement the elimination phase.

Avoiding Predictable Medical Issues

Before making changes to your diet, you should always check with your medical providers to ensure it is safe for you to do so and to see if you require any changes or monitoring based on your health status. This is especially true for those with a current or history of conditions that come with a higher risk of complications when implementing dietary changes like AIP. They include inflammatory bowel disease (Crohn's disease and ulcerative colitis), any history of bowel obstruction or bowel surgery, gallbladder disease, gastric bypass surgery, chronic kidney disease, diabetes, and blood clots, among others.

Even after your healthcare providers have cleared you to implement the elimination phase, clear communication and collaboration with them is necessary to prevent any adverse events that might occur due to your medical history, or even new challenges that come up during the implementation of the elimination phase.

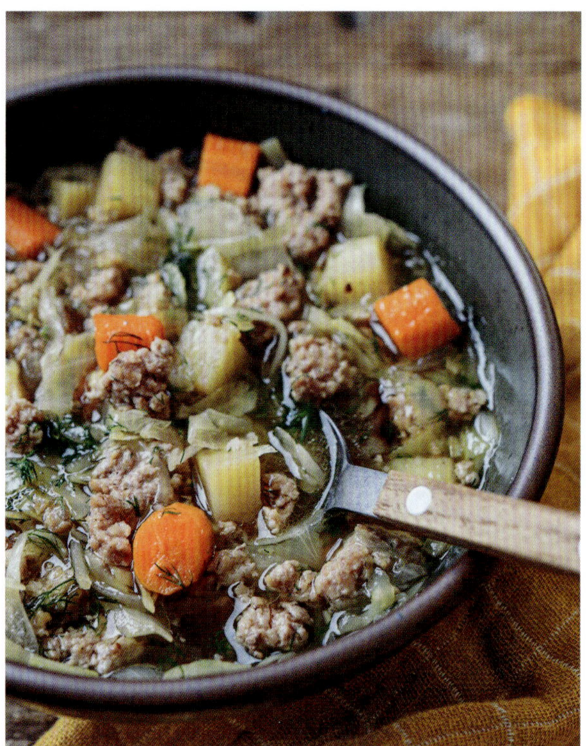

TRANSITION PHASE FAQ

Why isn't it recommended to just start the elimination phase immediately?

By jumping straight into the elimination phase without transition, you are likely to experience overwhelm and will be much less likely to be successful at maintaining compliance. In the early days of AIP, many people were unsuccessful in implementing the elimination phase not because it was too difficult, but because they didn't have a clear vision for why they were doing the protocol or gave up because they encountered a barrier (like lack of cooking skill, time, or support) without a plan in place.

Allowing yourself a comfortable transition phase gives you the opportunity to perform important tasks that will make implementing the elimination phase much easier and effective. Setting aside time to track baseline symptoms and develop your personal health vision will help you stay focused later in the process and accurately determine what is working for you. Additionally, the confidence assessment allows you to identify your largest potential barriers and address them proactively. Working through the transition phase ensures that you are fully prepared, mentally and practically, for the demands of the elimination phase, setting you up to implement it successfully and effectively. Don't skip it!

Are there other options for baseline tracking?

Yes! The sample journal pages provided on page 38 are just a suggestion for how you can structure your tracking and represent a minimum of what you'd want to track for a week as you capture your baseline. If you have a condition that presents with different types of symptoms that can be tracked in different ways or with more detail, feel free to adjust those pages or create your own to accurately track this data. We'll be discussing tracking more in Chapter 3, and after reading the guidance there, you might decide to adjust your baseline tracking to be the same as how you'll track during the elimination phase for consistency.

In addition, if you have a condition that relies primarily on biomarkers to assess progress, you might add an action item during your transition phase to see your medical team to get any baseline testing done before you start the elimination phase. This can also be a great time to inform them of your plans to try AIP and to see if they have any concerns, as everyone should be doing this before implementing a dietary change like AIP.

What if I decide to track during a week when I don't have many symptoms?

It is very common for autoimmune symptoms to fluctuate naturally over the course of weeks or months. If you have an autoimmune condition that ebbs and flows, you might expand your baseline tracking to cover two to three weeks to have a chance of capturing at a time of higher symptom burden, which will be important for assessing progress later in the elimination and reintroduction phases.

How do I know if I'm moving through the transition phase too quickly or slowly?

The length of your transition phase should be guided by your list of action items identified during the confidence assessment. If you start to feel stressed that you don't have enough time to complete these actions before your elimination phase start date, you can move that date a week or two into the future. It is always better to give yourself more time in transition, especially since many action items involve practice and familiarity, which tend to improve drastically with more repetitions.

On the flip side, if you find that your action items are not taking as long to complete as you originally thought, you can decide to move up your start date. In most cases, it is better to just stay the course and use that extra time to get some additional practice navigating potential barriers or simply planning for your elimination phase. If you find yourself being afraid to commit to picking a start date, you'll want to revisit action steps to increase your level of commitment on page 46 and your personal health vision.

Additionally, you might want to consider hiring an AIP Certified Coach to help you determine what needs to be done to make your transition successful.

What do I do about barriers to transitioning to AIP that I can't change?

If you experience barriers to adopting AIP that are not able to be modified or changed, start your focus on what you can control. Start by prioritizing small, actionable steps that move you closer to your goals without adding additional stress—like learning how to batch-cook if time is short or researching budget-friendly ingredients when finances are tight. Despite taking some actions, you might still struggle with getting to a point where you can implement the protocol—and in that case, you might have to modify it to work for you! Implementing AIP isn't about perfection, and many people have been able to use the protocol successfully despite facing considerable challenges. Focus on small ways that you can make progress in discovering sustainable ways to support your health despite these obstacles.

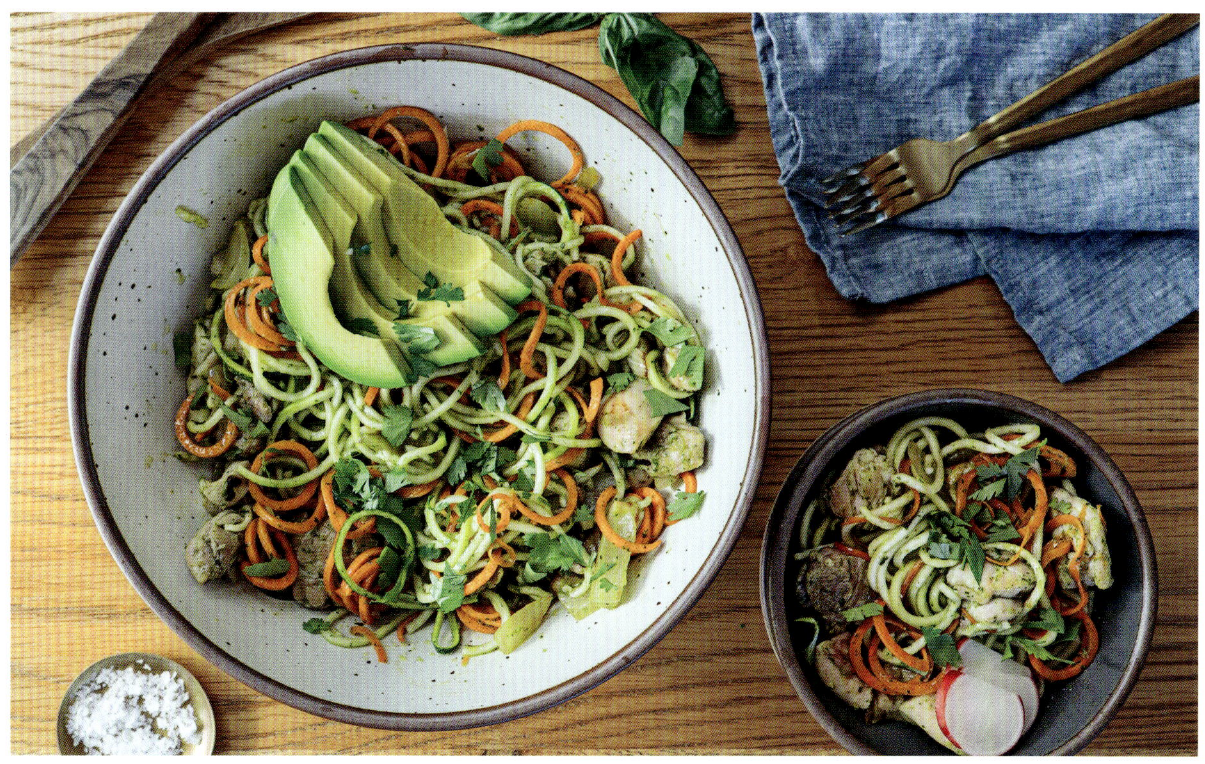

CHAPTER 3

Elimination Phase

It's time to discuss the most powerful part of the Autoimmune Protocol—the elimination phase. Using our road trip analogy, the elimination phase is the highway you'll use to get to your destination—designed for smooth, high-speed travel with minimal interruptions. For 30 to 90 days, you'll be strictly avoiding specific foods in accordance with your chosen elimination option, either Core or Modified AIP. This sets the stage for healing by removing foods that are most likely to cause inflammation or trigger your immune system and creates a supportive environment for your body to calm down, repair, and find balance. This chapter will teach you why the elimination phase is important, whether to use Core or Modified AIP, and give you exact guidance in how to implement this phase correctly.

Let's start by discussing elimination diets in detail. You already know that AIP is an evidence-based protocol that includes an elimination diet specifically designed for those with autoimmune disease. Elimination diets have been around for a long time; they were proposed in the 1920s and formally studied starting in the 1960s.[1] While exact protocols vary, elimination diets all require strict avoidance of specific foods for a set timeframe, followed by a period of reintroduction to determine if avoided foods are triggering symptoms. You've heard me say this already, because it's important—as advanced testing methods have come on the scene, elimination diets *remain* the gold standard for identifying food allergies and sensitivities.[2,3] Yes, this is why you can't replace doing the elimination phase with a food allergy test (sorry!).

I'll be the first to tell you that avoiding specific foods is *hard*. Many of us have good reasons why we are hesitant to give them up. You might be a foodie and love the flavor and texture of specific ingredients. Or you might be part of a family or friend group that frequently gathers to cook together and have food-centric celebrations. You might not be that interested in food, but as someone with a full schedule or not a lot of cooking skill, more convenient options provide most of your fuel (no judgment . . . we all must eat!). You may also suffer symptoms from your illness that impact your ability to source or cook meals from scratch or even influence the flavors and textures you find palatable. All these reasons, as well as the ones I haven't mentioned, are real and valid; I've also experienced them to varying degrees while shifting my diet to manage my health over the years. It is normal to be worried about undertaking an elimination diet. Remember that this process is in service to the personal health vision you set out on in embarking on AIP in the first place. These changes aren't forever, but they do help you identify what is working and what isn't so you can make a more informed decision about your health going forward.

As we discuss what implementing the elimination phase might look like for you, I'd like you to start by making a commitment to focus on all the foods you *can* eat during this time, instead of what you'll be avoiding. A quick look at the food lists starting on page 61 will show you how much longer the foods to include lists are than the foods to avoid lists. On the included food lists you'll likely find many delicious, nutrient-dense foods that are already your favorites (berries, avocados, and salmon are some of mine!). You are also likely to find foods that you already know you don't enjoy (okra and melons are on my personal "not a fan" list). That's fine, as you won't need to eat anything you aren't excited about, although I will encourage you to try some foods you haven't tried before or just aren't sure about yet! Starting with a focus on foods you already enjoy gives you areas of exploration when it comes to adding new foods to your routine. In my many years of coaching, I've noticed that people who choose to focus on the positives tend to find their rhythm with implementation more quickly and find more joy in the process.

Next, we'll discuss the details of how to implement the elimination phase, starting with your two options: Core and Modified AIP.

CORE AND MODIFIED AIP ELIMINATION PROTOCOLS

In 2024, based on the results of the AIP medical studies and reports from coaches trained in my AIP Certified Coach practitioner training program, the Autoimmune Protocol got a complete update. This included a new name for the original AIP elimination phase, as well as the addition of a second option for the elimination phase that is less restrictive, more accessible, but still effective. Before beginning, you'll need to choose which elimination is right for your circumstances. The two protocol options are as follows:

Core AIP Elimination

The original AIP elimination protocol is now known as Core AIP Elimination. This is the same protocol that has been in use in the AIP community for more than a decade, as well as used as an intervention in the AIP medical studies. Core AIP Elimination is the more restrictive of the two protocols, and may be most appropriate for those who have the highest burden of illness or risk of food sensitivity, as well as those who have high levels of cooking skill, prep ability, and/or outside support in implementation. Core AIP Elimination avoids all grains, legumes, dairy, eggs, nuts, seeds, nightshade-family vegetables, alcohol, and food additives (comprehensive list on page 61).

Modified AIP Elimination

The new option for the elimination phase is Modified AIP Elimination. In exploring the results from the AIP medical studies as well as feedback from medical researchers and AIP Certified Coaches, a less-restrictive, more accessible option was created that was still evidence-based but easier to implement due to the inclusion of key foods that are typically well tolerated by the autoimmune population. Modified AIP differs from Core AIP in that it includes ghee (but not other dairy), rice (but not other grains), pseudo-grains, legumes (except soy), and seeds (comprehensive list on page 66).

CHOOSING WHICH ELIMINATION PROTOCOL TO START WITH

There are many factors that go into deciding whether to start with Core AIP or Modified AIP. Let's be real—most autoimmune patients are looking to feel better quickly, and if that is you, going all-in on Core AIP might seem like your best option. A decade ago, I might have told you to just go for it, as that was what most of us in the autoimmune community were experiencing success with at the time. We've learned so much since then, though—now, my recommendation for most everyone is to start with Modified AIP. Let's unpack why.

While Core AIP has been the focus of all the AIP medical research to date, results indicate that the original protocol may be more restrictive than necessary for most autoimmune patients. You already know that the first AIP IBD study reported that 73 percent of patients reached clinical remission in just six weeks. If you look carefully at the study details, you'll notice that this was the week *before* the participants were due to complete their transition to the full elimination phase—indicating that those positive changes were likely due to the earliest eliminations (foods like gluten, grains, dairy, and eggs) and not the final ones (like nuts and seeds).[4] This is a big clue that it may not be necessary to eliminate so many foods, at least initially, to see beneficial results.

Additionally, feedback from AIP Certified Coaches also indicates that Core AIP is often more restrictive than necessary or too difficult to implement. An integral part of my training program with these coaches includes how to assess each client or patient and to modify AIP to suit the individual. This is a process I have developed with my collaborators working one-on-one, guiding health coaching clients through the details of AIP implementation. The reality is that Core AIP is not the best starting place for many people we've coached, for a variety of reasons—lack of finances, time, support, or simply being too extreme compared to their typical diet. In this case, we've long recommended customizing AIP to suit the needs of each individual. In my practice, I've been surprised at the excellent results I've seen despite using these adjusted protocols, and for those who don't see an improvement in the usual timeframe, we then still have some elimination ground to cover once their customized protocol becomes more sustainable.

When I interviewed AIP Certified Coaches who had many years' experience using AIP in their practices, I discovered that my experience as a clinician was ringing true for these coaches as well—they were reporting using customized AIP eliminations most often for their patients and clients. Like me, these providers were reporting good results with their clientele despite the modifications to the original protocol. Almost all

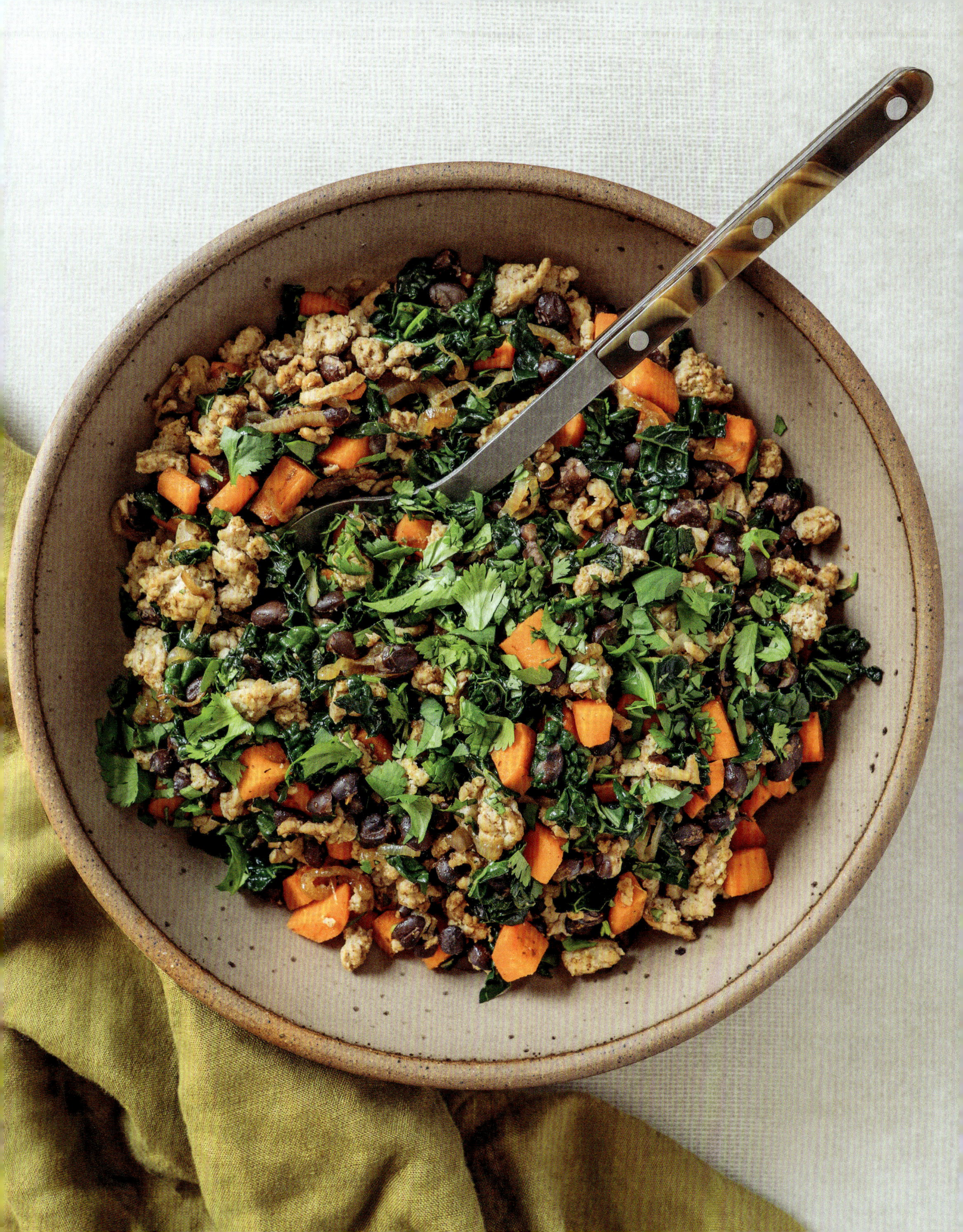

coaches reported still using Core AIP some of the time, but for a small, motivated, and supported subset for which clinical assessment determined this was still the ideal approach.

I've spent a lot of time discussing these findings and the rationale behind adding Modified AIP because I know the autoimmune community tends to think that stricter is always better, or that it will produce better results. In fact, a decade ago I thought the same. But new research and a wealth of clinical experience from providers across the natural and conventional healthcare spectrum shows us that a gentler approach can be just as effective, while at the same time more affordable, accessible, and easier to implement. If you are someone who has come across Core AIP in the past, and thought, *This is just too hard,* I am so happy that you are here now and can take advantage of this new shift toward Modified AIP so you can get started feeling better with the least number of eliminations.

If you are still exploring your decision on whether to start with Modified AIP or the original elimination protocol now known as Core AIP, you'll want to consider the following deeply before making your final decision:

- **Guidance from your healthcare providers:** While your doctor or specialist may not be familiar with AIP, they do know your health history and can give you advice on which protocol might be best for you (or they may bring up a reason why you should not attempt AIP—like an eating disorder history, or a dietary need due to your medical conditions that is not compatible with an elimination diet). If you are working with an AIP Certified Coach, they can absolutely assess your specific needs and recommend which protocol is best for you, as this is a major focus of their training using AIP.
- **Health conditions and disease severity:** Autoimmune disease and chronic illness can range from a mild annoyance to life-threatening. If you experience a higher burden of illness, you may be more motivated or have more support to implement Core AIP. This doesn't automatically mean that Core AIP will be most effective for you—in fact, it could be that Modified AIP is more effective due to less stress and more convenience (it goes both ways!). This is just a piece to think about and perhaps discuss with your healthcare providers when deciding on which protocol might work best for you.
- **Cooking skill and ability:** If you are a skilled cook and don't experience major barriers to cooking due to your health, or if you have supporters available to help you with these tasks, you may be better able to implement Core AIP successfully. If you are less skilled in the kitchen, or if you experience a lack of ability to perform cooking duties or stand because of your health, you might be more successful with Modified AIP.
- **Food access and budget concerns:** If you have limited access or budget for fresh fruits, vegetables, meat, and fish where you live, you would be better off with Modified AIP, which includes more ingredients that are accessible, affordable, and shelf-stable (like rice, pseudo-grains, legumes, and seeds).
- **Time and other implementation barriers:** If you are busy with work, caretaking, or other nonmodifiable commitments as you plan to be on your elimination, you should consider choosing Modified AIP, as it includes more convenient options (like rice, pseudo-grains, legumes, and seeds).
- **Vegetarians or vegans:** It is not possible to meet minimum protein and nutrient needs by implementing Core AIP as a vegan or vegetarian, but it is possible to implement Modified AIP with some planning. Additionally, those who eat less meat or fish in their diet should chose Modified AIP, as it provides some additional protein sources to help meet minimum protein and nutrient needs (like rice, legumes, pseudo-grains, and seeds).

COMPLIANCE DURING THE ELIMINATION PHASE

No matter which elimination option you choose, Core or Modified AIP, it is essential that you achieve and maintain 100 percent compliance during the elimination phase. In contrast to *diets*, which can be applied long-term and often have guidelines like "the 80/20 rule" or "cheat days," AIP is a *protocol* that needs to be followed precisely to clear the slate in preparation for reintroduction. Remember your goal: to set the stage for determining which foods are causing you inflammation and symptoms, so that you can make an informed choice on how to structure your diet long-term. Elimination diet research tells us that to achieve this, you need 100 percent compliance to allow the immune system to recover and rebalance before reintroducing foods.[5]

Think of it this way—you are at a party with loud music. There may be some people who you are trying to have conversations with, but they must yell to talk over the music, and you might not understand what they are saying. If someone turns down the volume, it is now easy to hear them clearly. Think of chronic inflammation as that volume being cranked up and making it impossible for you to listen to your body to determine subtle ways your diet and lifestyle are affecting you. Full compliance in the elimination phase turns down the volume on chronic inflammation, allowing you to then be able to listen to those signs that a food is triggering your symptoms. By only achieving partial compliance with the elimination phase, you're still at that loud party and much less likely to be able to "hear" what is causing your symptoms.

The importance of compliance to your success on AIP is why transition is now considered a complete phase in the New Autoimmune Protocol. Taking the time necessary to make a thoughtful, complete transition where you've set yourself up for navigating every aspect and barrier that could come up during this time will undoubtedly help you be successful. If you are still unsure that you can achieve 100 percent compliance with either Core or Modified AIP, be sure to revisit the guidance in Chapter 2 to ensure you have designed a transition phase that will set you up for success in achieving this goal.

DETERMINING IDEAL LENGTH OF THE ELIMINATION PHASE

Whether you decide on Core or Modified AIP for your elimination phase, you should plan to maintain it for a minimum of 30 days, and up to 90 days. Elimination diet research shows us that a minimum of 3 weeks is necessary for the immune system to recover from potential inflammatory foods or triggers. The elimination phase requires a minimum of 30 days to be sure that your hard work is productive at getting you past this immunological milestone.

Anecdotes and clinical experience of AIP Certified Coaches teach us that there are a range of elimination timeframes that autoimmune patients with specific conditions can expect to see results with AIP. Generally, those with autoimmune conditions affecting the digestive tract (Crohn's disease, ulcerative colitis, and celiac disease) report seeing improvements rather quickly, usually in a matter of weeks. Most autoimmune conditions, like rheumatoid arthritis, ankylosing spondylitis, Hashimoto's thyroiditis, and Graves' disease, take a little longer to see shifts, needing closer to the two-month mark. Last, a pattern has emerged for autoimmune skin conditions, like psoriasis, needing the longest amount of time in elimination, sometimes up to three months. Of course, your experience may vary—and I've seen results across the spectrum of timeframes, but as more autoimmune patients implement AIP, these patterns have emerged.

Before embarking on AIP, you should plan to stick with at least 30 days in your chosen elimination, but be prepared to extend that up to 90 days, if necessary. If you suffer from a condition that has more nebulous, hard-to-track symptoms, like Hashimoto's thyroiditis, or a skin condition like psoriasis, you might decide from the outset that you are going to prepare for 60 to 90 days in elimination. If you've already mentally prepared for the potential for extending your elimination, it won't be as difficult to make that decision should you need to at the end of your first month on the protocol.

Next, let's talk about the longer end of this timeframe. Remember, the elimination phase of AIP is not a diet and is not meant to be implemented long-term. You should not maintain these eliminations for longer than 90 days (unless you are receiving guidance from a medical provider or AIP Certified Coach that you should do so). This may contrast with what you've heard, especially in support groups online, where some less informed community members apply the elimination phase of AIP as a diet to prevent or maintain progression of their autoimmune diseases. Anecdotal and clinical evidence tells us that you are unlikely to see additional positive changes after continuing to eliminate foods after the 90-day mark, and that negative effects such as eating disorder risks, mental health challenges, and negative impacts on microbiome health, among other things, may crop up.

We'll be discussing this further in the next chapter when we cover reintroductions, as well as what to do when you don't see progress and need troubleshooting later in Chapter 6. For now, just understand that just as you plan to transition to the elimination phase, you also need to plan to enter the reintroduction phase, instead of stalling in elimination for an indefinite period.

Now we've arrived at the fun part—detailed lists of the foods you'll be avoiding and including while on your chosen elimination, either Core or Modified AIP. If you'd like printable copies of these lists to stick to your fridge or carry with you to the grocery store, head over to THEAUTOIMMUNEPROTOCOL.COM/PRINTABLES to download them—here we go!

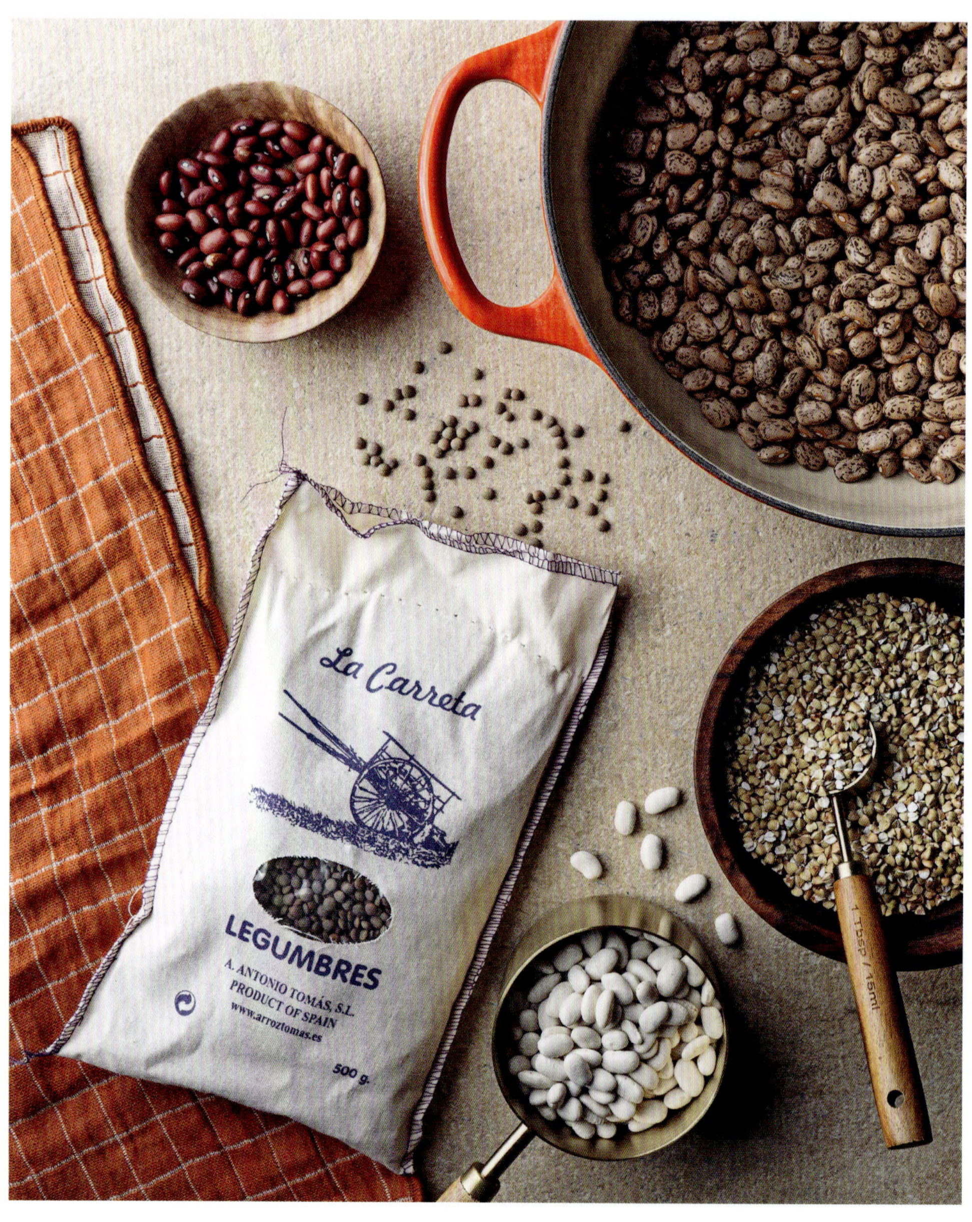

CORE AIP FOODS TO **AVOID**

GRAINS: Barley, bulgur, corn, durum, farro, fonio, Job's tears, Kamut, millet, oats, rice, rye, sorghum, spelt, teff, triticale, wheat (all varieties, including einkorn and semolina), wild rice, and all foods derived from these ingredients.

GLUTEN: Barley, bulgur, farro, rye, wheat, and all foods derived from these ingredients.

PSEUDO-GRAINS: Amaranth, buckwheat, chia, quinoa, and all foods derived from these ingredients.

DAIRY: Butter, buttermilk, butter oil, cheese, cottage cheese, cream, cream cheese, curds, dairy-protein isolates, ghee, heavy cream, ice cream, kefir, milk, sour cream, whey, whey protein, whipping cream, yogurt, and all foods derived from these ingredients.

EGGS: Chicken eggs, duck eggs, goose eggs, quail eggs, and any other type of egg.

LEGUMES: Adzuki beans, black beans, black-eyed peas, butter beans, calico beans, cannellini beans, chickpeas (aka garbanzo beans), fava beans (aka broad beans), Great Northern beans, green beans, Italian beans, kidney beans, lentils, lima beans, mung beans, navy beans, peanuts, peas, pinto beans, runner beans, split peas, soybeans (including edamame, tofu, tempeh, other soy products, and soy isolates, such as soy lecithin), and any other beans or legumes.

NIGHTSHADES (including spices derived from them): Ashwagandha, bell peppers, Cape gooseberries (ground cherries, not to be confused with regular cherries), cayenne peppers, eggplant, garden huckleberries (not to be confused with regular huckleberries), goji berries (aka wolfberries), hot peppers (chile peppers and chile-based spices), naranjillas, paprika, pepinos, pimentos, potatoes, tamarillos, tobacco, tomatillos, tomatoes.

PROCESSED VEGETABLE OILS: Canola oil (rapeseed oil), corn oil, cottonseed oil, grapeseed oil, palm kernel oil, palm olein, peanut oil, safflower oil, soybean oil, sunflower oil.

NUTS AND NUT OILS: Almonds, Brazil nuts, cashews, chestnuts, hazelnuts, macadamia nuts, pecans, pine nuts, pistachios, walnuts, and any flavors, flours, butters, oils, or other products derived from them.

SEEDS (including oils and spices derived from them): Allspice, anise seeds, annatto seeds, black caraway (Russian caraway, black cumin), cardamom, celery seeds, chia seeds, chocolate, cocoa, coffee, coriander seeds, cumin seeds, dill seeds, fennel seeds, fenugreek seeds, flax seeds, hemp seeds, juniper berries, mustard seeds, nutmeg, pepper, poppy seeds, pumpkin seeds, sesame seeds, sunflower seeds, and any other seeds. (For more information on spices, see the Core AIP Spice List on page 68.)

NONNUTRITIVE SWEETENERS AND SUGAR ALCOHOLS: Acesulfame potassium, allulose, aspartame, erythritol, mannitol, neotame, saccharin, sorbitol, stevia, sucralose, xylitol.

PROCESSED FOOD CHEMICALS AND INGREDIENTS: Acrylamides, artificial food color, artificial and natural flavors, autolyzed protein, brominated vegetable oil, emulsifiers (carrageenan, cellulose gum, guar gum, lecithin, xanthan gum), hydrolyzed vegetable protein, olestra, phosphoric acid, propylene glycol, textured vegetable protein, trans fats (partially hydrogenated vegetable oil, hydrogenated oil), yeast extract, any ingredient with an unrecognized chemical name.

ALCOHOL: Beer, liquor, mead, wine, or similar products.

CORE AIP FOODS TO **INCLUDE**

LEAFY VEGETABLES: Arugula, beet greens, bok choy, broccoli rabe, brussels sprouts, cabbage, carrot tops, celery, chicory, collard greens, cress, dandelion greens, endive, kale, lamb's lettuce, lettuce, mizuna, mustard greens, napa cabbage, purslane, radicchio, sorrel, spinach, Swiss chard, tatsoi, turnip greens, watercress.

NON-STARCHY VEGETABLES: Artichokes, asparagus, broccoli, capers, cauliflower, celery, fennel, nopal, rhubarb, squash blossoms.

ALLIUM-FAMILY VEGETABLES: Chives, garlic, green onions, leeks, onions, shallots, wild leeks (ramps).

ROOTS, TUBERS, AND BULB VEGETABLES: Arrowroot, bamboo shoots, beets, burdock, carrots, cassava, celeriac, daikon, ginger, horseradish, Jerusalem artichokes, jicama, kohlrabi, lotus root, parsnips, radishes, rutabaga, sweet potatoes, taro, tigernut, turnips, wasabi, water chestnuts, yacon, yams.

VEGETABLE-LIKE FRUITS: Avocado, bitter melon, chayote, cucumber, okra, olives, plantains, pumpkin, squash, zucchini.

BERRIES: Acai, bilberries, blackberries, blueberries, cranberries, currants, elderberries, gooseberries, grapes, huckleberries, lingonberries, loganberries, mulberries, muscadines, Oregon grapes, raspberries, salmonberries, sea buckthorn, strawberries.

ROSACEAE-FAMILY FRUITS: Apples, apricots, cherries, nectarines, peaches, pears, plums, quince, rosehips.

MELONS: Cantaloupe, honeydew, horned melon, melon pears, Persian melon, watermelon, winter melon.

CITRUS-FAMILY FRUITS: Blood oranges, Buddha's hands, clementines, grapefruits, key limes, kumquats, lemons, limes, makrut limes, mandarins, Meyer lemons, orangelos, oranges, pomelos, tangelos, tangerines, yuzu.

TROPICAL FRUITS: Acerola, bananas, cherimoya, coconut, dates, dragon fruit, durian, figs, guava, jackfruit, kiwi, loquat, lychee, mangos, mangosteen, papaya, passionfruit, pawpaw, persimmons, pineapple, plantains, pomegranates, quince, rambutan, star fruit, tamarind, vanilla.

EDIBLE FUNGI/MUSHROOMS: Chanterelles, creminis, morels, oysters, porcinis, portobellos, shiitakes, truffles.

MEAT: Antelope, bear, boar, buffalo (bison), caribou, cattle (beef, veal), deer (venison), elk, goat, hare, horse, kangaroo, moose, pig (pork), rabbit, sheep (lamb, mutton).

POULTRY: Chicken, dove, duck, goose, grouse, guinea hen, ostrich, pheasant, quail, turkey.

FISH: Anchovy, arctic char, bass, bonito, carp, catfish, cod, eel, gar, haddock, hake, halibut, herring, mackerel, mahi-mahi, marlin, monkfish, perch, pollock, salmon, sardines, snapper, sole, swordfish, tilapia, trout, tuna, turbot, walleye.

SHELLFISH: Clams, crab, crawfish, lobster, mussels, octopus, oysters, scallops, shrimp, squid.

SEA VEGETABLES: Arame, dulse, hijiki, kombu, nori, wakame.

ANIMAL FATS: Bacon fat, lard (rendered pig back fat), leaf lard (rendered pig kidney fat), pan drippings, poultry fat, salo, schmaltz (chicken or goose fat), strutto (clarified pork fat), tallow (rendered fat from beef, lamb, or mutton).

OFFAL: Bones, heart, kidney, liver, spleen, tongue.

PLANT FATS: Avocado oil, coconut oil, olive oil, palm oil, palm shortening, red palm oil.

PROBIOTIC FOODS (always check additional ingredients): Fermented meat or fish, kombucha, kvass, lacto-fermented fruits and vegetables, non-dairy kefir, sauerkraut.

LEAF, FLOWER, ROOT, AND BARK SPICES: Asafetida, basil leaf, bay leaf, chamomile, chervil, chives, cilantro (coriander leaf), cinnamon, cloves, curry leaf, dill weed, fennel leaf, garlic, ginger, horseradish (root), lavender, lemongrass, mace, makrut lime leaf, marjoram leaf, onion powder, oregano leaf, parsley, peppermint, rosemary, saffron, sage, savory leaf, spearmint, tarragon, thyme, truffles, turmeric, vanilla (whole-bean and extract).

BEVERAGES (always check additional ingredients): Black tea, coconut milk (without additives), coconut water, green tea, kombucha, mineral water, plain water, rooibos tea, sparkling water.

OTHER FLAVORINGS (always check additional ingredients): Anchovies or anchovy paste, apple cider vinegar, balsamic vinegar, capers, carob powder, coconut aminos (a soy sauce substitute), coconut concentrate, coconut milk and coconut cream, coconut vinegar, fish sauce, fruit and vegetable juices, jams and chutneys, red wine vinegar, salt, truffle oil, white wine vinegar.

SWEETENERS TO INCLUDE IN MODERATION: Coconut sugar, coconut syrup, honey, maple sugar, maple syrup, molasses.

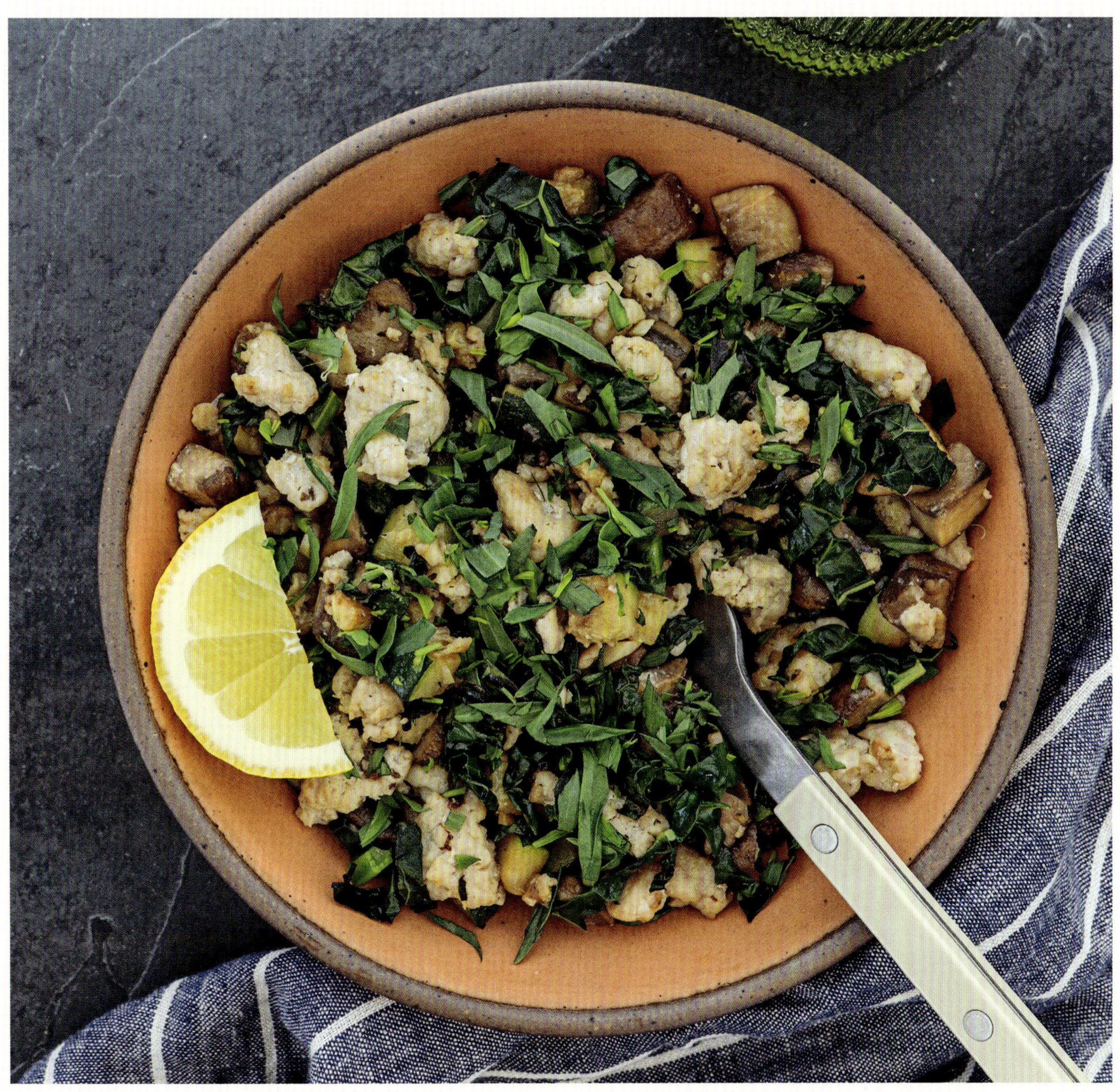

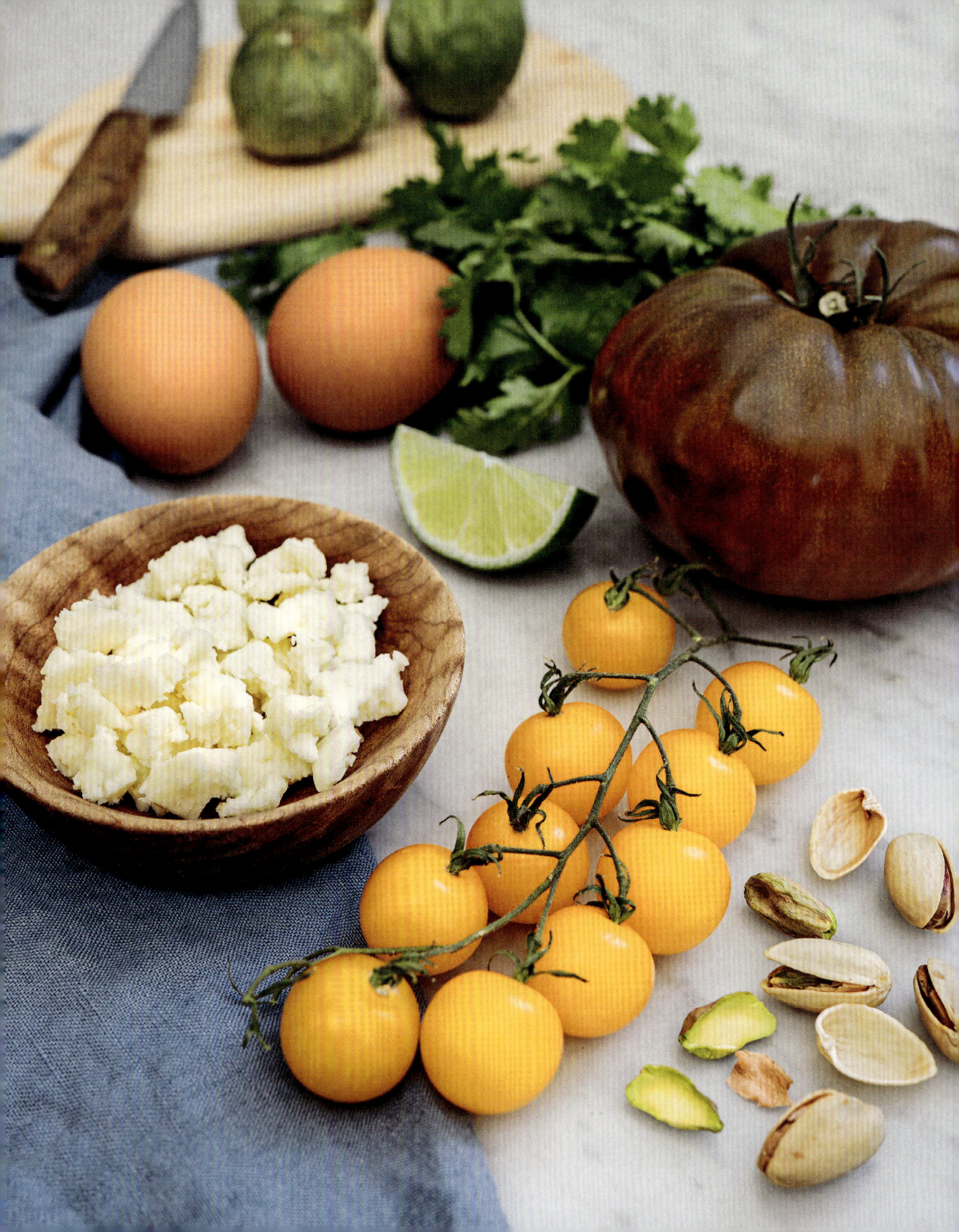

MODIFIED AIP FOODS TO **AVOID**

CEREAL GRAINS (EXCEPT RICE): Barley, bulgur, corn, durum, farro, fonio, Job's tears, Kamut, millet, oats, rye, sorghum, spelt, teff, triticale, wheat (all varieties, including einkorn and semolina), and all foods derived from these ingredients.

GLUTEN: Barley, bulgur, farro, rye, wheat, and all foods derived from these ingredients.

DAIRY (EXCEPT GHEE): Butter, buttermilk, butter oil, cheese, cottage cheese, cream, cream cheese, curds, dairy-protein isolates, heavy cream, ice cream, kefir, milk, sour cream, whey, whey protein, whipping cream, yogurt, and all foods derived from these ingredients.

EGGS: Chicken eggs, duck eggs, goose eggs, quail eggs, or any other type of egg.

NIGHTSHADES (INCLUDING SPICES DERIVED FROM THEM): Ashwagandha, bell peppers, Cape gooseberries (ground cherries, not to be confused with regular cherries), cayenne peppers, eggplant, garden huckleberries (not to be confused with regular huckleberries), goji berries (aka wolfberries), hot peppers (chile peppers and chile-based spices), naranjillas, paprika, pepinos, pimentos, potatoes, tamarillos, tobacco, tomatillos, tomatoes.

SOY: Edamame, miso, natto, tamari, tempeh, tofu, or other products derived from soy (including soy cheese, milk, protein, ice cream, sauce, and others).

TREE NUTS AND PEANUTS (including ingredients derived from them): Almonds, Brazil nuts, cashews, chestnuts, hazelnuts, macadamia nuts, peanuts, pecans, pine nuts, pistachios, walnuts, and any flavors, flours, butters, oils, or other products derived from them.

NONNUTRITIVE SWEETENERS AND SUGAR ALCOHOLS: Acesulfame potassium, allulose, aspartame, erythritol, mannitol, neotame, saccharin, sorbitol, stevia, sucralose, xylitol.

PROCESSED FOOD CHEMICALS AND INGREDIENTS: Acrylamides, artificial food color, artificial and natural flavors, autolyzed protein, brominated vegetable oil, emulsifiers (carrageenan, cellulose gum, guar gum, lecithin, xanthan gum), hydrolyzed vegetable protein, olestra, phosphoric acid, propylene glycol, textured vegetable protein, trans fats (partially hydrogenated vegetable oil, hydrogenated oil), yeast extract, any ingredient with an unrecognized chemical name.

ALCOHOL: Beer, liquor, mead, wine, or similar products.

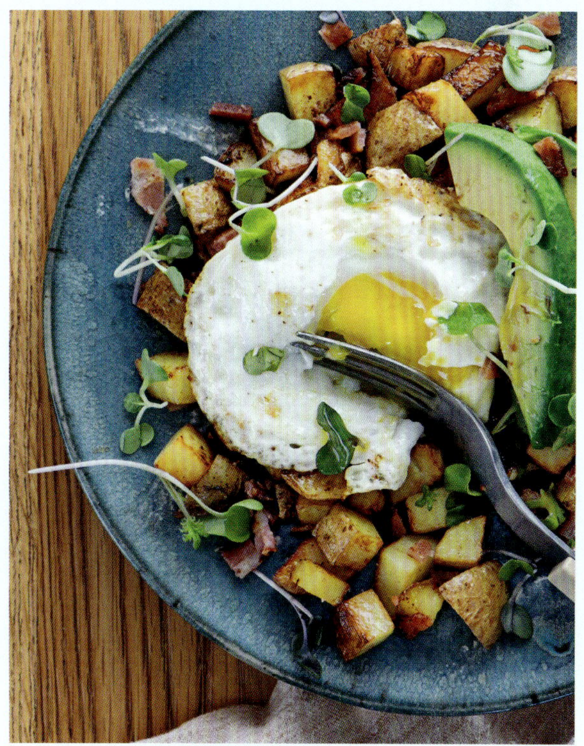

MODIFIED AIP FOODS TO **INCLUDE**

LEAFY VEGETABLES: Arugula, beet greens, bok choy, broccoli rabe, brussels sprouts, cabbage, carrot tops, celery, chicory, collard greens, cress, dandelion greens, endive, kale, lamb's lettuce, lettuce, mizuna, mustard greens, napa cabbage, purslane, radicchio, sorrel, spinach, Swiss chard, tatsoi, turnip greens, watercress.

NON-STARCHY VEGETABLES: Artichoke, asparagus, broccoli, capers, cauliflower, celery, fennel, nopal, rhubarb, squash blossoms.

ALLIUM-FAMILY VEGETABLES: Chives, garlic, green onions, leeks, onions, shallots, wild leeks (ramps).

ROOTS, TUBERS, AND BULB VEGETABLES: Arrowroot, bamboo shoots, beets, burdock, carrots, cassava, celeriac, daikon, ginger, horseradish, Jerusalem artichokes, jicama, kohlrabi, lotus root, parsnips, radishes, rutabaga, sweet potatoes, taro, tigernut, turnips, wasabi, water chestnuts, yacon, yams.

VEGETABLE-LIKE FRUITS: Avocado, bitter melon, chayote, cucumber, okra, olives, plantain, pumpkin, squash, winter melon, zucchini.

BERRIES: Acai, bilberries, blackberries, blueberries, cranberries, currants, elderberries, gooseberries, grapes, huckleberries, lingonberries, loganberries, mulberries, muscadines, Oregon grapes, raspberries, salmonberries, sea buckthorn, strawberries.

ROSACEAE-FAMILY FRUITS: Apples, apricots, cherries, nectarines, peaches, pears, plums, quince, rosehips.

MELONS: Cantaloupe, honeydew, horned melon, melon pear, Persian melon, watermelon, winter melon.

CITRUS-FAMILY FRUITS: Blood oranges, Buddha's hands, clementines, grapefruits, key limes, kumquats, lemons, limes, makrut limes, mandarins, Meyer lemons, orangelos, oranges, pomelos, tangelos, tangerines, yuzu.

TROPICAL FRUITS: Acerola, bananas, chayote, cherimoya, coconut, dates, dragon fruit, durian, figs, guava, jackfruit, kiwi, loquat, lychee, mangos, mangosteen, papaya, passionfruit, pawpaw, persimmons, pineapple, plantains, pomegranates, quince, rambutan, star fruit, tamarind, vanilla.

RICE, PSEUDO-GRAINS AND GRAIN-LIKE SUBSTANCES: Amaranth, buckwheat, chia, quinoa, rice, wild rice.

LEGUMES (except peanuts and soy): Adzuki beans, black beans, black-eyed peas, butter beans, calico beans, cannellini beans, chickpeas (aka garbanzo beans), fava beans (aka broad beans), Great Northern beans, green beans, Italian beans, kidney beans, lentils, lima beans, mung beans, navy beans, pinto beans, peas, runner beans, split peas.

EDIBLE FUNGI/MUSHROOMS: Chanterelles, creminis, morels, oysters, porcinis, portobellos, shiitakes, truffles.

MEAT: Antelope, bear, boar, buffalo (bison), caribou, cattle (beef, veal), deer (venison), elk, goat, hare, horse, kangaroo, moose, pig (pork), rabbit, sheep (lamb, mutton).

POULTRY: Chicken, dove, duck, goose, grouse, guinea hen, ostrich, pheasant, quail, turkey.

OFFAL: Bones, heart, kidney, liver, spleen, tongue.

FISH: Anchovies, arctic char, bass, bonito, carp, catfish, cod, eel, gar, haddock, hake, halibut, herring, mackerel, mahi-mahi, marlin, monkfish, perch, pollock, salmon, sardines, snapper, sole, swordfish, tilapia, trout, tuna, turbot, walleye.

SHELLFISH: Clam, crabs, crawfish, lobster, mussels, octopus, oysters, scallops, shrimp, squid.

SEA VEGETABLES: Arame, dulse, hijiki, kombu, nori, wakame.

ANIMAL FATS: Bacon fat, lard (rendered pig back fat), leaf lard (rendered pig kidney fat), pan drippings, poultry fat, salo, schmaltz (chicken or goose fat), strutto (clarified pork fat), tallow (rendered fat from beef, lamb, or mutton).

PLANT FATS: Avocado oil, coconut oil, olive oil, palm oil, palm shortening, red palm oil.

DAIRY: Ghee (only).

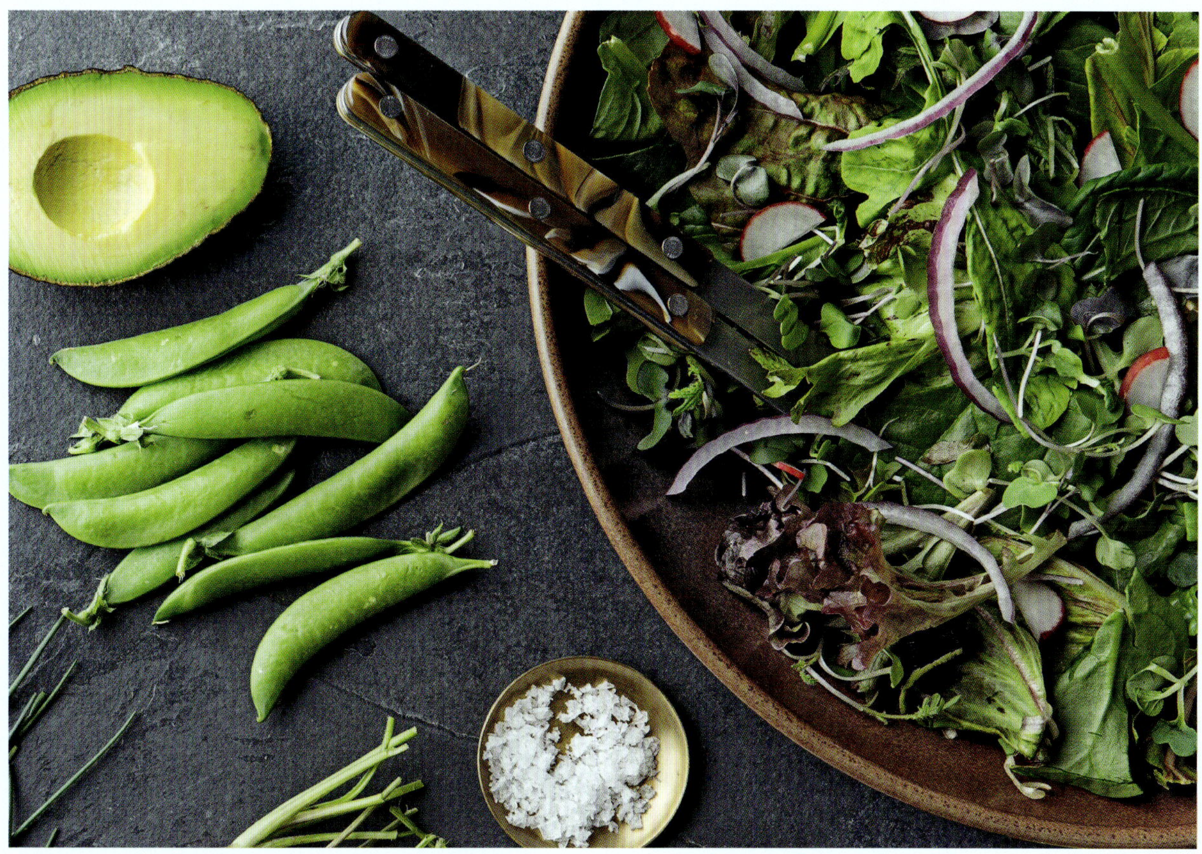

PROBIOTIC FOODS (always check additional ingredients): Fermented meat or fish, kombucha, kvass, lacto-fermented fruits and vegetables, non-dairy kefir, sauerkraut.

SEEDS (including oils and spices derived from them): Allspice, anise seeds, annatto seeds, black caraway (Russian caraway, black cumin), cardamom, celery seeds, chia seeds, chocolate, cocoa, coffee, coriander seeds, cumin seeds, dill seeds, fennel seeds, fenugreek seeds, flax seeds, hemp seeds, juniper berries, mustard seeds, nutmeg, pepper, poppy seeds, pumpkin seeds, sesame seeds, sunflower seeds.

LEAF, FLOWER, ROOT, AND BARK SPICES: Asafetida, basil leaf, bay leaf, chamomile, chervil, chives, cilantro (coriander leaf), cinnamon, cloves, curry leaf, dill weed, fennel leaf, garlic, ginger, horseradish (root), lavender, lemongrass, mace, makrut lime leaf, marjoram leaf, onion powder, oregano leaf, parsley, peppermint, rosemary, saffron, sage, savory leaf, spearmint, tarragon, thyme, truffles, turmeric, vanilla (whole-bean and extract).

BEVERAGES (always check additional ingredients): Black tea, coconut milk (without additives), coconut water, coffee, green tea, kombucha, mineral water, plain water, rooibos tea, sparkling water.

OTHER FLAVORINGS (always check additional ingredients): Anchovies or anchovy paste, apple cider vinegar, balsamic vinegar, capers, carob powder, coconut aminos (a soy sauce substitute), coconut concentrate, coconut milk and coconut cream, coconut vinegar, fish sauce, fruit and vegetable juice, jams and chutneys, red wine vinegar, salt, truffle oil, white wine vinegar.

SWEETENERS TO INCLUDE IN MODERATION: Coconut sugar, coconut syrup, honey, maple sugar, maple syrup, molasses.

CORE AIP SPICE LIST

It can be tricky to figure out which spices are in and which spices are out in the Core AIP elimination phase due to the exclusion of seeds and nightshades. Use this list to help you identify which spices to remove.

Spices to **avoid** on Core AIP:

BERRIES AND FRUIT: Allspice, caraway, cardamom pods, juniper berries, pepper (from black, green, pink, or white peppercorns), star anise, sumac.

SEEDS: Anise seeds, annatto seeds, black caraway (Russian caraway, black cumin), celery seeds, coriander seeds, cumin seeds, dill seeds, fennel seeds, fenugreek seeds, mustard seeds, nutmeg, poppy seeds.

NIGHTSHADES: Capsicum, cayenne, chile pepper flakes, chile powder, curry powder (typically contains red pepper), paprika, red pepper.

SPICE BLENDS: Chinese five-spice powder (can contain star anise, peppercorns, and fennel seeds), curry powder (can contain coriander seeds, cumin seeds, fenugreek seeds, and red pepper), garam masala (can contain peppercorns, cumin seeds, and cardamom pods), poultry seasoning (can contain peppercorns and nutmeg), steak seasoning (can contain peppercorns, chile pepper, cumin seeds, and cayenne pepper).

Spices to **include** on Core AIP:

LEAF SPICES: Basil leaf, bay leaf, chervil, chives, cilantro (coriander leaf), curry leaf, dill weed, fennel leaf, lemongrass, mace, makrut lime leaf, marjoram leaf, oregano leaf, parsley, peppermint, rosemary, sage, savory leaf, spearmint, tarragon, thyme, wasabi (additive-free).

BARK AND FLOWER SPICES: Chamomile, cinnamon, cloves, lavender, saffron, truffles, vanilla.

ROOT SPICES: Asafetida, galangal, garlic, ginger, horseradish (root), onion powder, turmeric.

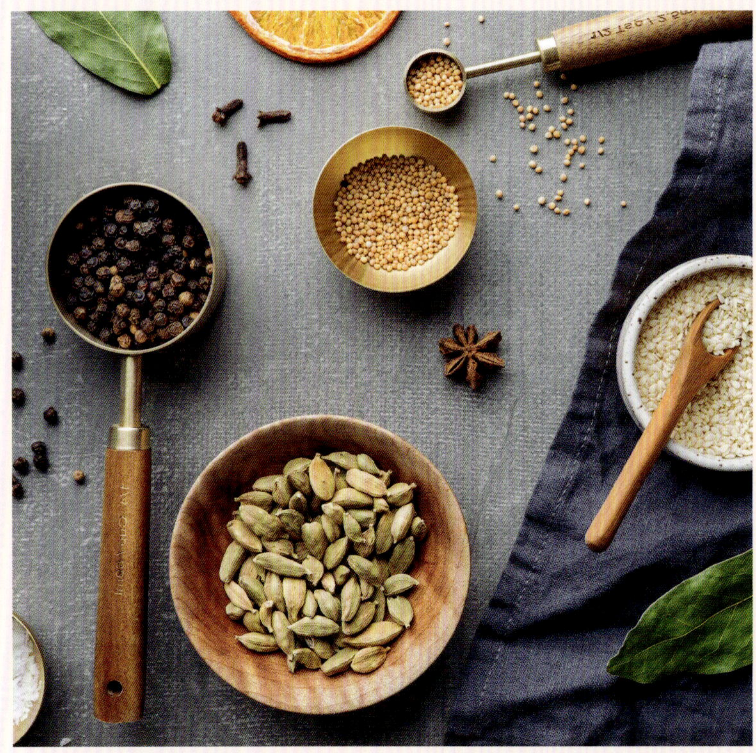

TRACKING DURING THE ELIMINATION PHASE

The final part of the elimination phase we need to discuss is tracking your progress. You're already familiar with tracking from our overview of baseline symptom tracking in the transition phase, but for the elimination phase, you'll be expanding this practice to capture data to track your progress during the entire time you are eliminating foods. Keeping a daily symptom journal is the best way to do this. The ways you can keep this journal are many, and very personal to your needs—you might prefer pen and paper, a text document on your computer or device, a spreadsheet, or an app specifically designed for symptom tracking on your smartphone (be sure to refer to the weekly symptom journal pages on page 38). It doesn't matter which tracking method you decide to use, as long as you are consistent and can glean the data to make informed decisions about the next steps in your journey. Here are the details on how to best use tracking to inform your progress on AIP.

Daily Symptom Journaling

In addition to the baseline tracking you completed during the transition phase, you should plan to track specific symptom metrics daily while in the elimination phase so that you can later assess your progress. Consider using the weekly symptom journal pages on page 38 or coming up with your own using the following guidance.

Areas to include in your symptom journaling:

- Energy levels
- Pain level
- Digestive changes
- Bowel movements
- Mood
- Skin changes
- Notable symptoms (especially those specific to your condition)

For many symptom metrics, using a scale of 1 to 10 (1 being the lowest and 10 being the highest) can make tracking fast and the data easy to analyze—compare "energy—7" to "I had a good amount of energy today." For metrics where you have a numerical value, you'll be able to see subtle trends and how they shift over time. For example, if your pain levels go from an 8 to a 6 over the course of a month—thinking back, you might not notice that subtle of a change, but upon analysis, you identify that is a 20 percent improvement! You can also use software to plot those numbers and create a graph of your progress (not necessary but might intrigue the data lovers!).

Other areas, like digestive changes, benefit from a "fill-in" style of reporting, such as noting when you experience gas, bloating, diarrhea, or constipation. Or, if those symptoms are daily occurrences and primary symptoms of your condition (such as for those with IBD), you can choose to use a 1 to 10 scale to notate severity and track that over time. For bowel movements, use the Bristol Stool Chart (reference online) for a simplified way of tracking eliminations. If you have a specific symptom that is related to your autoimmune condition, think of how you can track it in a way that will allow you to accurately assess your progress over time.

To avoid overwhelm, choose the metrics that are most relevant to your health and set yourself up with a system for capturing that easily. For example, if you are like me and have Hashimoto's thyroiditis, you might want to track energy levels (on a scale of 1 to 10), pain levels (on a scale of 1 to 10), digestive changes (fill in), bowel movements (fill in), and joint pain (on a scale of 1 to 10), plus leave yourself a designated space to add in anything notable that comes up (e.g., "cystic acne" or "unexplained anxiety"). I like to designate a small journal just for this purpose and check in at mealtimes to notate my symptoms throughout the day. Again, you might be a spreadsheet or app user, and if your tracking method is convenient and you do it regularly, it will work!

While it isn't essential that you complete your symptom tracking every single day, you should aim to complete it most days while in the elimination phase. Don't be worried if life gets busy, or if you forget a couple of days—what matters is overall consistency! This creates an accurate record of how your symptoms have changed and gives you important information that you'll need to decide how to proceed with the next phase.

Tracking in Other Areas

In addition to symptom journaling, you may decide to expand your tracking to capture other helpful information, like medication intake (especially if you have medication that you use on an as-needed basis), supplement intake, dietary intake, or body measurements. I'll add a note here, that some people find tracking overwhelming, and if this is you, please understand that you don't need to track in these "extra" areas. In fact, I have a couple of notes of caution on two of these points:

- **Tracking dietary intake:** A food and beverage journal can consist of writing down everything you eat and drink in a day and can be either simple (e.g., "Pork skillet with sweet potatoes") or extremely detailed ("4 oz ground pork, ½ sweet potato, avocado oil, and a scoop of fermented cabbage"). I generally don't recommend tracking dietary intake, as it is a lot of work and isn't useful to charting your progress in the elimination phase. An unnecessary focus on measuring and tracking intake can also increase the potential for disordered eating tendencies. If you decide that tracking your dietary intake may be supportive for managing your health, make sure to do so sparingly and with intention.
- **Body measurements:** We've already discussed that the goal of AIP is to help manage symptoms and increase quality of life, not to reach any specific goals with body size (and again, AIP is not a diet). This is why I specifically don't recommend tracking weight or body measurements while in the elimination phase. The exception might be for those who have an autoimmune condition for which weight gain is a primary symptom (like Hashimoto's thyroiditis) and can be helpful for big-picture analysis, or for those for whom unintentional weight loss is a potential symptom (like those with Crohn's disease or ulcerative colitis). In these cases, getting a baseline measurement and then checking in at regularly scheduled intervals (not every day!) can be helpful for determining if any concerning shifts are happening.

Tools and Technology for Tracking

There are some great tools out there that can help you track some of these metrics with ease. Before we discuss them, you should know that there is nothing wrong with the low-tech method of creating your own journal either on paper or digitally (again, a good old-fashioned journal is still my favorite choice!). Additionally, you might find that the extra work inputting data into your device or simply reviewing the large amount of data these programs create can cause unnecessary stress. My best advice here is to know thyself—if this additional information is likely to add to your stress levels, they aren't for you. On the other hand, you might be someone who finds metrics interesting and motivating, and so these options might be helpful in supporting your journey. If that is you, here is what you need to know:

- **Wearable trackers:** Today we have many options for wearable trackers, including rings, watches, and wristbands, all of which can be excellent for capturing data without needing input. Helpful information includes sleep duration and quality, heart rate variability (HRV, a marker of recovery), and exercise or movement tracking. While these wearables can't help you track your symptoms, they can help you assess your sleep patterns and quality and your recovery, and track your exercise or movement patterns and how you are recovering from them.
- **Symptom journaling apps:** These are software solutions designed to help you track symptoms over time, available on your device or computer. Many programs have been designed with autoimmune or chronic illness patients in mind and offer lots of flexibility in methods and types of tracking possible. Some also offer device notifications and check-ins to remind you to input your tracking for the day, as well as sleep analysis and reporting of your data over time. Because program offerings change over time, I recommend querying or searching autoimmune or chronic illness support forums for recommendations on which apps or programs other patients are finding most helpful.

ELIMINATION PHASE FAQ

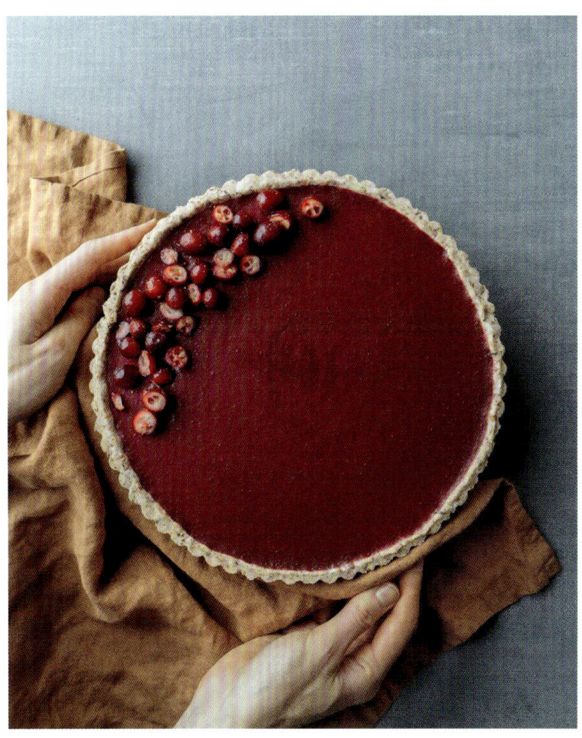

What if I mess up and eat a food that I'm supposed to avoid during the elimination phase?

If you eat a food you are supposed to be avoiding during your chosen elimination (either Core or Modified AIP), you should start over. Yes, this seems strict—but the point of the elimination diet is to allow your immune system the time to recover from potential triggers so that you can accurately identify them as problematic in the reintroduction phase. This is why taking the time to educate yourself about all the ingredients you could encounter during elimination and thoughtfully designing your transition phase is essential (revisit Chapter 2 for guidance if you need support here). Your success in the reintroduction phase depends on compliance during elimination, so make sure to prioritize that in your mental and practical preparation.

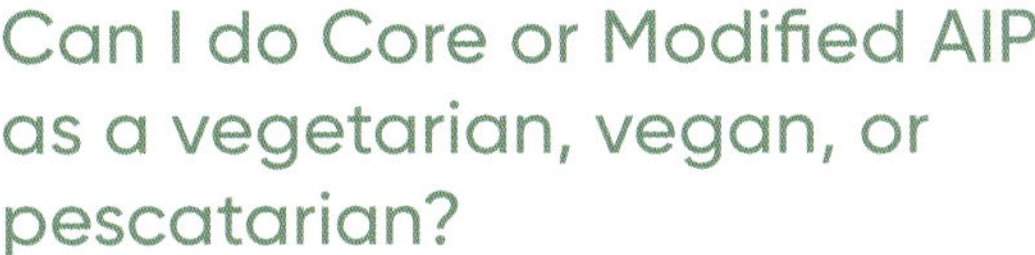

Can I do Core or Modified AIP as a vegetarian, vegan, or pescatarian?

It is important to note that both eggs and dairy are eliminated with both Core and Modified AIP (with the exception of ghee), so there are minimal differences between applying these protocols as a vegetarian or vegan (vegan diets differ from vegetarian ones in that they avoid eggs and dairy). It is not advisable to apply Core AIP as a vegetarian, as without grains, legumes, meat, fish, nuts, and seeds, it is impossible to meet minimum protein and micronutrient needs and is not safe (*please, do not do this!*). However, it is possible to apply Modified AIP as a vegetarian, as rice, pseudo-grains, legumes, and seeds are allowed. If this is what you'd like to do, I recommend working with a nutritionist to ensure that your elimination phase includes planning for adequate protein and micronutrients, as you may need to try to include foods in specific quantities to ensure adequate intake.

Pescatarians are those who eat fish and shellfish but not meat, and it is possible to apply either Core or Modified AIP using this approach provided you are eating enough seafood to meet your protein needs. This is more of a challenge on Core AIP and likely requires eating seafood at two meals per day to meet minimum protein and nutrient requirements. With Modified AIP, a pescatarian approach can be more flexible, as the inclusion of rice, pseudo-grains, legumes, and seeds allows for more non-seafood sources of protein. In fact, the high nutrient density of seafood makes this an especially anti-inflammatory and smart approach to healing and is highly recommended!

Can I combine dietary protocols (such as a low-FODMAP, low-histamine, or anti-candida diet) with AIP?

There are a lot of dietary protocols out there, and if you are highly motivated to get to the root of your symptoms, it might be tempting to think you can combine them all to "do it once" and heal your body. While I understand the thinking that leads people here, layering multiple approaches can backfire and cause problems.

First, AIP is the *only* complete protocol that has good evidence in medical research for patients with autoimmune disease. Many of these other protocols are designed to manage or treat specific issues that affect a minority of autoimmune patients. Second, executing an AIP elimination is already hard, and there is no reason to make it harder. And third, these protocols may be most appropriate for you to try at another time, separate from working the phases of AIP. By being able to devote all your time and energy to a specific protocol, you are more likely to be successful with achieving your desired outcome.

I'm not saying that these approaches don't have merit—in fact, many of them have good scientific evidence for efficacy in specific conditions (such as managing symptoms in the case of SIBO or histamine intolerance). Many of the conditions that these dietary protocols are designed to manage also require medical treatment (such as SIBO), and if you believe you need support in that area, it is important to ensure you are seeing a provider for diagnosis and treatment. Sometimes the smartest approach is to seek treatment to resolve these underlying issues before implementing AIP so that you can focus on one thing at a time (you'll learn more about this in Chapter 6 when we discuss troubleshooting).

I have one caveat here—you may be working with a medical provider who recommends that you layer a dietary protocol with AIP due to your specific medical history and/or conditions. You should always follow the advice of your healthcare providers, as they know your medical history and what your situation calls for.

What do I do about medication or supplement ingredients during the elimination phase?

It is important to always take all medications and supplements as prescribed by your medical providers. One tricky reality is the possibility that ingredients in these medications and supplements could cause trouble during the elimination phase, especially if they contain ingredients that are problematic for many autoimmune patients, like gluten or dairy. First, start by researching the ingredients in your prescriptions or supplements and identifying if there are any major ingredients that may be an issue. You can bring this to your medical providers to see if they have alternatives for you (for example, for some thyroid medications that contain gluten, it may be possible to have them compounded, or you may find a source of magnesium that does not include corn). Due to the prevalence of celiac disease and dairy allergies, it is likely your providers will at least be able to come up with options that are free from these major triggers—and you can simply not worry about the other ingredients that may not be specifically compliant with the elimination phase.

If you take supplements that are not prescribed by your medical providers, you can examine their ingredients for compliance with either Core or Modified AIP. If they are not compliant, you can either search for other compatible products to switch over to or eliminate them along with foods and reintroduce them later during the reintroduction phase. Many basic nutrient support supplements that are commonly used by the autoimmune community, like vitamin D, magnesium, and probiotics, are easily found in formulations that are compliant with both options for the elimination phase. It is not required or necessary to take any supplements while on the elimination phase of AIP, unless you have a condition or deficiency that has already been identified or are being advised to do so by a healthcare provider.

Do I have to eat organic fruits and vegetables, grass-fed or pastured meat, or wild-caught fish in to be successful in the elimination phase?

While you may choose organic, locally raised, grass-fed, and/or wild-caught ingredients for personal reasons relating to environmental impact or sustainability, they are not required for AIP implementation, as they do not have a significant impact on the nutrient density of the food itself.

Additionally, it's important to recognize that organic, grass-fed, or wild-caught options are not accessible or affordable for everyone, and this should not be a barrier to starting or succeeding on the AIP.

The medical studies conducted on the AIP did not require participants to use these ingredients, yet they still experienced significant improvements in their symptoms. The primary goal of the AIP is to identify and eliminate foods that may trigger inflammation, not to mandate a specific sourcing of ingredients. Prioritizing what works for your budget and accessibility is perfectly acceptable and can still yield excellent results.

Why shouldn't I stay in the elimination phase longer than 90 days?

I've seen two types of people who want to stay in the elimination phase long-term. First are those who see dramatic, positive improvements in the elimination phase—these autoimmune patients have often been suffering for so many years that once they discover the major impact of those food eliminations, they think they could easily maintain them forever just to continue those results (to be honest, this was my personal experience!). Additionally, they may be experiencing some fear that if they reintroduce foods, they will quickly regress back to the state they were in before beginning AIP. The second group are those who have not seen much improvement during their time in elimination. They are often tempted to think that time is the factor that is hindering their progress, and that if they just continued, at some point they would see the improvements or shifts they were looking for.

While these groups have opposite reasons why they want to continue the elimination phase, neither of them is correct in thinking that implementing the elimination phase long-term will help them achieve their goals. In fact, implementing for too long can cause issues like disordered eating, mental health challenges, nutrient deficiencies, and social isolation, among other things that can crop up, even if these were not previous concerns. Those who see great benefit from eliminations may need to work through their fears of reintroductions, and those who see a lack of progress need to begin troubleshooting. We'll discuss this more in Chapter 4 when we cover reintroductions in depth, as well as in Chapter 6 when we cover troubleshooting.

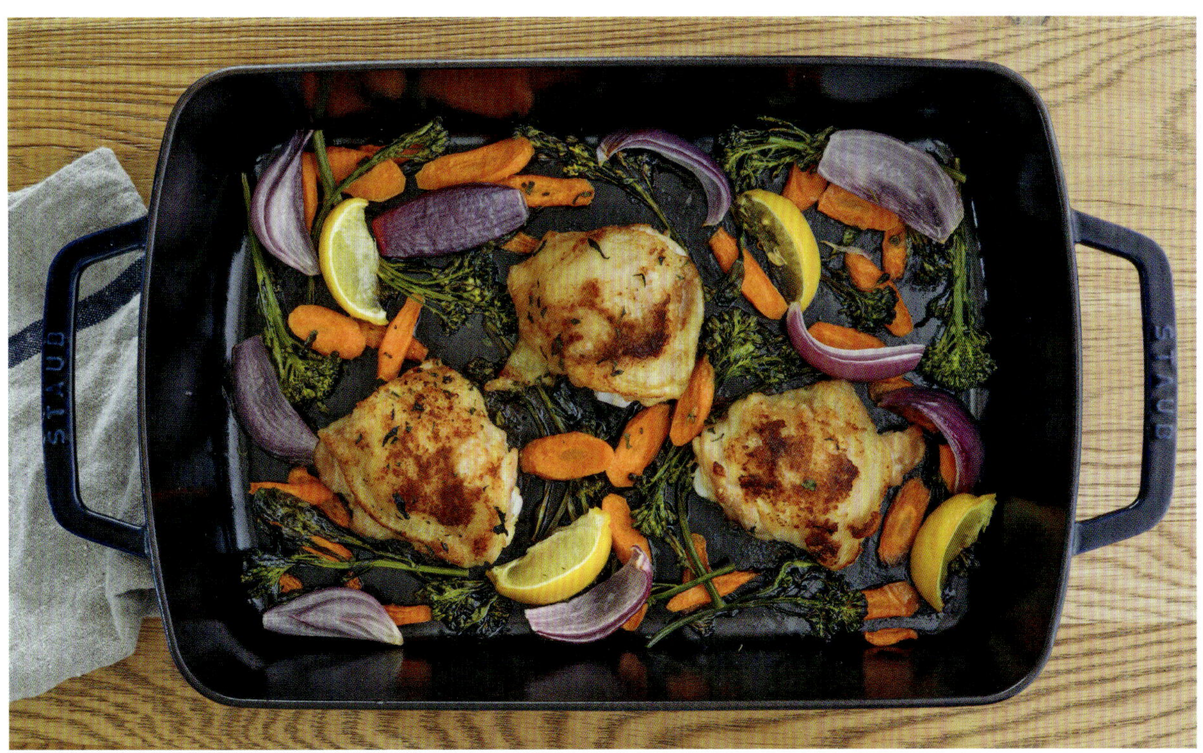

CHAPTER 4

Reintroduction Phase

Ready to discover exactly how those foods you've avoided are impacting your health? You've finally made it to the reintroduction phase, which begins as soon as you have maintained the elimination phase for your desired length of time and have had measurable improvements in your baseline symptoms. Using our road trip analogy, you're almost at your destination and ready to use the reintroduction phase as an off-ramp. Hooray! During this phase, each of the foods you've been avoiding are carefully and systematically reintroduced according to a specific procedure, and detailed journaling and tracking helps you identify which foods contribute to your symptoms. This chapter will teach you the purpose of the reintroduction phase, as well as give you guidance for how to navigate it carefully and successfully.

Because the point of reintroductions is to pinpoint how foods affect you, let's talk about what exactly could be happening when you have a reaction. Food allergy and sensitivity research shows us that there are many potential ways in which a food can cause negative reactions.[1] Food allergies are immune-mediated, meaning they are caused by various pathways of the immune system reacting to dietary triggers. Food intolerances cover an even broader range of causes that are non-immune, including those which have pathways that are are explained (like fructose or lactose intolerance) and those that are still mostly unknown. Additionally, components of foods (like bacterial or mold toxins) can be another cause of adverse reactions. Because of these many ways in which foods can trigger symptoms, it is impossible for food allergy or sensitivity testing to accurately pinpoint all the ways in which you could react to a food[2]—and why doing a food allergy test is not a replacement for careful elimination and reintroduction (again . . . sorry!). The takeaway here is that since there are many potential ways of reacting to foods, elimination and reintroduction is the best way for you to determine what works for you. Which is great news, because that is exactly what we are up to on AIP!

So, when can you go back to eating pizza? Unfortunately, the reintroduction phase *does not* mean that you automatically go back to including all the foods you avoided during the elimination phase (especially combined in one package—gluten, dairy, and nightshades, a sure recipe for disaster!). It *does* mean that you are now starting the process of carefully and systematically reintroducing the foods you've been avoiding, one by one, which can sometimes take even more focus and planning than implementing the elimination phase. I know this might not be what you want to hear, but it is important to take this part seriously!

In my years of coaching AIP implementation, the biggest mistake I see is rushing reintroductions; I've even done it myself. This can come in the form of reintroducing late-stage foods early, not spending enough time between reintroductions, or combining reintroductions (for example, the pizza). A lot of the time this comes from the assumption that the elimination phase is the hard part, and then reintroductions are the reward. The reintroduction phase requires continued diligent work to discover which foods are affecting your symptoms. After this period of discovery, the true reward is gaining information that can help you decide how to eat to support your best health.

Now that you know the reintroduction phase requires just as much, if not more, attention than the elimination phase, what exactly does it involve? You'll be reintroducing foods in a specific order according to the reintroduction stages list corresponding to your chosen dietary elimination, Core AIP or Modified AIP. These stages have been designed to set you up to ideally have some successful reintroductions early on, expanding your diet and making it easier to continue through the process until it is complete. Adding to your journaling practice in specific ways will help you make connections between food intake and symptoms, as well as identify which items you can include in your diet without problem.

Next, we'll discuss the finer details of implementing the reintroduction phase so you can start finalizing this journey of self-discovery.

THE GOAL OF THE REINTRODUCTION PHASE

You should already know by now that completing the reintroduction phase is an essential part of working through the Autoimmune Protocol, with the end goal being determining the least-restrictive diet that supports your healing process. Your results may be very different from mine, those of your friends, or from other autoimmune patients who may even share your history or conditions. Or they may line up neatly with what is reported by the autoimmune community and

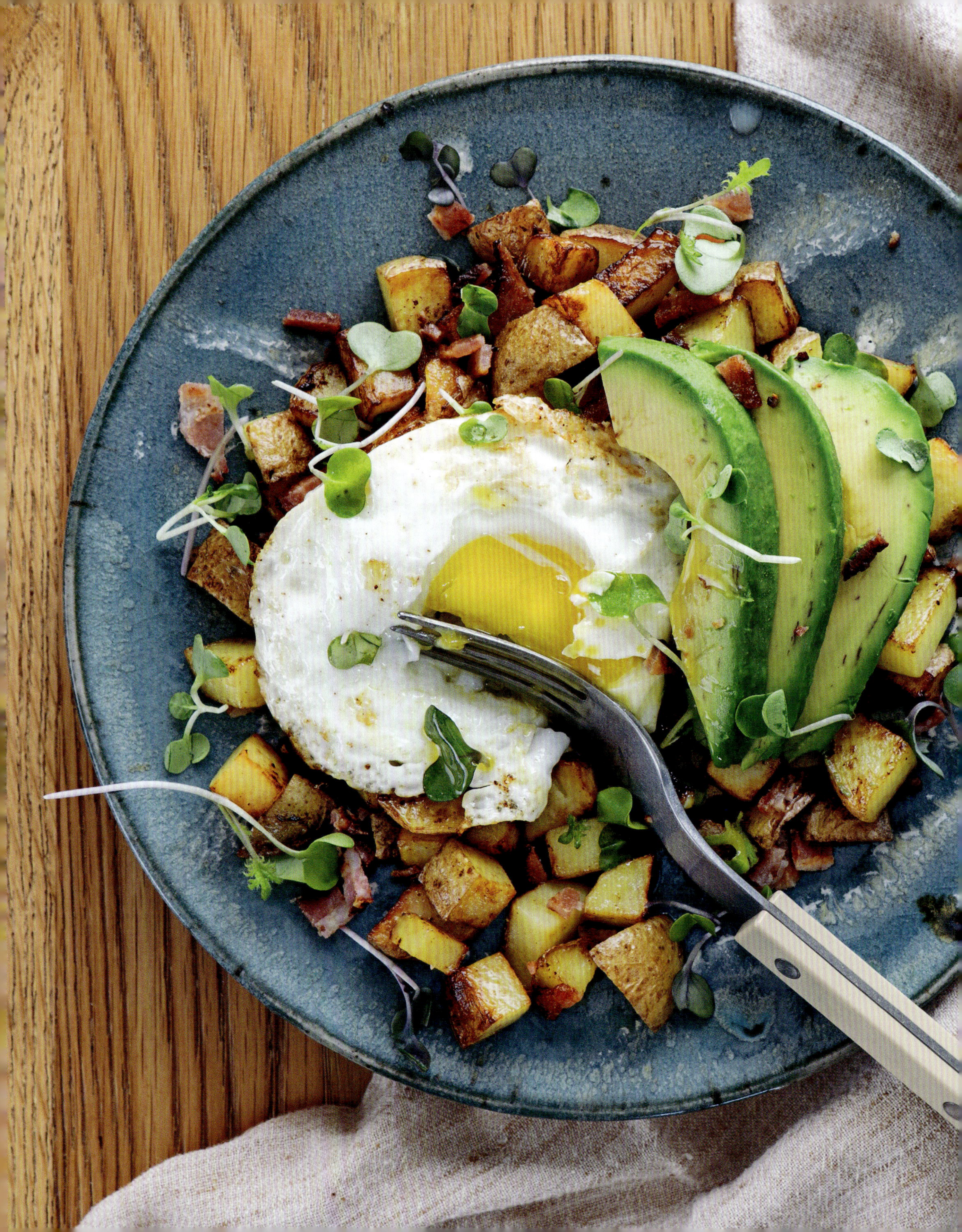

emerging AIP research. You have no way of knowing before you get started what results your experiment will yield—so best to be open to all the possibilities!

Reintroducing foods is important for many reasons. Some foods avoided during the elimination phase are nutrient-dense, affordable, and accessible, and can be excellent options for those who tolerate them. They can also make eating well practical and sustainable, and they increase your ability to socialize or travel. All these things are important to your ongoing health and finding ease with managing autoimmune disease or chronic illness.

Your experience navigating the reintroductions not only yields information about how food is affecting you in your current state of health but also gives you a tool to revisit should your health status change over time. If you've got some experience with autoimmune disease, you already know that things *will* change at some point. Through navigating the reintroduction phase, you learn how to tune in to the subtle changes your body makes in response to individual foods. This awareness also supports your navigating the ebbs and flows of managing your autoimmune disease the next time you sense a shift in your health status.

CORE AND MODIFIED AIP REINTRODUCTION PROTOCOLS

You might be curious how your choice of Core or Modified AIP affects navigating the reintroduction phase. The reintroduction procedure (found on page 83) is the same for both elimination options, so no matter which protocol you are using, you'll be following the same instructions to determine which foods might be causing you trouble.

What is different are the reintroduction stages. You'll notice that foods avoided during the elimination phase are grouped into stages to streamline the reintroduction process. It is ideal to attempt reintroductions of foods that are least likely to cause a reaction and most nutrient-dense first and wait to reintroduce foods that are most likely to cause a reaction and/or least nutrient-dense last. This sets you up for success in hopefully progressing through some successful reintroductions early in the process, expanding your diet and making it more sustainable as you work through some of the more difficult food reintroductions, which are often problematic for autoimmune patients (like gluten!). These reintroduction stage lists have been created from a mix of anecdotal evidence from the autoimmune community reporting reintroduction successes, feedback from AIP Certified Coaches about trends they see in their practices, as well as medical research in food reintroductions for those with autoimmune disease.[3,4]

Because there are two options for the elimination phase, Core and Modified AIP, there are two different starting places for the reintroduction phase. Core AIP eliminates more foods, and thus navigating reintroductions takes longer; for Core AIP, reintroductions are organized into four stages (see page 81). Modified AIP eliminates fewer foods, so reintroductions can progress more quickly; because there are fewer food groups, reintroductions are organized into two stages (see page 82).

DECIDING WHEN YOU ARE READY FOR REINTRODUCTION

You are ready to enter the reintroduction phase when you have maintained the elimination phase for 30 to 90 days and you've had measurable improvements in your symptoms from baseline captured during the transition phase. These improvements should be obvious when you assess data from symptom journaling, tracking, or even lab testing, if you are working with a healthcare provider as you navigate the phases of AIP. There is a big range of options inside the window of 30 to 90 days, so this section will help you understand the need for such a wide range of possibilities here.

In Chapter 3, we discussed the necessity of spending at least 30 days in the elimination phase—your immune system needs that amount of time to recover from potential food triggers. If you haven't spent the minimum 30 days, even if you are feeling major improvements, it is important to continue your elimination to meet that minimum threshold so you can ensure you learn everything possible from your reintroduction phase. Yes, this includes if you are experiencing quick, beneficial results (and I am so happy for you!).

What can measurable improvements look like? Ideally, they come as a relief of your primary autoimmune symptoms. If you have Hashimoto's thyroiditis, your symptom journals might show an average fatigue level of 8 at baseline, while your average after 60 days in elimination has improved to 5. If you have Crohn's disease, your bowel movement frequency might have shifted from six times per day to two. If you have psoriasis, your lesions may have decreased by 25 percent surface area. It is important to note that you don't need to experience a complete relief of symptoms to progress toward reintroductions. You simply need to experience a measurable improvement over your baseline, which you'll be able to discover from tracking your symptoms. (Remember from Chapter 2, part of developing your personal health vision means understanding that health exists on a spectrum, and perfectionism is a big hinderance to being successful with AIP. Be sure to revisit that chapter if you find yourself struggling!)

While not as easy to determine, these improvements can also come as changes in areas that are not your primary autoimmune symptoms. This might look like digestive improvements, where typical diarrhea or constipation, gas, bloating, or indigestion resolves or improves. Or other general indicators like better skin, hair, or clear eyes. Sometimes improvements in sleep, memory, focus, and mood are obvious and notable. Even if fatigue is not a primary symptom of your autoimmune disease, you may find that you have more energy or even perform better in your workouts, if you have a defined routine. It is possible that you could not see a large or meaningful improvement in your primary symptoms, but major changes in other areas—and those still qualify as measurable improvements to gauge your food reintroductions by!

If you have spent the maximum amount of time recommended in the elimination phase (90 days) and don't see a shift in either your primary autoimmune symptoms or more subtle general health changes, you should consider troubleshooting what might be hindering your progress. It is very unusual to not see any improvements, especially when general indicators are measured; if this is you, be sure to check out guidance on troubleshooting in Chapter 6.

Your ability to correctly determine when it is time to shift to reintroductions is why symptom tracking is an important part of navigating the elimination phase—you need good data to assess your improvements, both subtle and obvious, so that you can determine if you are ready to begin reintroductions. Be sure to revisit guidance on tracking during the elimination phase (page 69) to ensure you set yourself up for success here.

REINTRODUCTION TIMELINE

Just like with the transition phase (your on-ramp to the AIP), the timing of the reintroduction phase (your off-ramp) can vary. Unlike the transition phase, where you get to decide how long you'll take to implement AIP, you might not know exactly how long your reintroduction phase will last. This is because your reintroduction timeline is dependent on many factors—if you are starting with Core or Modified AIP, how many food reactions you have along the way, how long it takes you to recover from any food reactions, and how quickly you decide to proceed through the stages and individual food reintroductions.

While there is no official timeline for the reintroduction phase, if you are using Modified AIP, you should expect at least one month, and if you are using Core AIP, you should expect at least two months, as the more restricted protocol has more stages of food reintroductions and generally takes longer to work through. It is very common for a thorough reintroduction phase to last three months. If you happen to work through early-stage eliminations without an issue, or if you recover quickly from any failed reintroductions, this timeline can be shortened. If you have some early reactions, or if your reactions are more severe and require a lot of time to recover from, your timeline may be longer.

Although you may not know how long this phase will take you, it is important to ensure that you are mentally prepared to spend as much time in the reintroduction phase as necessary to determine which foods are problematic for you.

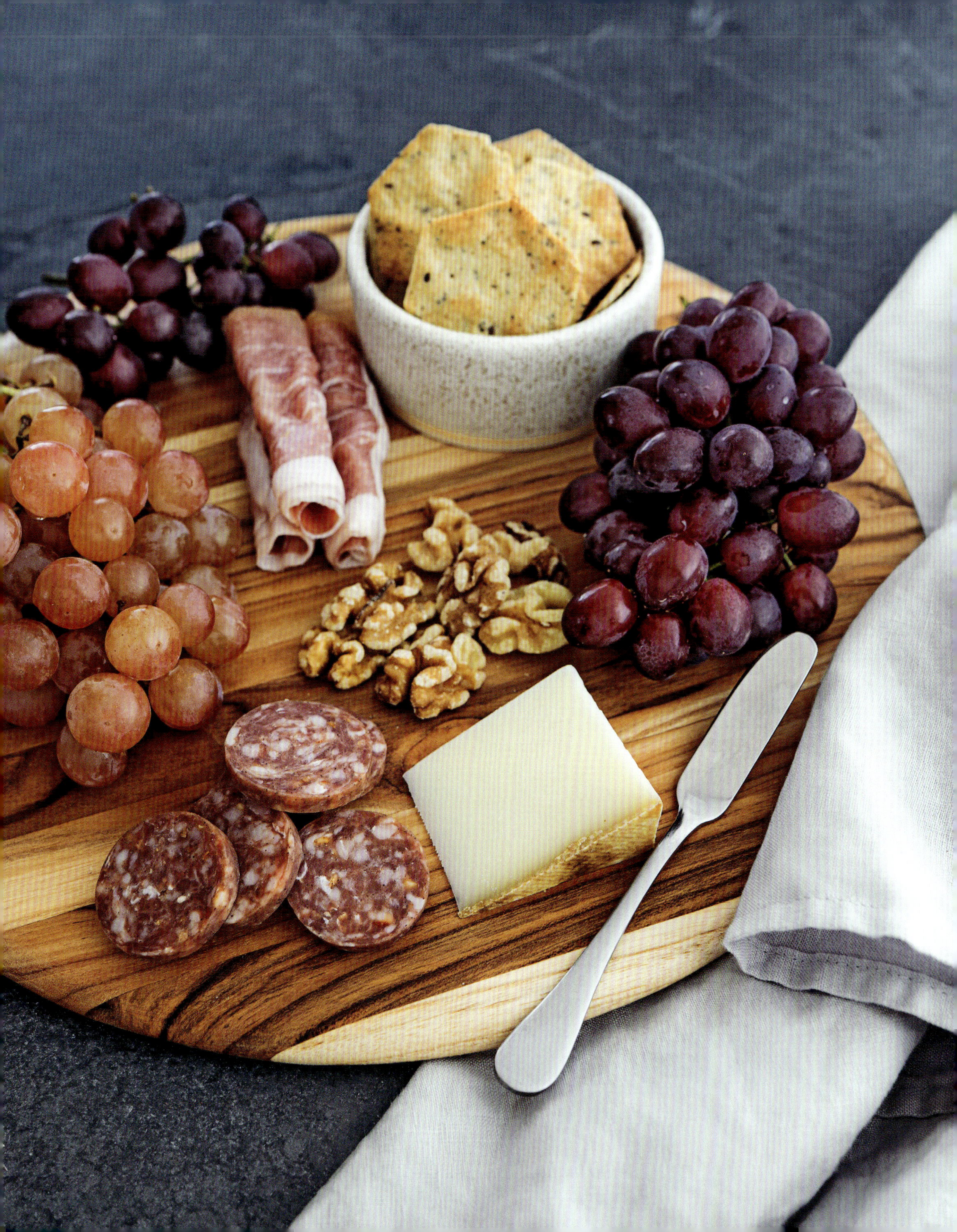

HOW TO REINTRODUCE FOODS

The procedure for reintroducing foods following the elimination phase of AIP is relatively simple, but it is important to follow it carefully to yield the best results.

First, once you've met the conditions for completing the elimination phase, you will pick a date on the calendar to begin. Congratulations, as this marks your official transition to the reintroduction phase! Second, you'll pick one food from stage 1 of the reintroduction stages list corresponding with either Core or Modified AIP. This will be your first trial, and you can either pick something you really missed during elimination (like chocolate) or something that will bring you specific nutritional benefits (like egg yolks). On that date, you'll begin the reintroduction procedure with that food as outlined on page 83. Each food reintroduction will take you anywhere from 3 to 7 days to complete.

So, what happens next? If you do not have a reaction to that food, great news, you can now include it in your diet! If you do have a reaction to that food, you now know how your body responds, and you can continue to eliminate it. When you have a successful reintroduction, you can simply move on to another food in stage 1 of the protocol. If at any point during this process you experience a reaction, you need to go back to how you were eating prior to that specific trial and wait until your symptoms improve back to baseline (this can take anywhere from a few days to weeks). It is at that point that you are ready to progress to the next food.

How long should you take between food trials? You'll quickly notice that if you devote a full 7 days to each food, your reintroduction phase is going to last many months. While you are most likely to see symptoms from food allergy, sensitivity, or intolerance crop up within 1 to 3 days of eating the specific food, elimination diet research shows us that delayed reactions of up to 5 to 6 days can happen to some people.[5] The official reintroduction procedure for AIP includes a range so that you can decide how to progress through reintroductions at a pace that works for you, understanding that you may decide to speed up (while still waiting a minimum of 3 days in between) or slow down should you need to.

Once you have completed your first food trial and have returned to the improved baseline you reached during the elimination phase if the response was negative, you are ready to trial the next food. Continue this way until you have reintroduced all the foods you desire to in the reintroduction stages for either Core or Modified AIP.

ORDER OF REINTRODUCTION

To determine the order of reintroduction, research on inflammatory potential and nutrient density of individual foods has been used to organize foods into stages for both Core and Modified AIP. The goal here is to promote successful reintroductions early in the process, as well as give you some additional ingredient options that add to the nutrient density of your diet.

Because Core AIP removes more foods during the elimination phase, it has foods organized into four stages. Modified AIP removes fewer foods, so there are only two stages. Stage 1 foods, for both protocols, are the least likely to be problematic and the most nutrient-dense. On the other hand, for those using Core AIP, stage 4 foods are the most likely to be problematic and the least nutrient-dense. Essentially, you are starting with foods that will hopefully help you expand your diet and continue to make it more sustainable, achievable, and nutritious as you work through the reintroduction process.

Just like during the transition phase, the reintroduction phase allows you the opportunity to design the process to suit your needs. Instead of reintroducing foods on an exact schedule, you get to pick the order of reintroduction within each stage. This is because each person has different wants and needs in terms of foods they miss or enjoy. Once you successfully reintroduce a few food groups from stage 1, you can move on to stage 2 and beyond. On the following pages, you'll find the reintroduction stages for both Core and Modified AIP, as well as the reintroduction procedure. If you'd like a printable version of these resources, be sure to visit THEAUTOIMMUNEPROTOCOL.COM/PRINTABLES to download.

CORE AIP REINTRODUCTION STAGES

Stage 1

EGG YOLKS (not the whites): Chicken, duck, goose, quail, or any other type of egg yolk.

LEGUMES (beans with edible pods and legume sprouts): Green beans, peas, runner beans, snow peas, sugar snap peas.

FRUIT- AND BERRY-BASED SPICES: Allspice, caraway, cardamom pods, juniper berries, pepper (from black, green, pink, or white peppercorns), star anise, sumac.

SEED-BASED SPICES: Anise seeds, annatto seeds, black caraway (Russian caraway, black cumin), celery seeds, coriander seeds, cumin seeds, dill seeds, fennel seeds, fenugreek seeds, mustard seeds, nutmeg.

NUTS AND SEEDS (oils only): Macadamia, sesame, walnut.

NUTS AND SEEDS: Chocolate, cocoa, coffee (occasional basis).

DAIRY: Ghee.

Stage 2

NUTS AND SEEDS: Almonds, Brazil nuts, chestnuts, chia seeds, coffee (daily basis), flax seeds, hazelnuts, hemp seeds, macadamia nuts, pecans, pine nuts, pistachios, poppy seeds, pumpkin seeds, sesame seeds, sunflower seeds, walnuts, or any other flavors, flours, butters, oils, and other products derived from them.

EGG WHITES (or whole eggs): Chicken, duck, goose, quail, or any other type of egg white.

DAIRY: Butter, butter oil.

ALCOHOL (small quantities): Gluten-free beer or hard cider (8 ounces or less), wine (5 ounces or less), fortified wine (3 ounces or less), liqueur (3 ounces or less), or spirits (1 ounce or less).

Stage 3

NIGHTSHADES (limited): Paprika and potatoes (peeled).

DAIRY: Buttermilk, cheese, cottage cheese, cream cheese, curds, dairy-protein isolates, heavy cream, ice cream, kefir, milk, sour cream, whey, whey protein, whipping cream, yogurt. (Grass-fed, fermented, or A2 dairy may be better tolerated.)

LEGUMES: Chickpeas (aka garbanzo beans), lentils, split peas. (Legumes may be better tolerated when soaked and/or fermented.)

Stage 4

NIGHTSHADES OR SPICES DERIVED FROM NIGHTSHADES: Ashwagandha, bell peppers (aka sweet peppers), Cape gooseberries (aka ground cherries), cayenne peppers, eggplant, garden huckleberries, goji berries (aka wolfberries), hot peppers (chile peppers and chile-based spices), naranjillas, pepinos, pimentos, potatoes, tamarillos, tomatillos, tomatoes.

GLUTEN-FREE GRAINS, PSEUDO-GRAINS, AND OTHER GRAIN-LIKE SUBSTANCES: Amaranth, buckwheat, corn, fonio, Job's tears, Kamut, millet, oats, quinoa, rice, sorghum, spelt, teff, wild rice. (Grains may be better tolerated when soaked and fermented.)

LEGUMES: Adzuki beans, black beans, black-eyed peas, butter beans, calico beans, cannellini beans, fava beans (aka broad beans), Great Northern beans, Italian beans, kidney beans, lima beans, mung beans, navy beans, peanuts, pinto beans. (Legumes may be better tolerated when soaked and fermented.)

ALCOHOL (moderate quantities): Gluten-free beer or hard cider, wine, fortified wine, liqueur, or spirits.

MODIFIED AIP REINTRODUCTION STAGES

Stage 1

EGG YOLKS (not the whites): Chicken, duck, goose, quail, or any other type of egg yolk.

NUTS: Almonds, Brazil nuts, chestnuts, hazelnuts, macadamia nuts, pecans, pine nuts, pistachios, walnuts, or any other flavors, flours, butters, oils, and other products derived from them. (Nuts may be more easily digested when soaked or sprouted.)

DAIRY: Butter, buttermilk, cheese, cottage cheese, cream cheese, curds, dairy-protein isolates, heavy cream, ice cream, kefir, milk, sour cream, whey, whey protein, whipping cream, yogurt. (Grass-fed, fermented, or A2 dairy may be better tolerated.)

NIGHTSHADES (limited): Paprika, potatoes (peeled).

Stage 2

EGG WHITES (or whole eggs): Chicken, duck, goose, quail, or any other type of egg white.

GLUTEN-FREE CEREAL GRAINS: Corn, fonio, Job's tears, millet, oats, sorghum, teff. (Grains may be better tolerated when soaked and fermented.)

NIGHTSHADES OR SPICES DERIVED FROM NIGHTSHADES: Ashwagandha, bell peppers (aka sweet peppers), Cape gooseberries (aka ground cherries), cayenne peppers, eggplant, garden huckleberries, goji berries (aka wolfberries), hot peppers (chile peppers and chile-based spices), naranjillas, pepinos, pimentos, potatoes, tamarillos, tomatillos, tomatoes.

ALCOHOL (small quantities): Gluten-free beer or hard cider (8 ounces or less), wine (5 ounces or less), fortified wine (3 ounces or less), liqueur (3 ounces or less), or spirits (1 ounce or less).

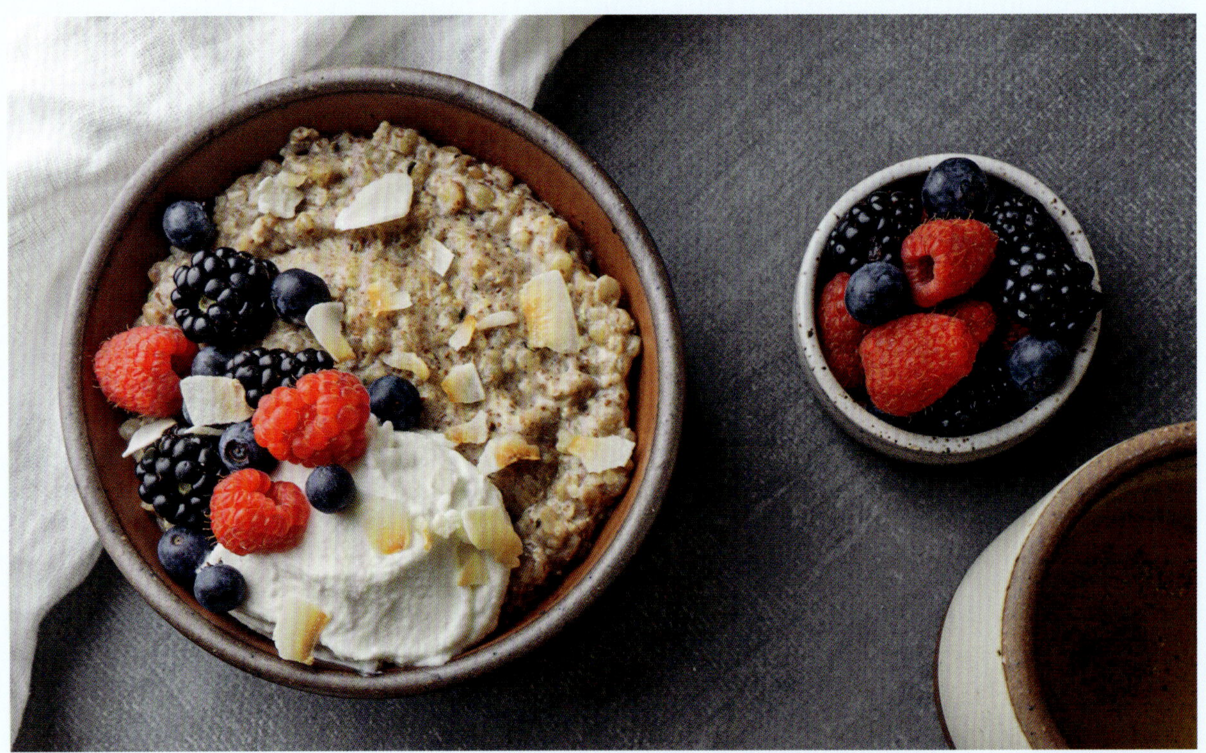

REINTRODUCTION PROCEDURE

1. Select a food you wish to reintroduce and prepare it in a manner that suits your taste and preferences. Take care that any other ingredients in the dish or meal are all foods you tolerate well, excluding any that you have not yet reintroduced or have only recently reintroduced.
2. Take a few moments to breathe and calm your mind.
3. Eat a small portion of the food as part of a regular meal. Do not eat any more of this food for at least 2 to 3 hours, or perhaps as long as 24 hours.
4. If you do not notice any unusual symptoms during this time (which could indicate an immediate reaction to this food), proceed to the next step. If you do notice symptoms, do not proceed to the next step and see page 84 for further guidance.
5. Eat a medium portion of the food as part of a regular meal. Do not eat any more of this food for at least 3 days, or perhaps as long as 7 days.
6. If you do not notice any unusual symptoms during this time (which could indicate a delayed reaction to this food), you may now bring it back into your diet as desired. If you do notice symptoms, see page 84 for further guidance.
7. Continue this process starting with step 1 for the next food you wish to reintroduce.

Notes:

- Consult the order of reintroduction section on page 80 for guidance on selecting foods to reintroduce.
- The exact size of a small or medium portion will vary depending upon the food and your personal preference. Here are some examples:
  - A small portion of paprika could be just a pinch sprinkled on top of a bite of other food; a medium portion could be a denser sprinkling on a bite, or a pinch sprinkled on multiple bites.
  - A small portion of butter could be just a small knob on top of a bite of other food; a medium portion may be a full tablespoon used to sauté a serving of vegetables.
  - A small portion of cashews might be 4 or 5; a medium portion might be a full handful.
  - A small portion of oats might be one or two spoonfuls; a medium portion might be ¼ cup to ½ cup.

IMPORTANT: If you know you have a severe allergy or a condition that prevents you from ever eating a particular food, do not attempt reintroduction of that food and always follow the advice of your medical providers.

NEGATIVE FOOD REACTIONS

You already know that it isn't only possible but likely that you will discover negative reactions to foods you might have previously enjoyed. Here is what you should do when you experience symptoms that indicate an immediate or delayed reaction to a specific food during the reintroduction phase. In addition to eliminating that food once again, you'll need to give your body time to recover from the reaction and reach the baseline you already achieved at the end of your elimination phase, so that you can accurately determine if your next trial is producing a reaction.

This looks like going back to eating Core or Modified AIP elimination plus any successful reintroductions you've already made until you reach this improved baseline once again. This can take as quickly as a few days for a subtle reaction, and up to a week or two for a stronger one. You'll need to listen to your body and use the symptom journaling skills you learned during the elimination phase to determine when your body is ready once again.

While frustrating to feel like you are taking a step backward, it is essential to do this before you begin the process again with a new food. If you do not, it will be difficult to gauge positive or negative reactions to the next reintroduction attempts. Although discovering a negative food reaction can be disappointing, especially if the food was on your favorites list, you now have valuable information about choices you can make to avoid the symptoms caused by eating that food in the future.

INCONCLUSIVE REACTIONS

Sometimes reactions are obvious, which makes it easy to connect the dots between a specific food and symptoms. Other times, reactions can be more subtle or due to other explanations, making accurately determining if they are due to a specific food tricky. Here are some guidelines on what to do if you

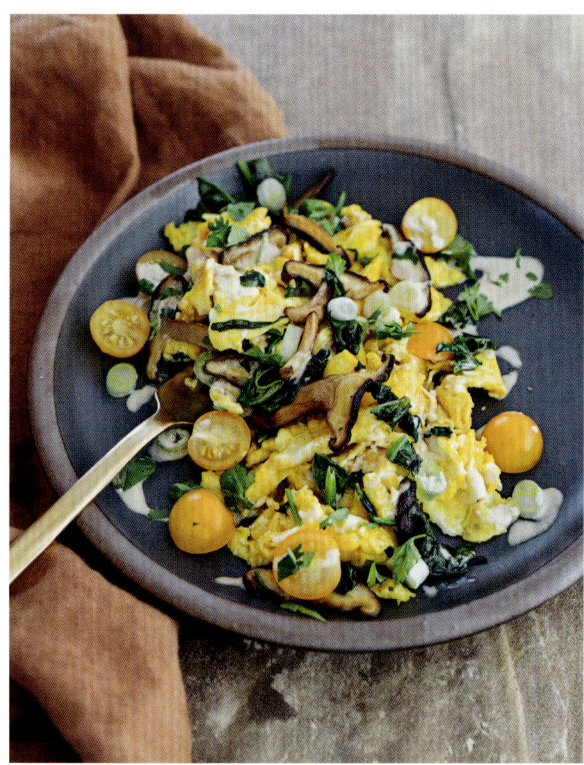

suspect this is happening during the reintroduction of a specific food.

First, examine if this reaction could be due to something other than food. Have you experienced a new stressor, lack of sleep, or something else in your routine that could have caused the symptom? Don't be afraid to slow down and start over again with the same food. Just as with a negative reaction, go back to your elimination plus well-tolerated foods for a few days to a week to return to your baseline. If you eliminate the other potential culprit, it may be more obvious what was the real cause of the reaction.

Second, it could be that you are experiencing a subtle or delayed reaction. If you aren't sure that your reaction is due to the reintroduced food, try again, this time giving yourself extra time and perhaps pay more attention to tracking to determine if you are experiencing a delayed reaction. You can also try increasing the quantity by eating a larger portion of the food or eating it on consecutive days to make that reaction more obvious.

TRACKING DURING THE REINTRODUCTION PHASE

Tracking is essential to your success in the reintroduction phase. While in elimination, the goal of tracking is to determine when you've reached a measurable improvement over baseline, in reintroduction, the goal of tracking is to make those connections between which foods cause your symptoms. While you will be familiar with tracking at this point, you'll want to shift your practice to accommodate what will serve your reintroduction phase of AIP.

In addition to the metrics you decided to track during the elimination phase, you'll want to begin tracking each food reintroduction in detail, including the date, which food you are trialing, and the time and form you consumed it, and allow space to notate any physical, emotional, or symptomatic changes you notice in the days following consumption.

TYPES OF REACTIONS TO LOOK OUT FOR

You may be surprised to find out the range and types of reactions and symptoms you can experience following the reintroduction of a specific food. Our brief overview of the immunology of food allergies, sensitivities, and intolerances has given you an understanding of why these reactions are likely to be heightened during the reintroduction phase (and is, in fact, part of what we're after, as uncomfortable as it can be sometimes!).

During the reintroduction phase, you'll be putting your detective hat on and expanding your awareness in many areas to see if you can discover any connections. Here are the most common areas to look for changes:

1. **Return or worsening of primary symptoms:** If you were lucky enough to see a direct improvement of your autoimmune or other primary symptoms during the elimination phase, look for signs that they may be returning following a food reintroduction.
2. **Classic allergy symptoms:** These can include a range of mild to life-threatening levels of shortness of breath, racing pulse, runny nose, coughing, headaches, dizziness, rashes, and swelling. Always seek immediate medical attention if you have trouble breathing or symptoms ramp up quickly following a food reintroduction, as sometimes allergic responses can be life-threatening.
3. **Digestive changes:** Note any changes to your digestion and elimination habits, from upper gastrointestinal symptoms like acid reflux, nausea, or burping, to bloating, stomach cramps or pain, and lower gastrointestinal symptoms like diarrhea, constipation, or excess gas. These are usually key indicators of dietary sensitivity or intolerance.
4. **Joint or muscle stiffness and/or pain:** If they are not your primary symptoms, be aware of the new onset of joint pain or changes in muscle stiffness and/or recovery as you reintroduce foods. This is often an area where autoimmune patients discover they were living with a low level of stiffness or pain until unexpected improvement during the elimination phase.
5. **Skin changes:** Some classic allergy symptoms involve the skin, such as the appearance of flushing, itchiness, or rashes. Other more subtle skin reactions include various types of acne and even dry skin. Pay attention to your skin health and note any changes, both immediate and delayed, as you reintroduce foods.
6. **Fatigue:** Ensure you are checking in with your energy levels as you reintroduce foods. While fatigue can often be caused by lifestyle factors (such as sleep, exercise, or stress), excess fatigue can be a more subtle food reaction, so be on the lookout for any increases in that area.
7. **Sleep changes:** A range of sleep issues can be caused by subtle food reactions, including trouble falling asleep or staying asleep, or waking up throughout the night.
8. **Mood changes:** Similarly, increase in anxiety, depression, or mood swings unrelated to other lifestyle factors can be tied to food sensitivities.

AFTER THE REINTRODUCTION PHASE

What does your diet look like after successfully navigating the reintroduction phase? First, you will have identified any obvious food allergies, sensitivities, or intolerances, and your time in the elimination phase may have helped to produce a heightened response, making it clear those foods are producing a negative reaction for you. You now have the information you need to move forward excluding these foods and/or ingredients long-term to support your health. By removing them strictly for the long haul, you allow your body to continue at that baseline level of improved health you achieved during the elimination phase.

You may have also discovered some more subtle sensitivities or intolerances that didn't produce major reactions but were still connected to your symptoms. I like to call these "gray area" foods—those that cause symptoms but can be tempting to include sometimes, as the reaction is milder. A gray area food might only be problematic if you eat a lot of it, if you eat it in combination with specific foods, or if you consume it when you haven't slept well or are particularly stressed out. Reactions to gray area foods are also easier to recover from. You may choose to exclude gray area foods strictly, or you may include them if you are willing to put up with their effects.

I'll use myself as an example here to share how someone might navigate integrating what they've learned using AIP: I have serious allergies to gluten and dairy (even ghee!), and I go to great lengths to avoid them at a cross-contamination level. I also have a sensitivity to nightshade-family vegetables that is specific to certain species and not others (tomatoes are a major trigger for me, followed by bell peppers and eggplant, but I have no reaction to potatoes). While I don't need to avoid them to a cross-contamination level, I strictly avoid tomatoes and peppers. Next are my gray area foods, which cause me comparatively milder symptoms but I've still identified as problematic. They include eggs and legumes, which are only an issue if I eat them often (threshold tolerance), alcohol, and some nuts. I don't strictly avoid these gray area foods, but I usually don't include them in my cooking or consuming at home. I've also noticed that if I have alcohol along with another food from this category (especially eggs), I get a much larger reaction than if I had either of them on their own. I'll usually reserve eating these gray area foods for special occasions, such as eating out or while traveling, but only if I can minimize the potential of a negative reaction to disrupt my plans to celebrate or on a vacation!

After completing the reintroduction phase, what you have is valuable knowledge. You know how your body can change over a (relatively!) short period of time when you shift what you eat, and how specific foods cause or contribute to your symptoms. You also know about which nutrient-dense and anti-inflammatory foods you love and how they support your best health. You are an expert in listening to your body and tracking how you feel over time. All this knowledge can be used to make informed choices about how you want to eat long-term. Remember, AIP is not about perfection or implementing a restricted diet forever. It is about taking joy in discovering what works and what doesn't work so you can make choices about how to navigate your future, despite autoimmune disease. And that is empowering!

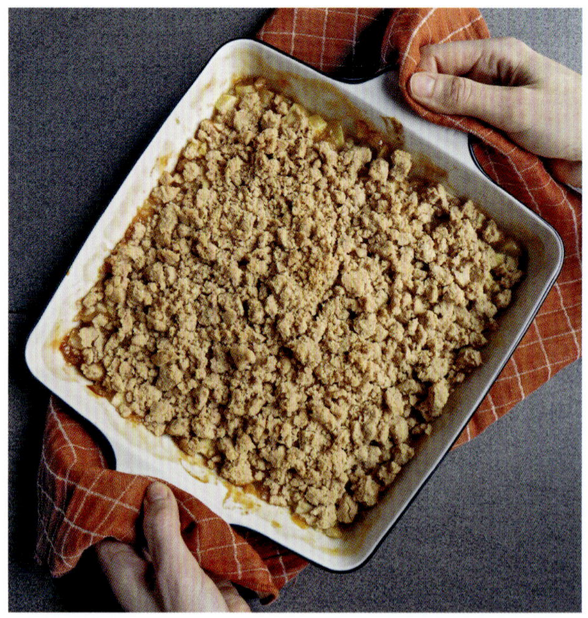

REINTRODUCTION PHASE FAQ

Do all my symptoms need to be reversed before I start reintroductions?

No! It is a misconception that symptoms need to be completely reversed during the elimination phase before beginning reintroductions. While it is necessary to experience a measurable improvement over your baseline to clear the slate for reintroductions, it is not necessary to experience "complete" healing before beginning this process (*complete* is in quotes, because as autoimmune patients, this concept is elusive to us). After identifying which foods cause your symptoms to worsen during the elimination phase, you can move on to a dietary approach that allows long-term healing due to the removal of these foods.

In my many years' experience walking people through AIP, I have come to see the progress made in the reintroduction phase to encapsulate the beginning, not the end of the process of learning how to live well with autoimmune disease. In fact, a study by Dr. Terry Wahls and her team found that a six-month elimination and reintroduction protocol was effective at improving fatigue and quality of life in patients with multiple sclerosis, even though reintroductions were implemented at the three-month mark.[6] Healing progress can and does continue to happen post-reintroductions!

Can I still reintroduce foods if I don't feel any better?

If you are still in the elimination phase and haven't noticed any measurable improvements over your baseline, then you are unlikely to have a productive reintroduction process. One thing to keep in mind is that if you don't see improvements in your primary symptoms, but you do see measurable improvements in other areas (like energy levels, digestion, or skin health), you may be able to start reintroductions. Be sure to see the guidance on page 59 for extending your elimination if under 90 days, as well as Chapter 6 for troubleshooting if you have reached the 90-day mark.

How long do I need to go back to the elimination phase if I have a bad food reaction?

If you are trialing your first food after the elimination phase and have a negative reaction, you'll go back to the elimination phase until your symptoms improve to the baseline you achieved before your first reintroduction. In most cases, this takes a few days to a week but can last longer for more severe reactions. This is always frustrating, as it can feel like you are going backward in the process, when you've done what you set out to do in the first place—identified a source of your food-driven symptoms!

If you have successfully reintroduced other foods but encounter one later in the process that produces a negative reaction, you'll go back to the elimination phase *plus* any of those successful reintroductions until your symptoms improve to that same baseline. There is no need to return to the full elimination phase if you are confident that the previously reintroduced foods are not causing you trouble. If your reintroduction process got messy at any point and you aren't sure (it happens!), try to return to the last point where you were confident that you were still at your improved baseline. As you gain experience through working the reintroduction phase, it will become clear when you have recovered enough to try again.

If I react to a food in an early stage, can I progress to the later stages of reintroduction?

It is recommended to start reintroductions with stage 1 foods, as these foods are most nutrient-dense and least likely to cause reactions. If you have a reaction to a stage 1 food, pick a new stage 1 food from a different food family to try once you've recovered to your improved baseline. For example, for someone on Modified AIP, this might look like failing a reintroduction of butter. Next, they could try other stage 1 foods—egg yolk, almonds, or potatoes. While it isn't required to attempt all stage 1 foods before moving on to stage 2, it is a smart approach to get some early stage attempts before moving on to foods that are more likely to cause a reaction. You may want to move on to other food families because you are excited about introducing those foods or avoid specific reintroductions because you don't like that food at all (this is the case for me and peanuts!).

Do I need to reintroduce all foods in a group separately?

Yes, each food in a group should be reintroduced separately. For example, say you try almonds as a stage 1 reintroduction, and it is successful. You still need to trial each other nut separately, as this gives you the opportunity to learn if you have a sensitivity to specific nut varieties, versus all nuts (and a side note—individual nut sensitivities are among some of the most common discoveries on AIP, so take your time!).

Similarly, each form of dairy needs to be introduced separately. It is common for many people to find that they tolerate certain forms of dairy, such as ghee, butter, or yogurt, but not others, like milk or ice cream. Additionally, you might find that you tolerate dairy from different species animals, and products from goat, sheep, A2 cows, or others can be trialed as well. Separating these reintroductions ensures that you learn which forms work for you, and if you have those that you need to avoid.

If I react to an early-stage form of a food group, can I progress to the other forms of that food group that follow?

If you have a negative reaction to a specific form of a food found in the earliest stages of reintroduction, you do not progress to reintroduce other forms of that food. This is most often the case with dairy, as it is a diverse food family with many derivative products and types of potential reactions. For example, on Core AIP, if you successfully reintroduce ghee in stage 1, you will then progress to butter in stage 2. If you do not tolerate butter, you won't move on to reintroduce cheese and other forms of dairy in stage 3. For Modified AIP, which includes reintroduction of all forms of dairy in stage 1, you'll need to trial each form separately to determine if there are any differences between the various forms.

Can preparation method or food quality affect reintroduction?

Any foods for which preparation method affects potential tolerance are notated in the reintroduction stages. For example, some people find soaked, sprouted, or fermented nuts, grains, and seeds more tolerable than modern preparations of the same ingredients. Similarly, dairy can be separated out into species to test tolerance, with some people finding that dairy products from sheep or goat[8] are more tolerable.

Achieving this level of specificity of your testing is not required, and I don't recommend exploring it until you discover you don't tolerate a food that you'd like to enjoy. This might look like exploring a goat cheese reintroduction after you recover from a failed attempt at reintroducing cow's milk cheese.

Can I react to quantities or specific combinations of foods?

If your symptoms are due to more traditional food allergy or sensitivity, even a small amount is likely to produce a reaction. If your symptoms are due to a food intolerance, it is likely that you may discover a threshold of tolerance whereby a small amount doesn't cause a reaction, but a larger amount does. As you navigate through the reintroduction process and start to eat larger quantities of reintroduced foods, you might notice new symptoms crop up, and this is a great opportunity to take a step back and consider quantity of any foods you might be suspicious about.

People also report being sensitive to some foods only in specific combinations with other foods. A great example of this is alcohol, which can cause symptoms in and of itself, but can also heighten the response to other foods when consumed in combination. If you notice that you tolerate certain foods on their own, but not in combination with other foods, this is an indicator that these may be "gray area" foods for you, and you can make an informed decision to continue eating them separately or be careful about combining them in your meals going forward.

If I don't tolerate a food now, do I need to avoid it forever?

Your need to avoid a food long-term is dependent on the type of adverse food reaction. If your reaction is due to a classic allergy or other immune-mediated reaction, it is likely that will not change and you will need to take precautions to remove that from your diet forever, as well as manage exposure through cross-contamination (meaning, you'll need to always be extremely careful if you'd like to avoid those symptoms). Intolerances due to genetic deficiencies in enzyme production (such as lactose or fructose intolerance) are also unlikely to change over time.

Some types of reactions, however, may be modifiable dependent on your gut and microbiome health. These are usually reactions that are in the sensitivity or intolerance categories, which are due to unknown factors. I can tell you from my experience coaching that sometimes a food produces a reaction during the reintroduction phase, and the person goes on to try to reintroduce it again months, sometimes even years later, to find that they tolerate it. My theory is that in those early reintroductions, the person might still be in a phase of deep healing and recovering their health. Once they navigate reintroductions and increase their level of health, especially that of their microbiome, their resilience may increase, and tolerances can change. There is no way to know if you will be able to successfully reintroduce a food someday, but it is important to understand that health status is constantly fluctuating, especially with autoimmune disease, and you may be able to revisit those failed reintroductions later.

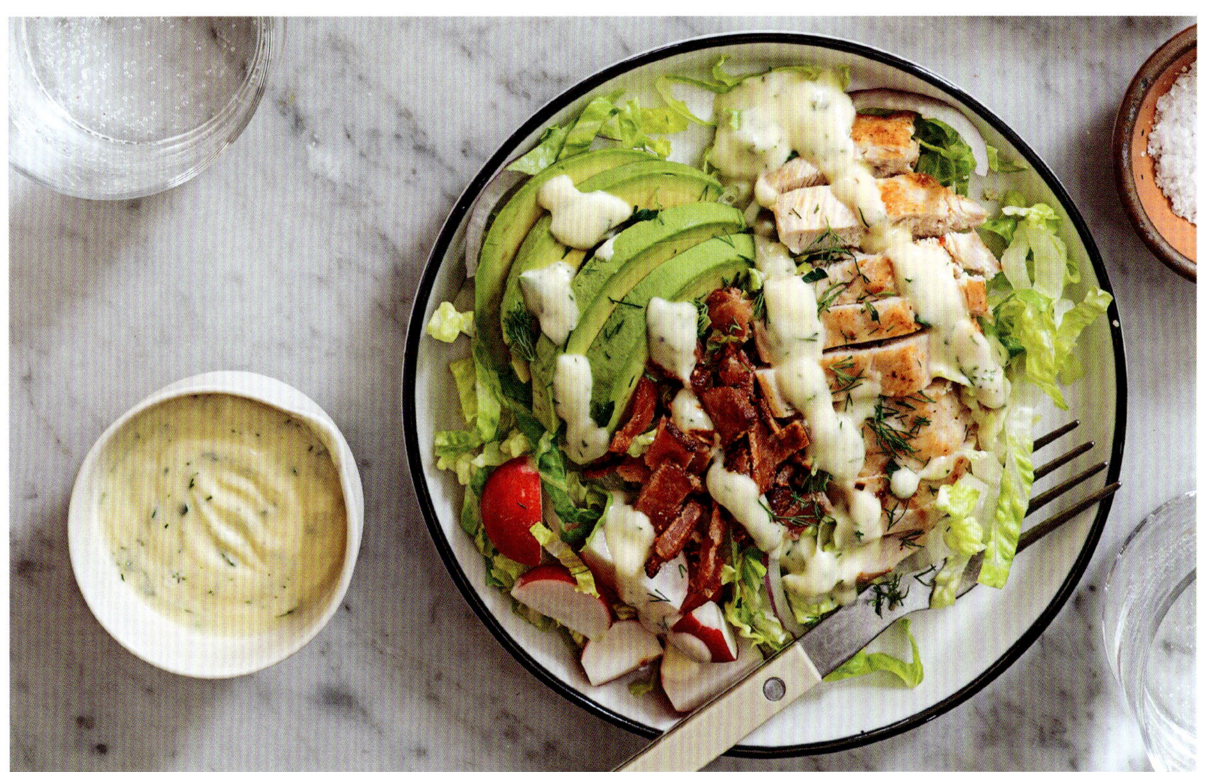

CHAPTER 5

Nutrient Density and Lifestyle

In addition to implementing the three phases of the Autoimmune Protocol, there are four areas you'll need to focus your attention on throughout the entire process: eating nutrient-dense foods, prioritizing sleep, managing stress, and getting the right amount of movement (exercise). Improving habits in these areas are foundational for supporting health for everyone, but especially those with autoimmune disease. Not only do they support healing while you implement AIP, but they are likely to be important to you long after you complete AIP. Over the years I've seen many people overlook these parts of the protocol even though they have always been an integral part of AIP, both in practice and in research. In fact, the medical studies investigating AIP for IBD and Hashimoto's incorporated specific actions to increase nutrient density and implement changes in the areas of sleep, stress management, and exercise in the interventions.[1,2] Don't make the mistake of thinking that attention to nutrient density or lifestyle factors is optional—it is very possible that changes in these areas could be more impactful to your progress than dietary eliminations.

Before we get started, you need to know that there is a lot of individuality and nuance in how you decide to implement changes in these areas. You might come to AIP having some great routines to support sleep, stress management, or managing your activity levels—which is great! Or, one of these lifestyle areas might be one that you continually struggle with. Because of this, you'll find the approach in this chapter less prescriptive and more open. While reading each section, take note of any areas you suspect might have a key role in your healing journey and make a commitment to experiment with changes that might help you make improvements. Shifting your routine in these areas can easily be overlooked, but my experience observing thousands of people implement AIP has taught me that these are often the areas that differentiate those who have a mildly positive response to the protocol and those who have a life-changing one. Be sure not to underestimate their value!

NUTRIENT DENSITY

We'll begin by discussing a dietary focus that is important to consider through all phases of AIP: nutrient density. Simply put, "nutrient density" refers to the amount of nutrients in a food relative to the energy it contains. Nutrients include macronutrients, which are necessary in large amounts for the proper functioning of the body and include carbohydrates, proteins, and fats; micronutrients, which are required in much smaller amounts and include vitamins and minerals; and other specific compounds such as phytonutrients, fatty acids, and fiber that confer health benefits to us when we consume them in our meals.

So, what is a "nutrient-dense" food? These foods have high amounts of nutrients relative to the calories they contain. Deciding which food is the *most* nutrient dense is a matter of opinion, as there is no official standard ranking for nutrient density. Some foods contain extremely high quantities of specific nutrients, like kombu, a seaweed that contains 2,000% of the recommended daily intake (RDI) for iodine per gram. Other foods contain good amounts of many nutrients, like chicken liver, which provides over 100% of the RDI for vitamins A, B2, B5, B12, biotin, and folate, as well as over 50% of the RDI for iron, copper, selenium, and vitamins B3 and B6 in just one 3½-ounce serving—wow, right? We can also consider nutrient-dense foods that contain good amounts of nutrients that are otherwise difficult to obtain in our diets, such as cold-water, fatty fish; sardines and salmon are great examples with a uniquely high source of omega-3 fatty acids.

Before you get too hung up on the specifics of identifying which foods are most nutrient-dense—one of the benefits of AIP is that it naturally encourages you to consume a diet that is more nutrient dense than the way you were eating previously. By cutting out processed and convenience foods and replacing them with whole foods, especially fruits and vegetables, you increase the nutrient density of your diet. This happens automatically as you transition to the elimination phase just by the nature of what is included on the protocol. An easy win in this area is recognizing that by simply making those ingredient swaps, you are already taking major steps to improvement!

So how nutrient dense is AIP, exactly? The medical study using AIP for patients with Hashimoto's out of Poland incorporated a detailed comparison of the patients' prior diets and their prescribed AIP meal plans. They found that despite energy density being similar before and after the study (a mean of 2,067 calories before and 1,997 during AIP), there was a broad increase in nutrient density of the diet. Specific nutrient intake increases included beta-carotene (550%), fiber (162%), folates (198%), long-chain fatty acids (262%), potassium (196%), vitamin A (341%), and vitamin C (886%), with other nutrients like B vitamins, iron, zinc, and magnesium also showing considerable increases.[3] This is a perfect demonstration of nutrient density, as calorie intake remained consistent but the participants consumed a much higher amount of nutrients once they transitioned to the elimination phase of AIP.

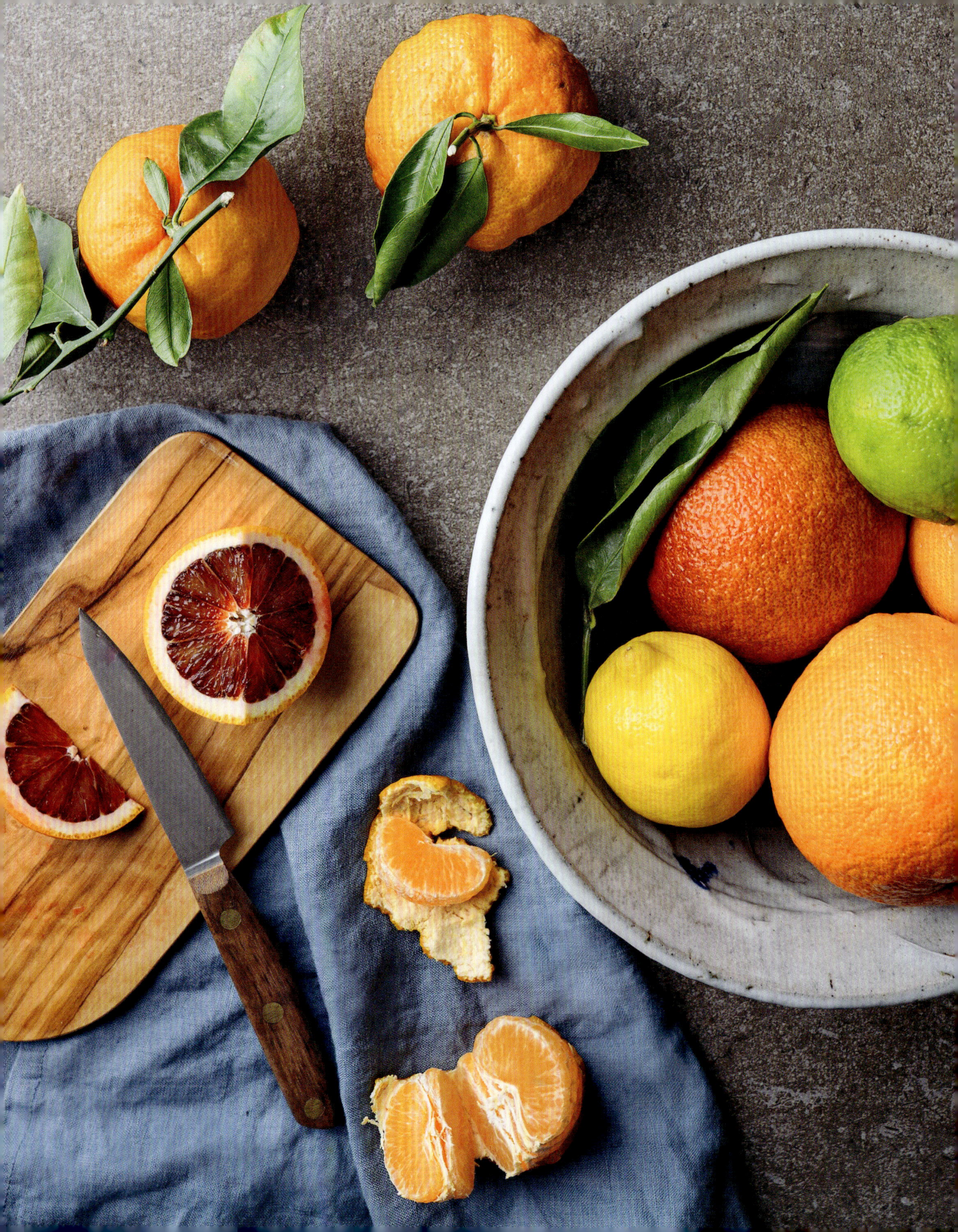

In addition to the detailed comparison of nutrient density in the Polish study, we also know that in two of the pilot studies using AIP as an intervention for IBD and Hashimoto's thyroiditis, patients were encouraged to add in specific nutrient-dense foods as a part of the study protocols.[4,5] One of the leading theories for the efficacy of AIP for improving symptoms and quality of life in autoimmune disease is the increased consumption of these nutrient-dense foods, which support deep healing and balance immune function. This is why during all phases of AIP (transition, elimination, and reintroduction), nutrient-dense foods are emphasized, as they are crucial for success and compounding healing. We'll discuss the specifics of which foods you'll want to incorporate later in this chapter, but first, we'll cover what happens when you don't meet your body's needs for a specific nutrient.

NUTRIENT DEFICIENCY

A nutrient deficiency occurs when you have a lack of an essential nutrient due to lack of intake in your diet or an issue with your body's ability to absorb it. Nutrient deficiencies can cause a wide range of symptoms due to their ability to impair essential bodily functions like energy production, immune response, and tissue repair.[6] To best manage your health with autoimmune disease or chronic illness, it is important to do everything you can to prevent nutrient deficiency in the first place as well as correct any known nutrient deficiencies as quickly as possible.

Research shows a lack of nutrient intake in typical diets is a major problem, with many people simply not eating enough nutrients to meet their needs. An analysis of the National Health and Nutrition Examination Survey data from 2005 to 2016 revealed that among adults, 84% had inadequate vitamin E intake, 45% lacked sufficient vitamin A, 46% did not consume enough vitamin C, and 15% were deficient in zinc intake.[7] Beyond those figures, dietary deficiencies are also common in vitamin B6, folate, zinc, copper, vitamin B12, and iron. In addition to inadequate intake, nutrient deficiencies can occur due to issues with digestion and absorption or as a side effect of medications, both of which can be common in those with autoimmune disease. For example, vitamin B12, iron, calcium, and magnesium can be impacted by altered pH in the digestive tract. This can come from low stomach acid, or as a side effect of medications like steroids or antacids that alter stomach pH over time.

A lack of nutrients due to insufficient intake or poor absorption is problematic because the immune system needs specific amounts of essential micronutrients to function to its fullest potential. Vitamins critical to immune function include A, C, D, E, B6, B12, and folate; important minerals include iron, copper, magnesium, selenium, and zinc. These micronutrients play essential roles in the immune system, including the maintenance of structural barriers like the gut lining and skin, proper structure and functioning of immune cells, direct antimicrobial effects, resolving inflammation, regulating the immune response, and antibody production and development.[8] It should go without saying that we all need to do our best to ensure that our intake of essential nutrients easily meets these needs for optimal health. While transitioning to AIP is likely to increase the nutrient density of your diet and help prevent nutrient deficiencies, if you have a known or suspected nutrient deficiency, it is important to prioritize troubleshooting this with your doctor. Your approach may include a focus on specific foods to help resolve any deficiencies, or supplementation as recommended by a healthcare provider.

NUTRIENTS AND DEEP HEALING

Now that you understand nutrient density, your action item is this: In all phases of AIP, you should prioritize specific foods to promote deep healing—bone broth, colorful fruits and vegetables, fermented or cultured foods, organ meats, fish, and shellfish. These foods have the highest amount of nutrients that not only prevent deficiencies and support the immune system but also help manage inflammation and repair tissues commonly damaged by autoimmune disease. Simply transitioning your diet to the elimination phase is likely to increase the nutrient density of your diet, but this *extra* focus can expand your healing and progress on AIP. This specific list of nutrient-dense additions has a long history of use in the AIP community, and the foods

NUTRIENT-DENSE FOODS LIST

BONE BROTH: A nutrient-rich liquid made from simmering animal bones and connective tissues for a long time to extract beneficial compounds important for deep healing, like minerals and collagen.

COLORFUL FRUITS AND VEGETABLES: Plant foods that come in a variety of vibrant colors, such as red, orange, yellow, green, and purple, which indicate the presence of diverse phytonutrients, vitamins, and minerals essential to good health.

FERMENTED OR CULTURED FOODS: Produced through controlled microbial fermentation, these foods offer enhanced flavor, preservation, and a source of prebiotic and probiotic compounds that support digestion and microbiome health.

ORGAN MEATS: Also known as offal, these include organs such as liver, kidney, and heart, which offer highly concentrated and absorbable sources of nutrients that can be difficult to come by in standard diets.

FISH AND SHELLFISH: Seafood options like fish and shellfish offer unique nutrient profiles for those on a healing diet, including high levels of anti-inflammatory omega-3 fatty acids and minerals essential to immune function.

on it are often credited by those who have experienced deep and profound healing. Personally, my original AIP implementation included daily broth intake, a scoop of fermented vegetables at breakfast, a few ounces of liver pâté per week, and as many vegetables and as much seafood on my plate as I could source and cook. On the following pages, you'll find the list of nutrient-dense foods to prioritize as well as some information about their specific benefits, tips on how to include them, and where to source them to help you focus on nutrient density as you implement all phases of AIP.

USING AND SOURCING NUTRIENT-DENSE FOODS

Bone Broth

BENEFITS: Long-simmered bone broth contains a wealth of amino acids and minerals that are supportive of deep healing. It contains good amounts of collagen, gelatin, and their components—the amino acids glycine and proline, which are important for connective tissues like tendons, ligaments, skin, and bone. Bone broth also contains glutamine, an amino acid that is used by the immune system and is a preferential fuel for the cells lining the intestinal tract.[9] Minerals like calcium, phosphorous, magnesium, and potassium are also found in broth. While human studies using bone broth as an intervention are lacking, a mouse model using bone broth as an intervention for ulcerative colitis demonstrated an anti-inflammatory effect.[10] Bone broth has a long history of use in the AIP community, with many patients reporting daily use and consumption as key to their success on the protocol.

HOW TO INCLUDE: Consume bone broth on its own as a healing beverage or simply use it as a regular ingredient in your cooking (see my recipe on page 119). Aim to consume about 1 cup per day either as a beverage or in soups or stews. You'll notice many of the recipes in this book include bone broth as an ingredient to add both nutrient density and flavor. I recommend always stocking frozen broth in your freezer to use as you implement all phases of AIP.

SOURCING: You can purchase bone broth premade or make your own (the first will save you time, the second will save you money). If you purchase premade, ensure that the product is true long-simmered, nutritious bone

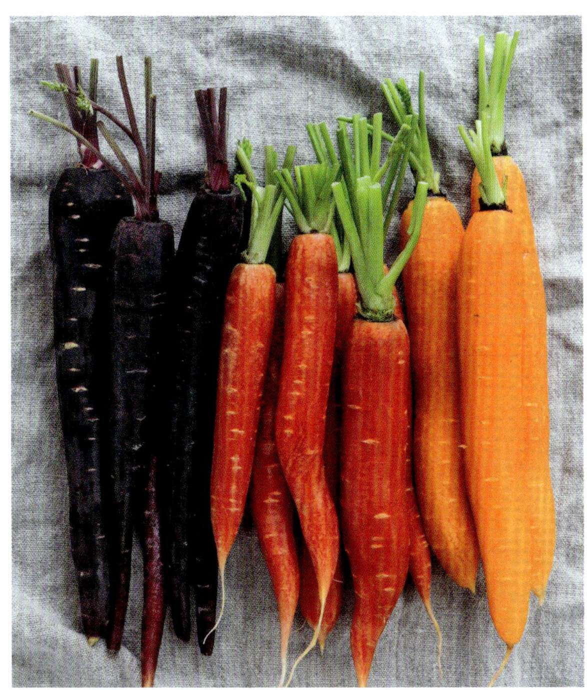

broth and excludes any ingredients you are avoiding. Look online, at farm stores or farmers' markets, or in the frozen section of your grocery store (check Resources on page 288 for recommendations). To make your own, you'll need to find a source of bones—they are usually not expensive or difficult to find. Cooking bone-in meats can provide an ample supply of leftover bones to make broth. Keep them in a bag in your freezer, ensuring you always have some when it is time for broth-making. If purchasing bones, ask for beef knuckle bones or poultry backs and necks at your butcher counter—they are usually easy to find for a good price.

Colorful Fruits and Vegetables

BENEFITS: Phytonutrients are chemicals made by plants that have health benefits when we eat them. Plants make phytonutrients for rich color, disease resistance, strength, and supporting reproduction. In humans, the phytonutrients we eat can function as antioxidants, which slow down damage to the body by free radicals and other compounds. Some of the most well-researched phytonutrients include carotenoids, polyphenols, and glucosinolates, which have been shown to improve health in a variety of ways.[11] In addition to phytonutrients, fruits and vegetables are rich sources of vitamins, minerals, and fiber. Fiber specifically is an often-overlooked dietary component, with both soluble, insoluble, and fermentable fibers being important to microbiome health and managing inflammation. Including ample colorful fruits and vegetables in your diet is a key component to success on AIP.

HOW TO INCLUDE: To start, aim to fill two-thirds to three-quarters of your plate with fruits and vegetables. Try to include as many colorful fruits and vegetables as you can, like berries, green leafy vegetables, and root vegetables, focusing first on the colorful fruits and vegetables you know you love before branching out to try new ones. If you can, rotate between raw and cooked forms of these foods to maximize intake of different types of fibers.

SOURCING: Fruits and vegetables with the most vibrant pigments often provide the richest source of phytonutrients. Seek a variety of colorful ingredients at the peak of their growing season. Some great unique examples you might find in-season are purple sweet potatoes, golden cauliflower, rainbow carrots, and purple artichokes—plus seasonal berries, which are always a treat. Anytime you see a local food in a new, vibrant color, it is an opportunity to add some extra nutrient density to your plate! This can be trickier in the winter months, so keep a supply of berries (like strawberries, blueberries, raspberries, and/or blackberries) in your freezer. If you have a hard time sourcing unique colorful fruits and vegetables, don't forget about the most accessible colorful vegetables—carrots, winter squash, broccoli, spinach, and berries!

Fermented or Cultured Foods

BENEFITS: Fermented foods have a long history of use in many cultures and come with many health benefits when consumed regularly. The process of fermentation breaks down components of food, often making them more digestible and can increase the concentration of certain nutrients due to microbial activity. They also serve as a source of probiotics and prebiotics, with potential to improve the microbial ecosystem

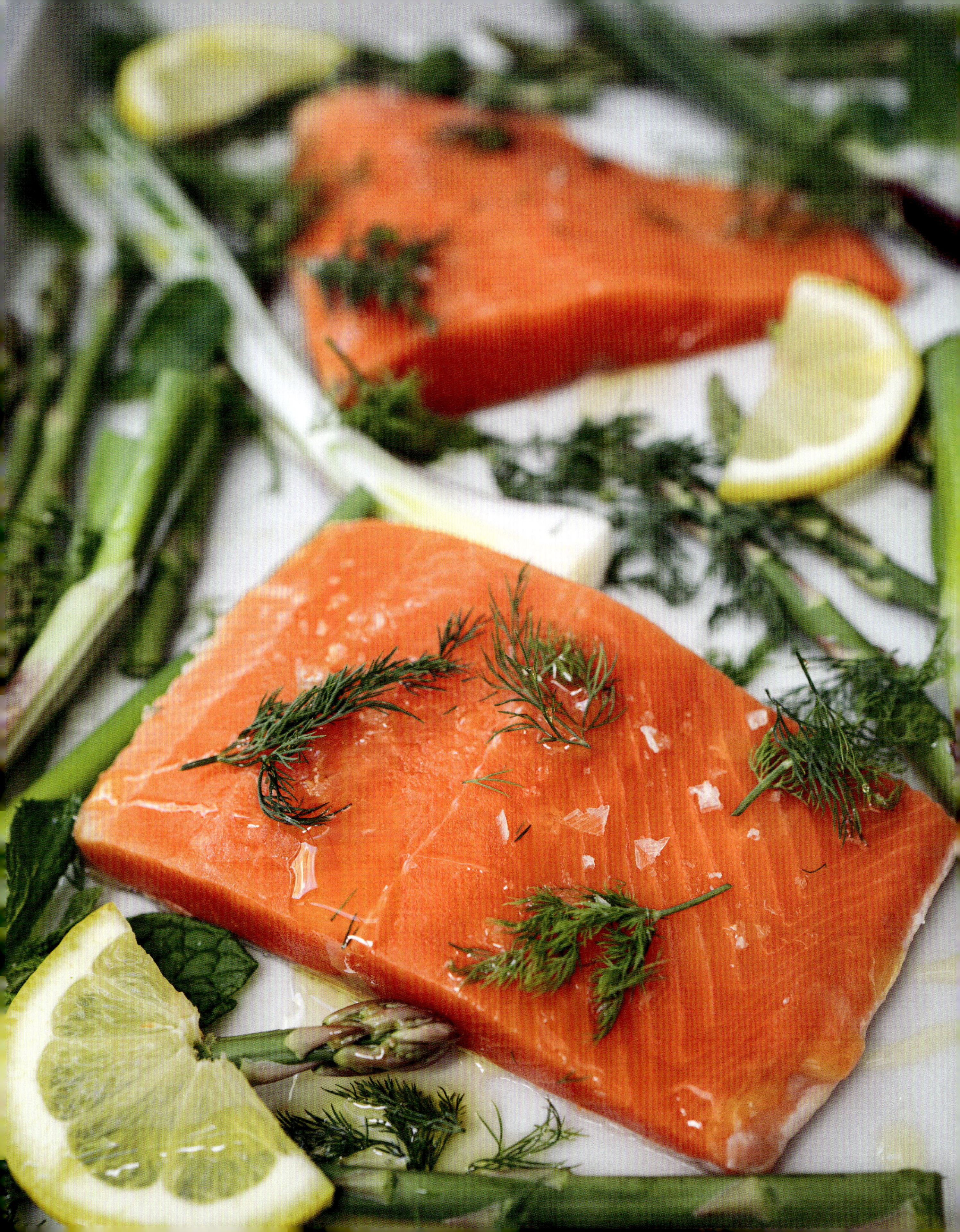

by supporting species associated with good health. Microbial by-products can also increase antioxidant content and provide compounds that further support a healthy gut microbiome.[12]

HOW TO INCLUDE: Plan to consume some fermented or cultured foods every day while on AIP. This might look like including a scoop of fermented vegetables with one meal a day, having some coconut yogurt with your breakfast, or drinking a probiotic beverage like kombucha or kvass between meals. If you are trying to get used to the flavor, try stirring a scoop of fermented vegetables into a soup or diluting your probiotic beverage with some sparkling water.

SOURCING: You can purchase premade fermented foods or make your own (see my recipe on page 120). I recommend starting with premade, especially if you are short on time or unsure about how to oversee a fermentation project (it isn't difficult, but it also might not be your cup of tea!). Ensure ingredients are compliant with your chosen AIP elimination and that it is live cultured (meaning it hasn't been pasteurized, which kills the probiotics). A good start is plain sauerkraut, with only cabbage, salt, and perhaps other ingredients that are compliant with your way of eating. Similar products made with other vegetables such as beets and carrots are available as well. Fermented beverages such as kombucha, water kefir, and beet kvass are also good options. Last, coconut yogurt is a newcomer on the cultured product scene with multiple companies offering products with live cultures and excluding any additives or thickeners that are avoided in the elimination phase.

Organ Meats

BENEFITS: Organ meats (also known as offal) are some of the most nutrient-dense foods available, providing high-quality protein, vitamins, minerals, and essential fatty acids. Organ meats are especially high in nutrients that can be otherwise difficult to obtain in the diet, including preformed vitamin A (retinol), B vitamins (including B1, B3, B5, folate, and B12), and highly absorbable forms of minerals such as iron, zinc, manganese, copper, and selenium. Organ meats also contain other bioactive substances in higher quantities than muscle meat, including creatine, taurine, coenzyme Q10, and glutathione.[13] Last, organ meats are incredibly affordable due to their low demand. Organ meats have a long history of use in the AIP community because of their rich nutrient density and affordability and can be especially helpful at quickly shoring up nutrient supplies for those who are depleted.

HOW TO INCLUDE: For those new to eating organ meats, I recommend making one batch of liver pâté (see my recipe on page 124), portioning it into quarters for the freezer, and eating one portion weekly on AIP-compliant crackers or apple slices during transition or elimination. If you are more adventurous or already know you enjoy eating these foods, you can include up to 1 pound per week of organ meats (including liver, kidney, heart, tongue, or others) in your meal planning. This is the only category where you'll want to be careful not to overdo it, especially in the case of liver, which can provide toxic amounts of vitamin A if regularly eaten in quantities higher than 1 pound per week.

SOURCING: Low demand for organ meats in the marketplace means you may need to work a little harder to find them, but be sure to ask, as many grocers can order them for you. If you can't find them at your usual grocer, check at your local farm or farmers' market, if accessible to you, or purchase online (check Resources on page 288 for recommendations). Some butchers and online retailers make things easy by offering ground meat with 10 to 30 percent organs so that you can benefit from the additional nutrient density while using ground meat in common recipes.

Fish and Shellfish

BENEFITS: Seafood options including fish and shellfish provide a unique set of nutrients that can support deep healing, like omega-3 fatty acids, iodine, selenium, and vitamin D, in addition to being a source of high-quality protein. Like organ meats, fish and shellfish represent some of the most nutrient-dense foods. Specifically, cold-water, fatty fish like sardines, mackerel, and salmon offer the highest food sources of omega-3 fatty acids, which are anti-inflammatory and difficult to obtain in other foods.[14] Including these foods regularly can help increase nutrient density and promote the anti-inflammatory nature of AIP.

HOW TO INCLUDE: If you enjoy seafood, aim to include 5 to 7 servings of fish or shellfish in your meal plans every week, prioritizing smaller, cold-water, fatty fish, like sardines, mackerel, and salmon, when possible. If you are new to eating seafood, start by including 1 to 2 servings of milder-flavored fish per week, like cod or sole, working your way up to including different types of seafood as your palate allows.

SOURCING: If you are lucky enough to live in a coastal area with high-quality fresh fish markets, these are likely the best places for you to purchase fish and shellfish, but you should also have some good options at your local grocer (although make sure to check your options, as stores vary in types of offerings and handling). Some types of fish, like wild salmon, can be purchased frozen in bulk from either a CSA or online from companies that specialize in selling frozen seafood. You can also stock up on BPA-free canned salmon, tuna, sardines, and oysters at your local grocery or specialty store (be sure to double-check those ingredients!).

LIFESTYLE FACTORS

In addition to taking steps to increase the nutrient density of your diet while on AIP, you'll also want to act in key lifestyle areas that can compound healing: improving your sleep, managing your stress, and ensuring you get the right amount of movement. Like nutrient density, the AIP medical studies used small but meaningful actions in each of these areas as part of study interventions; you should be sure to include them if you are hoping for similar results. The following sections will teach you about each of these lifestyle areas in detail as well as share ideas of how to start making changes to improve them.

OPTIMIZING SLEEP

Proper sleep is important for everyone, but especially those who are undertaking a healing protocol like AIP. If you experience signs that your sleep is not optimal, including having trouble falling asleep, staying asleep, waking up tired, or feeling sleepy or fatigued during the day, this area is one where you'll need to prioritize action.

First, let's discuss how sleep affects those with autoimmune disease. Research shows there is a bidirectional relationship between sleep issues and autoimmune disease, meaning that sleep issues are linked to the development of autoimmune disease, and sleep issues can also be worsened by existing autoimmune disease. Additionally, poor sleep and sleep disorders have been linked to higher levels of inflammation and autoimmune disease progression. Of those with chronic pain (a common autoimmune symptom), 88% report their pain as interfering with their ability to sleep.[15] This is one of the tricky realities of dealing with sleep and autoimmune disease—sleep issues are often worsened or caused by autoimmune disease, and those sleep issues can cause autoimmune disease to progress. This is why it is important to get control of any sleep problems early in the healing process.

What does research say about sleep quality and autoimmune disease? One assessment of ninety-five patients with rheumatoid arthritis found that those reporting optimal sleep showed less functional disability, higher rates of remission, lower levels of disease activity, lower levels of inflammatory markers, and lower levels of pain compared to patients who reported sleep issues.[16] A second study of 3,173 patients with inflammatory bowel disease found that a subset of Crohn's disease patients in clinical remission with sleep disturbances demonstrated a twofold increased risk of active disease in six months.[17] Improving your sleep quality is likely to help improve the course of illness and expand the healing you experience on AIP, and I've seen this ring true time and time again in my practice helping individuals implement the protocol.

So how much sleep do you need? Most research agrees that a range of seven to nine hours of uninterrupted sleep each night is optimal. If you are sleeping less than this, it is extremely important to troubleshoot underlying barriers to bring yourself up to this optimal range. But beyond sleep duration, what is most important is how you feel in the morning after you wake up. Do you feel refreshed and restored, ready to tackle a new day? Or do you feel tired and groggy, perhaps after a long sleep, like ten hours? This is a measure of sleep quality, which is a little harder to pinpoint than sleep duration. If you feel unrested even if you are getting the right amount of sleep, your focus is going to be on how to improve that quality so that you wake up feeling restored. Here are some areas to consider when coming up with an action plan to improve your sleep:

- **Try a sleep schedule:** Setting regular sleep and wake times helps your body find a consistent rhythm instead of having to constantly adjust to changing sleep patterns. In addition to setting a wake-up alarm, you should set a bedtime that allows you to get enough sleep despite known challenges like falling or staying asleep. A smart addition to your schedule could be a wind-down period of about an hour that allows you to perform any screen-free routines that help you transition to sleep, like reading a book, journaling, light stretching, or engaging breath work. Sometimes it can be tricky to remember to start a wind-down routine; setting an alarm just as you would for waking up can be helpful here.
- **Adjust your sleep environment:** The room you sleep in should be dark, cool, clean, and quiet, and your bedding should be comfortable. If there is too much light coming in from windows or appliances, you might try blackout shades, covering lights with tape, or using an eye mask. Sometimes noise is a challenge, so a white-noise machine, fan, or earplugs can be helpful. Make sure your devices are set to minimize or hold notifications.
- **Manage food and beverage intake:** Caffeine intake can disrupt sleep rhythm, even if it is only consumed in the early part of the day. While AIP is not a caffeine-free protocol (and coffee is allowed in Modified AIP), if you suspect that your caffeine intake could be negatively impacting sleep, you may want to reduce your use gradually to see if sleep improves. Next, highs or lows in blood sugar can also disrupt sleep rhythm. Some people find that having some starchy carbohydrates at dinner or a balanced snack before bed helps them avoid waking in the night. Last, if you have trouble holding your bladder at night, you might stay away from liquids an hour or two before bed to avoid this disruption to your sleep. This might involve some experimentation, but learning how to adjust your habits around food and beverage intake can lead to major improvements.
- **Consider daytime impacts:** There are changes you can make to your daytime habits that may improve your sleep. If you experience a lot of unmanaged stress, any effort you can take to improve that can also benefit the quality of your sleep. This might look like modifying or eliminating any stressors that are able to be changed or engaging in stress-management practices that help you feel resilient. Additionally, getting the right amount of exercise can improve sleep. We'll discuss both areas in later sections, but for now just understand that any improvements you make to manage your stress and improve your movement routine are also likely to benefit your sleep.
- **Rule out underlying conditions:** If you've made a good effort to troubleshoot your sleep and aren't making any progress, you'll want to get evaluated by your medical team to rule out sleep disorders or any other causes of your poor sleep.

MANAGING STRESS

Chronic stress is problematic for nearly everyone in our modern society, but especially those with autoimmune disease. Autoimmune patients often have higher levels of stress due to the symptoms we experience from our disease, challenges accessing care and navigating the healthcare system, impacts on ability to work and finances, not to mention all the additional practices we need to implement to manage our health. Worse yet, stress itself can cause worsening symptoms or lead us into flares, which gets us into a cycle that can be tricky to break. Getting control of and learning how to manage this stress is essential to learning how to live well with autoimmune disease, and why it is important to prioritize this during the healing process.

Does better managing our stress help improve autoimmune symptoms? We know that having a stress-related disorder puts a person at a higher risk for developing an autoimmune disease,[18] and stress has been shown to trigger flares or worsen symptoms of common autoimmune diseases like Crohn's disease and rheumatoid arthritis.[19,20] One randomized-controlled trial of patients with Hashimoto's thyroiditis found that after following an eight-week stress management program, patients demonstrated lower antibodies, lower levels of stress, depression, and anxiety, and higher lifestyle scores compared to the control group.[21] Another study of patients with rheumatoid arthritis found that a ten-week stress management program led to improvements in quality of life compared to the control group.[22] So, yes, implementing stress-management techniques may help you better manage your autoimmune condition, and I have seen great success in working with individuals in my practice who took this area seriously.

While embarking on AIP, you'll want to ensure that you are taking steps to manage your stress to expand your healing. Here are some action steps you can take to assess yourself and come up with a personalized routine to keep your stress levels down throughout this process:

- **Identify sources of stress:** Take some time to sit down and create a complete list of all the stressors in your life, both big and small. This list can include things like unexpected life events, caretaking, chronic health issues, intense exercise, allergies, family issues, financial stress, legal problems, child-rearing, emotional difficulties, relationship stress, employment, education, or changes in living situation. This list isn't meant to be overwhelming, but to help you work through some of the next steps.
- **Eliminate nonessential sources of stress:** When faced with the perspective of seeing all your stressors in a list, some might pop out to you as completely unnecessary—such as starting your day scrolling social media, overcommitting to nonessential obligations, or taking on tasks that others could or should be doing. If anything can simply be taken off your list, this is the time to do so.
- **Modify some sources of stress:** Can you make any changes to the way you currently handle your current stressors to help make them more manageable? This might look like setting better boundaries with coworkers who demand too much of your time or dialing down your high-intensity workout routine. Sometimes we can't eliminate stressors, but we can adjust our approach to them to minimize their impact on our lives.
- **Accept or reframe unmodifiable sources of stress:** Many stressors can't be eliminated or modified, but we can change how we think about them and give them less power over us. If you are experiencing extreme stressors that can't be modified, talk therapy can be a great tool for learning how to manage inner dialogue about unmodifiable stressors.
- **Identify what helps you manage your stress:** Make a list of which activities help you feel relaxed and restore your energy. They could include creative activities like art, music, or writing, exercising, self-care, playing games, being around certain people, unstructured time, mindfulness, or spiritual practice.
- **Develop a stress-management routine:** Using your list of practices that help you manage your stress, create a routine that includes these items in your calendar at regular enough intervals to help find balance and manage stress in your life.

MOVING WELL

If you have an autoimmune disease, you may face specific barriers to meeting your body's need for physical activity. Getting the right amount of movement is helpful for staying healthy, and you'll want to find balance in this area during your time on AIP. You'll notice that I prefer the term "movement" over "exercise," as it also includes activities that aren't traditionally considered exercise but still count, like gardening or play!

While getting the right amount of movement is important for everyone, there are specific benefits for patients with autoimmune disease. A review of research on exercise and autoimmune disease shows that moderate exercise interventions are effective at balancing the immune system, specifically in decreasing antibody production and supporting an anti-inflammatory state. Additionally, studies of physical activity and specific autoimmune conditions show that exercise interventions have been successful at helping manage conditions—including a milder disease course and improved mobility in patients with rheumatoid arthritis, improved cognitive ability and decreased fatigue in patients with multiple sclerosis, and decreased fatigue in patients with lupus.[23] It is important to stay active in our quest to live well with autoimmune disease!

Movement is one of those areas where more is not always better, and the highest levels of benefit are usually seen at a point of balance. You may be someone who experiences high levels of fatigue or disability due to your illness, so simply getting moving is a challenge for you. On the other hand, you may be someone who engages in an extreme exercise routine to manage your stress or the unwanted symptoms of your autoimmune condition (like weight gain). Addressing movement while embarking on AIP involves assessing your current habits surrounding your movement routine and identifying which steps you can take to find balance. Use the following lists to come up with ideas of how to shift your movement routine to be most supportive of your healing journey.

Ideas for those who aren't exercising enough:

- Start slow; increase volume slowly
- Emphasize enjoyable activities that are movement-oriented (gardening, playing with children or pets)
- Engage a supporter to make it a social activity
- Have backup plans in case of weather or flares
- Try multiple small movement routines throughout the day instead of a long workout (such as walks, stretching, or yoga)
- Enroll in classes designed for beginners
- Employ the help of an autoimmune-friendly personal trainer
- Act on psychological and physical barriers (such as engaging a talk therapist or physical therapist)

Ideas for those who exercise too much:

- Swap high-intensity workouts for more moderate workouts
- Schedule rest and recovery days
- Look for more appropriate ways to manage stress than intense exercise
- Let go of achievement in exercise or body composition
- Consider disease implications in weight loss resistance (such as Hashimoto's thyroiditis)
- Seek help for exercise addiction, body dysmorphia, or obsessive tendencies

PUTTING IT ALL TOGETHER

Incorporating the principles of nutrient density and making lifestyle modifications are key to your success on the Autoimmune Protocol. By prioritizing nutrient-dense foods like bone broth, colorful fruits and vegetables, fermented foods, organ meats, fish, and shellfish, you provide your body with the essential vitamins, minerals, phytonutrients, and other important factors it needs to promote healing and reduce inflammation. Alongside the dietary approach, incorporating supportive lifestyle practices to promote quality sleep, stress management, and a good movement routine can amplify these benefits.

It can be overwhelming to consider these layers in addition to what you've learned about implementing the phases of AIP; start slow, perhaps choosing one area per week and trying some new practices or foods. As these changes become habits and you discover what works for you, layer in additional adjustments over time, remembering that AIP is not a quick fix but a journey of discovery. By embracing both dietary and lifestyle factors, you are taking proactive steps toward improved health that will serve you a long time!

CHAPTER 6

Troubleshooting

Here's the scenario: You've prepared yourself completely to navigate AIP, only to have an unexpected challenge crop up along the way. First—don't panic, this happens to everyone! Using our highway analogy, this is like a flat tire, traffic jam, or bad weather disturbing your road trip. Some of these challenges might cause a short delay before you resume traveling to your destination. Others, especially if early warning signs are ignored, might leave you needing to delay or cancel your trip altogether. While you can't foresee all challenges you are likely to encounter during your time on AIP, my experience coaching has taught me that many of the issues that come up during implementation can be solved by simple modifications or adjustments in real time. This chapter serves as a resource to return to anytime you meet a new or unexpected challenge in any phase of implementing AIP. Make a note to review it if things go sideways, so that you can gain control of the situation before you need to abandon your plans!

Having witnessed thousands of people implement AIP, I've seen the same problems crop up time and time again. Common mistakes are usually to blame, like attempting to transition too quickly, skipping steps, or starting reintroductions too soon. This is human nature—most attempting AIP are doing so to help realize their personal health vision, and who doesn't want to take a shortcut to feeling better? The reality is that following the longer path to wellness often comes with greater clarity, more predictable outcomes, and better sustainability in managing changes over the long-term (darn!).

Other challenges to AIP implementation can include factors that we have less control over, like the accessibility of specific foods, budget or time constraints, and physical capabilities due to disability or disease. Similarly, they can come in the form of health concerns or changes, like different or worsening symptoms, complications due to existing medical issues, or a general lack of progress despite careful elimination. These factors can be incredibly frustrating and more difficult to navigate, but there are still steps you can take to lessen their impact on your ability to work toward your goals.

Here is what to do: As soon as you notice that you are struggling with a challenge that affects your ability to move forward in any phase of AIP, it is time for troubleshooting (don't wait!). Identify the problem and why it might be occurring, determine if you need to modify or change something about your plan, and then act on resolving it so that it doesn't present a further disruption to your ability to implement the protocol. This chapter will provide a detailed resource for how to navigate these challenges as they arise, so that you can continue the path to realizing your personal health vision.

COLLABORATION WITH MEDICAL AND HEALTHCARE PROVIDERS

It is essential that you collaborate with your medical and healthcare providers—not only are they an important resource for managing your health with autoimmune disease, but often troubleshooting problems that come up on AIP involve medical concerns that are within their scope of practice to help you tend to. You already know that before embarking on AIP, you should inform your medical providers of your intention to try the protocol, ask if there are any reasons why it might not be appropriate for you, and see if there are ways they can support you in your efforts. Even if you are working with a provider who is not familiar with AIP, this is an important step in building a working relationship with them and making sure you have your bases covered in terms of managing risks.

Another reason your medical providers need to be informed about AIP implementation is that dietary changes can result in an altered need for medications, especially those that affect lipids or blood pressure or that manage blood sugar. It is essential that if you are on a medication that can cause symptoms if not dosed precisely (such as blood pressure medication, thyroid medication, or insulin) that you are being monitored carefully so that your providers can make necessary changes to minimize unwanted symptoms. A little effort here can go a long way in preventing predictable medical events from occurring!

Troubleshooting can also highlight the need for further testing and/or treatment in specific areas, like obtaining another autoimmune diagnosis, identifying latent or hidden infections, or further exploration of areas that are specifically impacting your ability to implement the protocol, such as sleep or mental health. Engaging your providers in troubleshooting in these areas can help uncover root causes of your inability to experience improvements or make progress while attempting AIP elimination or reintroduction. We'll be discussing more specifics of troubleshooting in these areas later in this chapter, but for now, just understand that proactively seeking out a collaborative relationship with your healthcare providers is essential for your success here—don't wait until you are having a problem to begin building these important relationships!

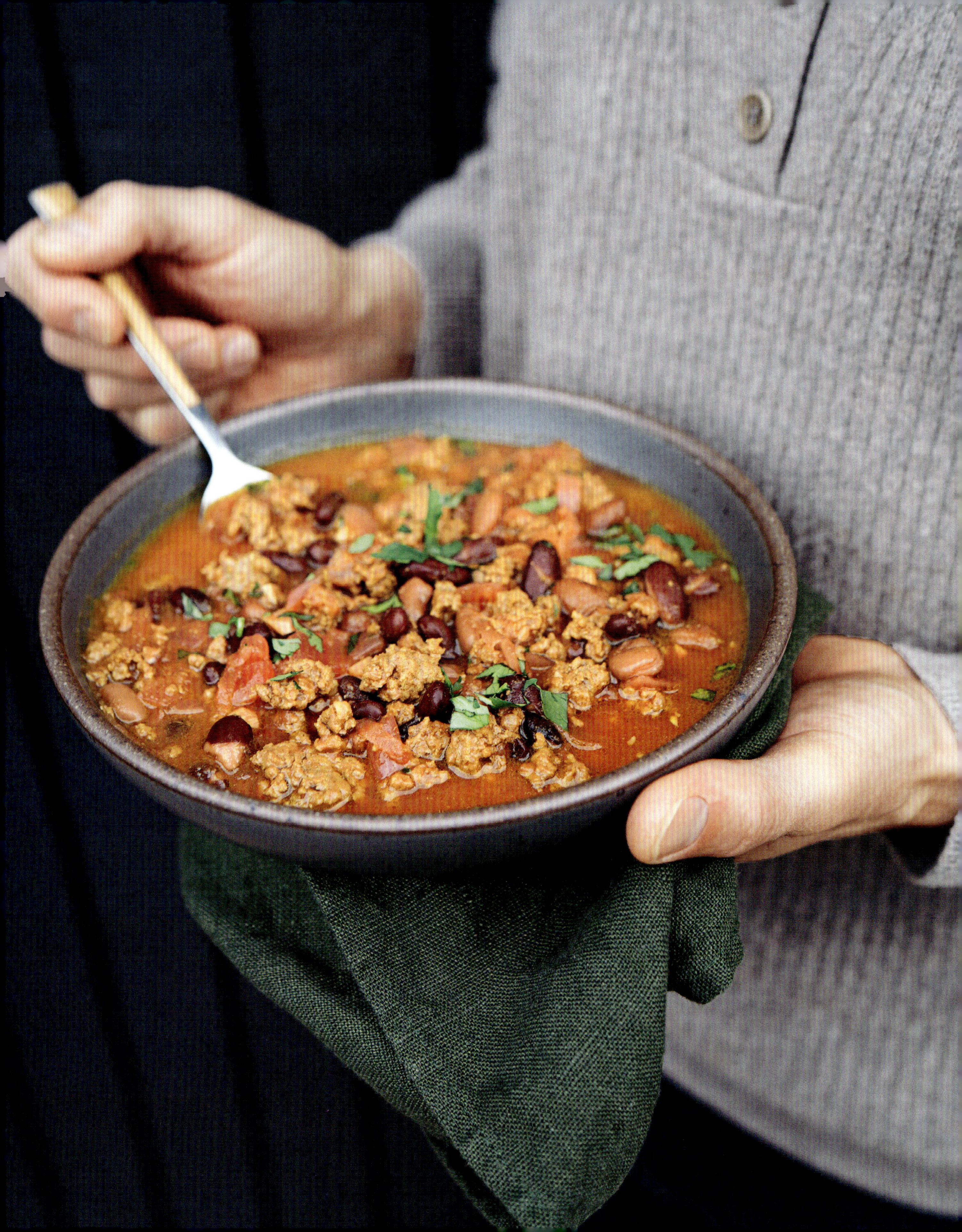

Now that you understand the importance of collaborating with your medical and healthcare providers during your time on AIP, we'll discuss troubleshooting as it applies to each phase of AIP—transition, elimination, and reintroduction.

TRANSITION PHASE TROUBLESHOOTING

Any issues that come up during the transition phase are likely to grow into ones that impair your ability to implement the elimination phase, so it is important to act on them right away. The transition phase is designed to help you make the shift to the elimination phase with as much ease as possible, but it still isn't easy—don't get discouraged if you notice yourself struggling! This section will highlight some of the most common issues that crop up during the transition phase and how to resolve them.

First, what can go wrong? The most common issues during the transition phase arise from simply rushing through the process to get to elimination. They include:

- Inadequate baseline tracking
- Skipping the personal health vision or confidence assessment exercises
- Attempting to transition too quickly
- Not enough confidence in key areas of implementation
- Not committing to a start date

By failing to address these issues during the transition phase, you run the risk of them becoming bigger problems later on during elimination. Consider the following in your troubleshooting:

- **Follow all the transition phase steps in sequence:** The transition phase is designed to prepare you for success in implementing the elimination phase with as much ease as possible. Each step builds on the prior work that you've done. Make sure to follow each step carefully before moving on.
- **Spend adequate time on tracking, visioning, and assessment:** These steps are not optional, and following them carefully will set the stage for how you approach the rest of the protocol. Give yourself adequate time to mindfully work through these exercises.
- **Schedule enough time acting on specific preparation tasks:** Your confidence assessment should have revealed which areas need action to successfully implement the elimination phase. Be honest about how much time it will take you to act in those areas before moving forward with the elimination phase.
- **Wait to begin the elimination phase until confidence in each area is adequate:** If you reach your elimination phase start date and you still don't feel ready, take additional time as needed to continue working through these barriers. It can be helpful to give yourself a couple more weeks (or even a month!) to thoughtfully work through some of these preparation tasks, as this is going to prevent problems later in the process. An exception might be those who feel prepared to implement the elimination phase but are experiencing fears about starting the process. This might be a good time to engage the support of an AIP Certified Coach or a mental health provider for personalized guidance.

ELIMINATION PHASE TROUBLESHOOTING

During the elimination phase it is essential that you maintain compliance for your chosen protocol, so it is important to begin troubleshooting as soon as you notice the first signs of new problems appearing. There are many types of issues that can come up during the elimination phase, and this section will teach you how to successfully navigate them.

What are the most common challenges during the elimination phase?

- Motivation or willpower aren't enough to maintain compliance
- Life obligations or other barriers impede cooking or other implementation tasks
- Support from family and/or friends is lacking

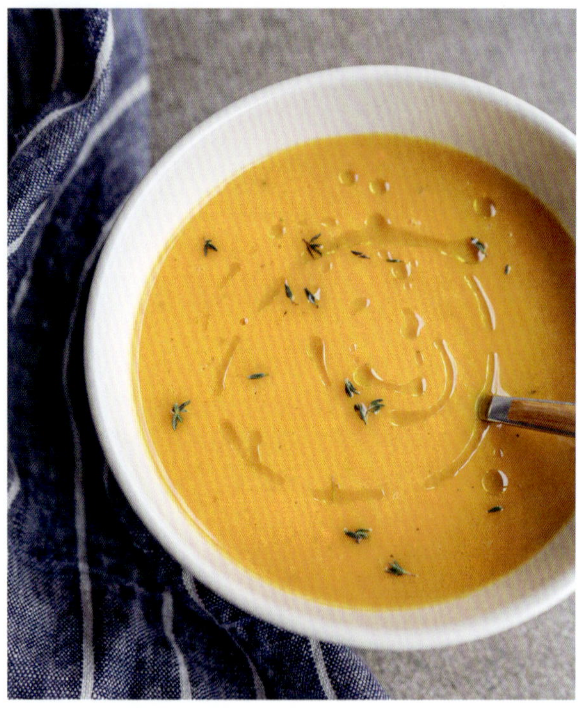

- New symptoms appear due to rapid dietary changes
- Coexisting or underlying medical needs are not being met

If these issues are not addressed promptly, they are likely to affect your ability to maintain compliance or sustainability to reach the reintroduction stage. Read on to learn more about troubleshooting in these key areas.

Issues with Compliance

If you have attempted to transition to the elimination phase and you can't maintain 100 percent compliance for your desired elimination protocol, you have a compliance issue. Some questions to ask yourself if you are having a difficult time maintaining compliance:

1. Do I understand why compliance is important to my success?
2. Am I fully prepared to make this change, or did I make it too quickly?
3. Do I have something unexpected going on in my life impacting my ability to make this change?
4. Are there any other barriers that were not understood during the transition phase that are impacting my ability to make this change? (This includes relationships, caretaking, mental health, and others.)

Compliance issues are usually solved by investigating these reasons underlying the lack of compliance and making changes to solve them, if possible. Solutions might include education, support, or modification. You might need a deeper understanding of why compliance is important to be motivated to make it happen. Or you might need support in a specific area, such as hiring an AIP Certified Coach to help you navigate transition. You could even need to modify your original plan, changing from Core to Modified AIP for ease of implementation. Whatever you decide, it is important not to cycle through short stints of starting and stopping your plans, as this adds undue stress and can lead to mental health challenges later. If you can't sustainably maintain compliance, revisit the action items revealed by your confidence assessment in the transition phase and continue making progress on them until implementing the elimination phase becomes achievable for you.

Issues with Sustainability

If you can implement the elimination phase successfully but you feel extremely stressed about your ability to maintain eliminations and are counting the days until it is over, you have a sustainability issue. This is problematic, as there is no guarantee that the minimum 30 days elimination is going to be effective, and you will still need to maintain eliminations throughout the reintroduction phase. While the elimination phase is not easy, you should not feel like every day you are hanging on using willpower alone. If this is the case, the chances that you will give in to temptation or make a mistake due to the high level of stress this mindset can cause are very high.

So, what do you do if you recognize a sustainability issue during the elimination phase? The root cause of this issue is the same as compliance, but harder to recognize because you may have had some success implementing the protocol for a short period of time ("I've already been hanging on for two weeks—I can definitely make it a month!"). This type of thinking can get you into trouble, as continuing without modifications is likely to increase stress, further impacting your ability to see progress. Here are some tips for navigating two types of sustainability issues:

- If you are noticing milder signs of a sustainability issue, such as feeling generally stressed by the elimination phase, but you still feel it is achievable, revisit the action items revealed by your confidence assessment in the transition phase to see if any of those solutions might make your elimination more sustainable. This might look like asking a friend or partner for support cooking for you a couple of times a week, purchasing premade ingredients or meals to save you time with food preparation, or any other changes that are accessible to you and will help you increase confidence in your ability to complete the required amount of time in elimination and reintroduction.
- If you are noticing signs of a larger sustainability issue, such as counting down the days or relying purely on willpower to stay on your plan, consider abandoning the elimination phase for now. Give yourself a week or two to regroup and then revisit the exercises in the transition phase, taking a hard look at your confidence assessment to see which areas need major work. Your goal is to bring up your confidence to a level that when you try again, you are more likely to be successful without as much stress or discomfort. If you are still struggling, consider hiring an experienced AIP Certified Coach to help assess your situation and make recommendations that help bridge the gap and make the elimination phase achievable for you.

Negative Changes or New Symptoms

Among the most frustrating challenges during the elimination phase include experiencing negative changes or new symptoms. After all, you are doing AIP to improve your health—what happens when you start to feel worse? While this can be demoralizing, it is important not to push through or ignore these changes or symptoms—they can be important indicators that you need to modify or seek professional guidance for what to do next.

This is where I put to rest another big misconception about AIP: There is no "detox phase" where you should expect to feel bad when implementing your eliminations. While it is possible that you feel some subtle changes, especially in the first few weeks as your body adjusts, you should not feel miserable or need to suffer through unpleasant symptoms as you transition to a new way of eating. Mild changes are expected as your body adjusts to altered macronutrient ratios (that's the balance of carbohydrates, fats, and protein you are eating) as well as the increased fiber and other nutrients in your diet. Beyond this, a new onset of more severe symptoms is often a sign that you need to transition more slowly, make modifications, or engage your healthcare providers in short-term solutions like digestive support as your body calibrates to your new way of eating.

Here are some common signs that you may need to adjust early on in implementing the elimination phase:

- **Fatigue, light-headedness, or headaches:** A new appearance of these symptoms (usually within days of starting the elimination phase) can indicate that you may not be eating enough carbohydrates for your needs, especially if you ate a diet particularly high in carbohydrates before (think processed or convenience foods). While the elimination phase is not a low-carbohydrate protocol, because of the excluded foods, some people may inadvertently implement in a way that lacks enough carbohydrates. If you suspect this could be the case, start including some AIP-friendly starchy carbohydrates, like sweet potatoes, winter squash, or plantains, at one to two meals per day, as well as making sure you are not avoiding other carbohydrate sources, like fruit.
- **Digestive changes:** A new onset of symptoms such as bloating, gas, diarrhea, or constipation when transitioning to the elimination phase might indicate that your body is struggling to adjust to certain components of your diet. If you are

experiencing these new symptoms, consider the following areas in your troubleshooting:

- **Raw/cooked vegetables:** If you haven't included many vegetables in your diet in the past, the increase in fiber when adopting AIP may initially cause you trouble. If you suspect this, be sure to ramp up your vegetable intake slowly, starting with slow-cooked vegetables and later moving on to raw vegetables, which can be harder to digest. As you include more vegetables in your diet, your digestion and microbiome can shift to adapt to this new intake and your symptoms may improve. Take it slow!
- **Fat intake:** If you have a history of eating a low-fat diet, your body may need time to adjust to the relative increased fat intake during the elimination phase. While AIP is not a high-fat protocol, quality fats are components of many nutrient-dense foods you will be eating during this time (like salmon and avocados) and increasing them too quickly can cause digestive symptoms. You may need to slowly increase your fat intake to manage them as your body adjusts.
- **Symptoms caused by new foods:** It is possible that you might experience symptoms after eating a food that you previously haven't consumed before the elimination phase (this happens commonly with coconut, but it can happen with other foods, too). If you notice new symptoms after eating a specific food, try eliminating it just as you would the other exclusions during the elimination phase. There are foods included in the elimination phase that can still cause symptoms for some people, so when in doubt, don't be afraid to leave them out.

- **Working with your medical or healthcare providers:** Sometimes troubleshooting a new onset of digestive issues involves collaborating with your providers. If you've made some of the above modifications to troubleshoot new digestive symptoms without results, it is important to seek guidance from a healthcare provider who may be able to help you with the following, if appropriate:
    - **Digestive support:** Your provider may determine that you need short-term digestive support (in the form of supplements or medications) to help you adjust to the elimination phase.
    - **Further testing:** Your new symptoms may indicate that you should be tested for other conditions, like small intestine bacterial overgrowth (SIBO) or histamine intolerance.
- **Worsening of autoimmune symptoms:** It is really frustrating to implement the elimination phase only to find your symptoms get worse. This is unusual, but it happens sometimes. You already know that there are no guaranteed results with AIP, and the nature of autoimmune disease is that it usually ebbs and flows in periods of better health and periods where your symptoms ramp up. There are many reasons why, ranging from the stress of implementing the protocol having a bigger negative impact than the dietary changes themselves to the natural fluctuations of your disease. If you feel meaningfully worse and basic troubleshooting does not yield early results, it is important to return to your prior routine and engage your medical and healthcare providers in a discussion of next steps. AIP is not a replacement or alternative to necessary healthcare, and you may need to spend some time getting your medical needs met before it is appropriate for you to attempt AIP again.

Experiencing a Lack of Progress

What happens if you've been diligent about implementing the elimination phase for the recommended 30 to 90 days and nothing has changed about your health status or symptoms, as evidenced by your baseline and elimination symptom journaling? This can be incredibly frustrating, but before you give up completely, be sure to explore all points in this section so you can be sure you aren't missing something.

If you are experiencing a lack of progress, begin troubleshooting by asking yourself the following questions:

1. **How is your progress or success being measured?** Your perceived lack of progress may be due to a mistake in tracking, such as not capturing accurate baseline symptoms, tracking the wrong metrics, or tracking inconsistently. Similarly, you may have entered the elimination phase with an unrealistic expectation of what success means to you (for example, expecting all your psoriasis lesions to disappear in thirty days, versus noticing that they have decreased in surface area by 10 percent in the same timeframe). Troubleshooting here might look like some self-exploration or hiring professional support to help you determine what to track and how to set realistic goals.
2. **Are you seeing progress or success in an area outside your primary goals?** My coaching experience has taught me that most people who report no beneficial changes during the elimination phase are often using their primary autoimmune symptoms as their only benchmarks. Upon further interview, just about everyone notices changes in general health, such as energy levels, sleep quality, skin health, digestion, and elimination. If you are noticing an uptick in general health indicators but not your primary autoimmune symptoms, often this can be enough improvement to base a successful reintroduction phase from if those metrics have been tracked properly.
3. **Have you only implemented the minimum of 30 days in the elimination phase?** If so, you should consider extending your elimination up to 90 days, as some people need a little longer to see those benefits more clearly.
4. **If you have implemented Modified AIP, would you be willing to shift to Core AIP?** While Modified AIP is an ideal starting place for most people, Core AIP is the approach that has been studied in medical research, is most nutrient-dense, and eliminates the most potential food triggers for those with autoimmune disease. If you are experiencing a lack of progress on Modified AIP, you might consider shifting to Core AIP to see if there are any additional benefits from those exclusions.
5. **Have you been implementing the principles of nutrient density in your approach to the elimination phase?** There is a tendency to focus mostly on the foods avoided during the elimination phase, instead of prioritizing nutrient-dense additions. If you are experiencing a lack of progress and you haven't been including foods like bone broth, fermented foods, seafood, or colorful fruits and vegetables in your routine, you might consider significantly increasing the nutrient density of your diet to see if that has an impact on your healing.
6. **Could you need more attention paid to lifestyle areas, like sleep, stress management, or movement?** For some autoimmune patients, specific factors in these lifestyle areas can trigger symptoms just as powerfully as dietary ones. If you've been focusing only on the dietary side of AIP and not adding in changes to these lifestyle areas, troubleshooting might look like planning to better address these lifestyle factors in your routine.
7. **Are there other options to explore on the medical side of managing your conditions?** A lack of progress while implementing AIP can also be due to a medical need that is unmet or unmanaged. This is a big reason why it is not appropriate to simply continue in the elimination phase without progress, as many of these medical needs require treatment for resolution. Troubleshooting here might look like further testing and treatments that might support your healing journey. Here is a list of some common areas that you might explore in collaboration with your healthcare providers:

- Gut infections (small intestine bacterial overgrowth, parasites, fungal infections, bacterial infections)
- Genetic alterations (methylation defects)
- Hormone imbalances (thyroid disorders, polycystic ovarian syndrome, menopause)
- Nutrient deficiencies
- Chronic viruses or infections (Epstein-Barr, long COVID)
- Structural or physical conditions
- Mental health or eating disorders
- Medication needs (flares not under control)
- Environmental exposures (mold, heavy metals, or allergies)
- Sleep disorders

There are experts out there who can help you troubleshoot a lack of progress during the elimination phase. Check out the AIP Certified Coach directory (AIPCERTIFIED.COM) for more information on how to gain the support of a qualified coach.

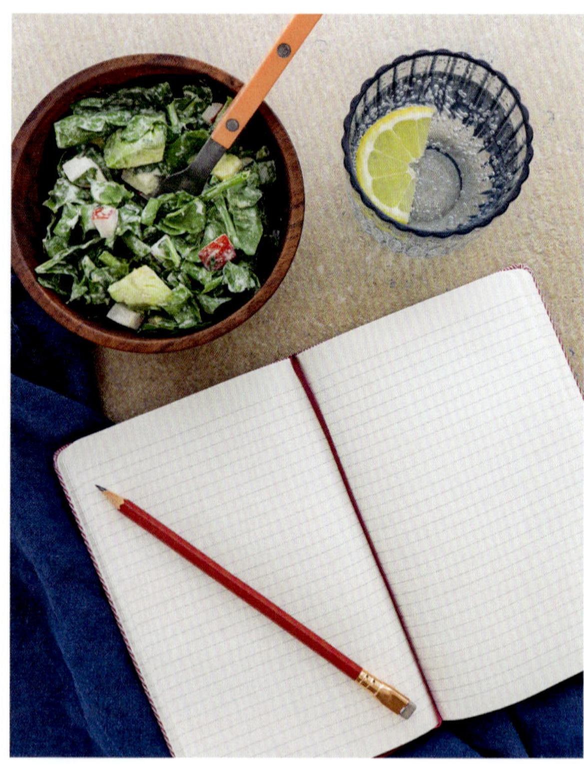

REINTRODUCTION PHASE TROUBLESHOOTING

The reintroduction phase differs from the elimination phase in that it can be much more variable in both your approach and your body's response, so there are more places where problems can arise. Fortunately, my coaching experience has given me a deep understanding of where this process usually goes wrong and how to course-correct. This section will help you navigate any problems that come up during this time.

What can go wrong during the reintroduction phase?

- Not spending enough time in the elimination phase
- Progressing too quickly through reintroductions
- Not following the reintroduction procedure carefully
- Lifestyle or other factors preventing smooth reintroductions
- Issues with expectation versus reality
- Mindfulness and body-awareness issues
- Food fears or mental health struggles

As the final phase of AIP, the reintroduction phase is the last piece to discover what dietary and lifestyle components are supportive of your best health. At this point, you've put a considerable amount of time and energy into maintaining compliance, so you'll want to get at the root of any problems quickly so that you don't lose any progress you've made. The following is a list of how to prevent most reintroduction phase issues.

Timing Issues

It is essential that you follow guidance for spending 30 to 90 days in elimination and experience measurable improvements over your baseline before beginning reintroductions. By entering the reintroduction phase too soon or without measurable improvements as evidenced by symptom journaling or other tracking, you will not be set up to accurately determine which foods are problematic for you. The timing for the reintroduction phase is one of the biggest decisions you'll make during your time on AIP, and it is important to ensure these conditions have been met before making plans to formally enter this phase.

Here is a list of conditions that need to be met before beginning reintroductions:

- You've spent 30 to 90 days compliant with your chosen elimination protocol with measurable improvements over your baseline as evidenced by tracking.
- You have solidified good habits and routines surrounding the lifestyle factors for good sleep, stress management, and movement.
- To the degree possible, you expect the next one to two months to be stable and predictable in terms of schedule and lifestyle factors that might impact this process.
- You are ready in terms of your medical monitoring or needs—this might look like having routine labs drawn for comparison, or if medication changes are a near-term possibility, that you negotiate timing with your healthcare providers, if appropriate, so that you can accurately rule out side effects or other changes.

Rushing Reintroductions

If you progress too quickly through the reintroduction process, you may find that you are unable to determine which foods are causing your symptoms. Rushing can look like not spending enough time between each individual reintroduction or moving to later stage reintroductions too early in the overall reintroduction process. In my years observing people implement AIP, the biggest mistake people make during reintroductions is simply rushing—which is natural, because everyone wants to return to eating some of their favorite foods as quickly as possible! Remember, all the hard work during the elimination is to set the stage for the reintroduction process, so it is important to treat this phase with as much dedication and careful planning.

How do you ensure you aren't rushing reintroductions? While it is normal to feel unsure about some food reintroductions and need a second attempt for confirmation, you should not move on to your next attempt until you are reasonably sure that the food you just reintroduced is working for you. Additionally, if you experience a negative reaction, it is important not to expedite the recovery period to get your level of health back to your improved baseline. If at any point you feel confused or unsure you've reached the improved baseline you achieved after elimination, give yourself more time. This could mean waiting a matter of days or even weeks until you are confident you are feeling good enough to resume the process.

Missing Key Reintroduction Details

Navigating the reintroduction process requires you to shift your planning and organizing routine to accommodate a more exploratory mindset. The reintroduction phase is full of nuance, and you will have many opportunities to decide what to do next—such as which food you'll try next, or how long to wait between each reintroduction. This makes it easy to overlook some key details about the process, such as following the exact reintroduction procedure, how to select foods for the order of reintroduction, how to gauge what is a food reaction, and when you are ready to move on to the next food. Revisit the reintroduction phase instructions often to ensure that you are planning the next steps of your protocol in a way that sets you up for success. If you are having trouble following the process or staying organized, print the reintroduction procedure and stages for handy access (downloads available at THEAUTOIMMUNEPROTOCOL.COM/PRINTABLES).

Other Factors Impacting Reintroductions

Sometimes you might have a hard time identifying if a symptom you are experiencing is due to a recently reintroduced food or something else. By accounting for these factors, you can become more skilled at interpreting your body's responses to food as you navigate the reintroduction phase.

Here is a list of non-dietary factors that could impact your ability to judge reintroductions:

- **Stress levels:** If you are experiencing chronic or acute stressors, they can cause symptoms that might skew your reintroduction results.
- **Sleep disturbances:** Poor sleep impairs immune function and worsens symptoms, masking the effect of reintroduced foods.
- **Physical activity:** Typically, intense exercise can induce symptoms similar to food reactions (like fatigue or joint pain), but sometimes a lack of exercise can be an issue as well.
- **Hormonal changes:** Menstrual cycles, pregnancy, or other hormonal changes affect the immune system and can complicate reintroductions.
- **Environmental factors:** Seasonal allergies or exposure to chemicals (such as cleaning or personal care products) can trigger symptoms that may overlap with food reactions.
- **Medications or supplements:** Starting, stopping, or changing medications or supplements can affect how your body responds to food reintroductions.
- **Illness or infection:** Having an active illness or infection can alter immune function and make it impossible to gauge food reactions.
- **Social or lifestyle habits:** Disruptions to your routine, such as travel, staying up late, or irregular mealtimes can affect reintroduction assessments.

Difficulty Navigating a Lack of Clarity

You might be expecting that during food reintroductions you will have either a clear negative reaction or a positive successful reintroduction. The reintroduction process can be confusing, and feeling unsure if a food is successful or not is a very normal and expected part of this process (I promise!). Some food reactions are subtle, occur only when a certain quantity threshold has been reached, or are more likely to occur when you have another factor impacting you, like a lack of sleep or feeling overly stressed out. Additionally, what you might consider a food reaction could be from something unrelated to your diet, like an environmental sensitivity.

If you are feeling stressed out by a lack of clarity during the reintroduction process, it is important to allow yourself more time between reintroductions and step back to reattempt any foods that were not conclusive later. If you are struggling to find clarity as you navigate reintroductions, keep three lists: one of foods you've reintroduced successfully, one of foods you've had a reaction to, and one of foods you've tried with inconclusive results. You'll avoid the second and third lists for now, but you can revisit the inconclusive foods again later.

Mindfulness and Body Awareness Issues

Many people with chronic illnesses have become skilled at disconnecting from their body as a coping mechanism, making it more difficult to determine if foods are causing symptoms during the reintroduction process. If you struggle with failing to notice or feeling unsure if foods are causing symptoms, you can try strategies to increase body awareness and sensitivity. Some options include mindfulness practices such as breath work, guided meditation, or biofeedback.

Gray Area Foods

It is possible for you to not tolerate foods in specific quantities, frequencies, preparations, or in combinations with other foods. These are called "gray area" foods, as opposed to the "black" and "white" distinction between foods that clearly are and are not tolerated in any quantity. If you attempt a food reintroduction and feel like your tolerance is conditional on some other factor or inconsistent, you may be encountering a gray area food.

Examples of ways gray area foods can manifest:

- The food can be eaten once or even for several days in a row, but not daily.
- The food is tolerated alone, but if accompanied by other reintroduced foods, it produces symptoms.
- Certain cooking preparations that make the food more easily digested allow it to be tolerated.
- Factors that increase food reactions, like vigorous exercise, prolonged stress, lack of sleep, or even

alcohol consumption may create a situation where a reintroduced food is temporarily not well tolerated.

This awareness of your personal tolerance level may unfold over a long period of time—even years! It can also change as you move through the stages of healing, or if other factors like your lifestyle change over time. If you identify any gray area foods, I recommend excluding them until your reintroduction phase is complete. At that point you can make an informed decision about how and when to integrate these foods into your diet long-term. Personally, I like to keep my gray area foods out of my diet when eating at home, but I will have them when eating out or traveling for ease of convenience, without going overboard to minimize potential symptoms.

Food Fears, Mental Health Struggles, and Eating Disorders

Sometimes people experience such great progress during the elimination phase that they become afraid to reintroduce foods, thinking that they will lose all their progress or that their symptoms will return with a vengeance. This happens most often to people who come to AIP with a high burden of illness as the discovery of something that works to help manage their symptoms is such a relief that they will "do anything" to capture those gains and manage their health long-term. I personally felt this way in my own experience with AIP and spent way too long in the elimination phase because of it! If you find yourself with similar feelings, it is important not to let food fears take root and avoid reintroductions. While reintroducing foods can cause you to experience some of your symptoms once again, it is an important and essential part of completing AIP; it helps you identify the foods you'll need to avoid long-term and which ones you can safely include in your diet, making your way of eating as practical, accessible, nutrient-dense, and easy to implement as it possibly can be.

By avoiding reintroductions and implementing the elimination phase "forever," you run the risk of developing unhealthy behaviors around food. For some, this can lead to disordered eating patterns, especially if this is an area they've struggled with in the past. If you notice that you are feeling especially anxious or unwilling to begin reintroducing foods, consider seeking professional support to work through these fears to begin this important and final phase of AIP.

CONCLUSION TO PART I

It's time for a pep talk! You now have a solid foundation of the New Autoimmune Protocol and its key components. From understanding what autoimmune disease is to learning about the essential phases of AIP—transition, elimination, and reintroduction—you're equipped with the knowledge needed to decide whether Core or Modified AIP is right for you and embark on this journey with confidence. You understand deeply that AIP isn't a one-size-fits-all approach but rather a dynamic process, tailored to your unique needs.

By integrating foundational dietary principles with lifestyle factors such as stress management, sleep, movement, and connection, you've learned that healing is a holistic endeavor. Nutrient density plays a pivotal role in supporting your body through the different stages of AIP, and we've touched on the importance of troubleshooting and refining your approach as you move through the protocol.

Staying committed to AIP might feel daunting at times, but remember why you started in the first place. Every small choice you make is an investment in discovering what best supports your future health and vitality. Celebrate the wins—big and small—and know that progress isn't about perfection but about persistence. The road to healing isn't linear, and setbacks don't define your success. Each meal, each mindful decision, and each step forward is a testament to your strength and resilience. You have the tools, the knowledge, and the power to reclaim your well-being. Keep going—you've got this!

It is now time to take a delicious approach to healing. In Parts II and III, you will find collections of Core and Modified AIP recipes, meal plans, and shopping lists to help you put your plan into action—let's go!

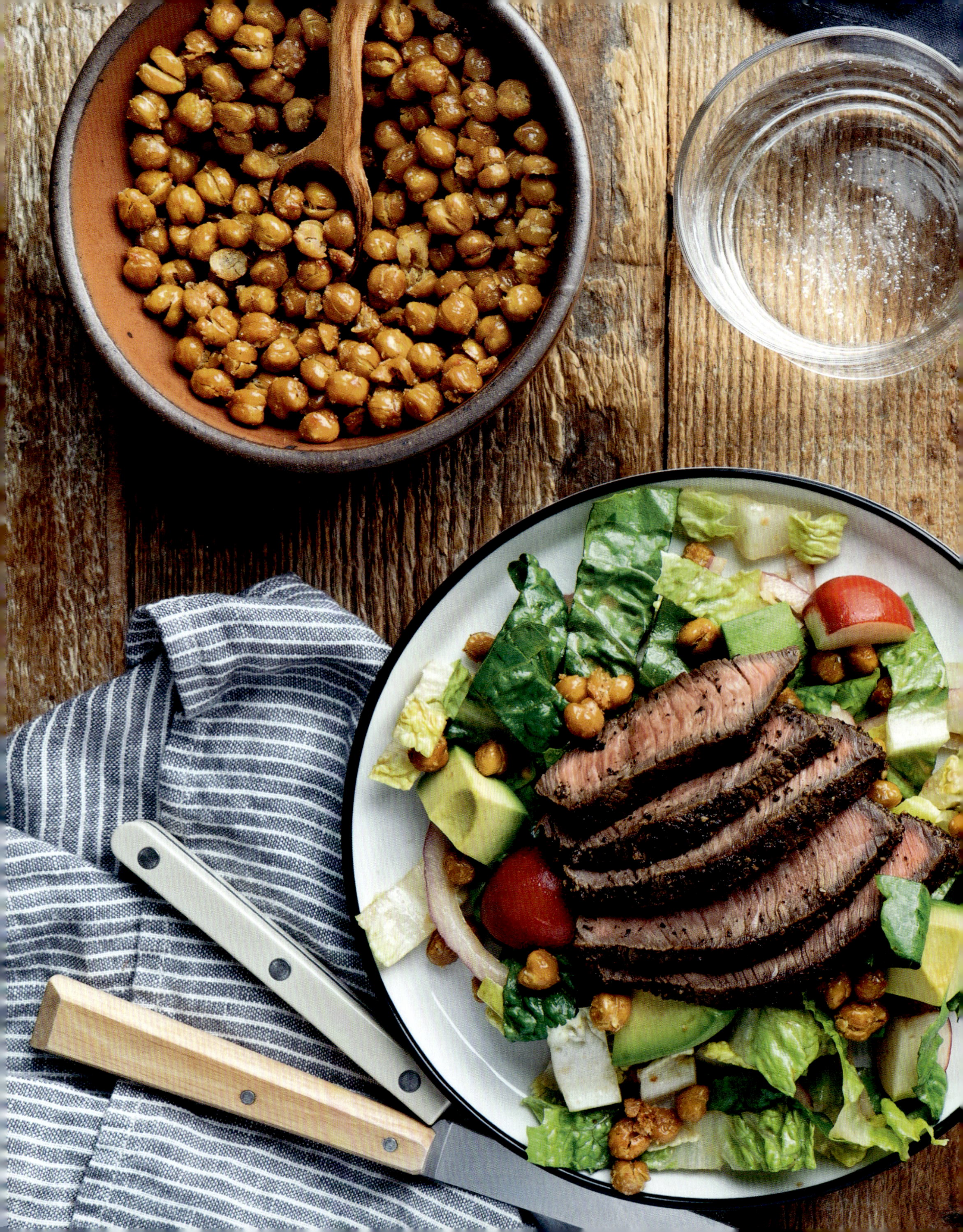

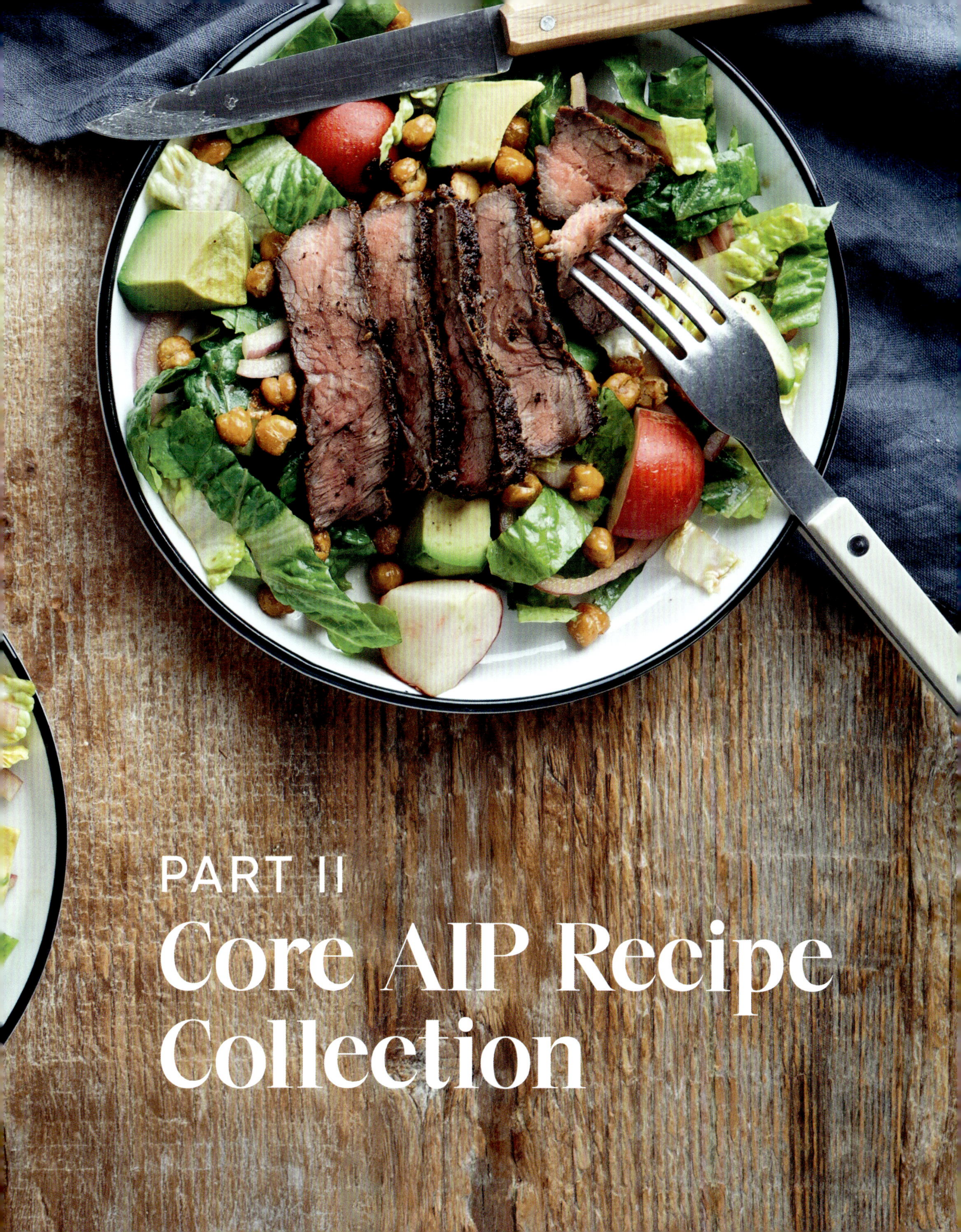

PART II

Core AIP Recipe Collection

If you've decided that Core AIP is right for you, this recipe collection has been curated to support your healing journey with nutrient-dense, anti-inflammatory meals that are free from all grains, legumes, dairy, eggs, nuts, seeds, and nightshades. You'll notice there is a heavy focus on flavorful basics, like *Healing Bone Broth* (page 119) and *Basic Sauerkraut* (page 120)—essential for gut health and immune support—as well as lots of sauces and dressings—like *Golden Curry Sauce* (page 128) and *Tangy Green Sauce* (page 123)—to bring vibrant flavors and powerful nutrients to any meal. These staples form the backbone of your Core AIP elimination.

Moving beyond the basics, I've included recipes that are flexible and adaptable, from satisfying soups like *Nourishing Core Chili* (page 150) to flavorful mains such as *Chicken Noodle Pesto Bowl* (page 169). Whether you're craving a hearty, comforting dish like *Curried Beef Vegetable Pie* (page 171) or seeking a light, refreshing meal like *Herb Roasted Salmon with Asparagus and Cauli Steaks* (page 180), this collection is designed to meet your needs and palate while following Core AIP. These recipes provide you with the flexibility to explore new flavors and textures while healing your body, and with detailed 4-week meal plans and shopping lists (page 196), it is easy to stay organized and on track.

A reminder: All Core AIP recipes also apply to those following Modified AIP.

CHAPTER 7

Core Basics

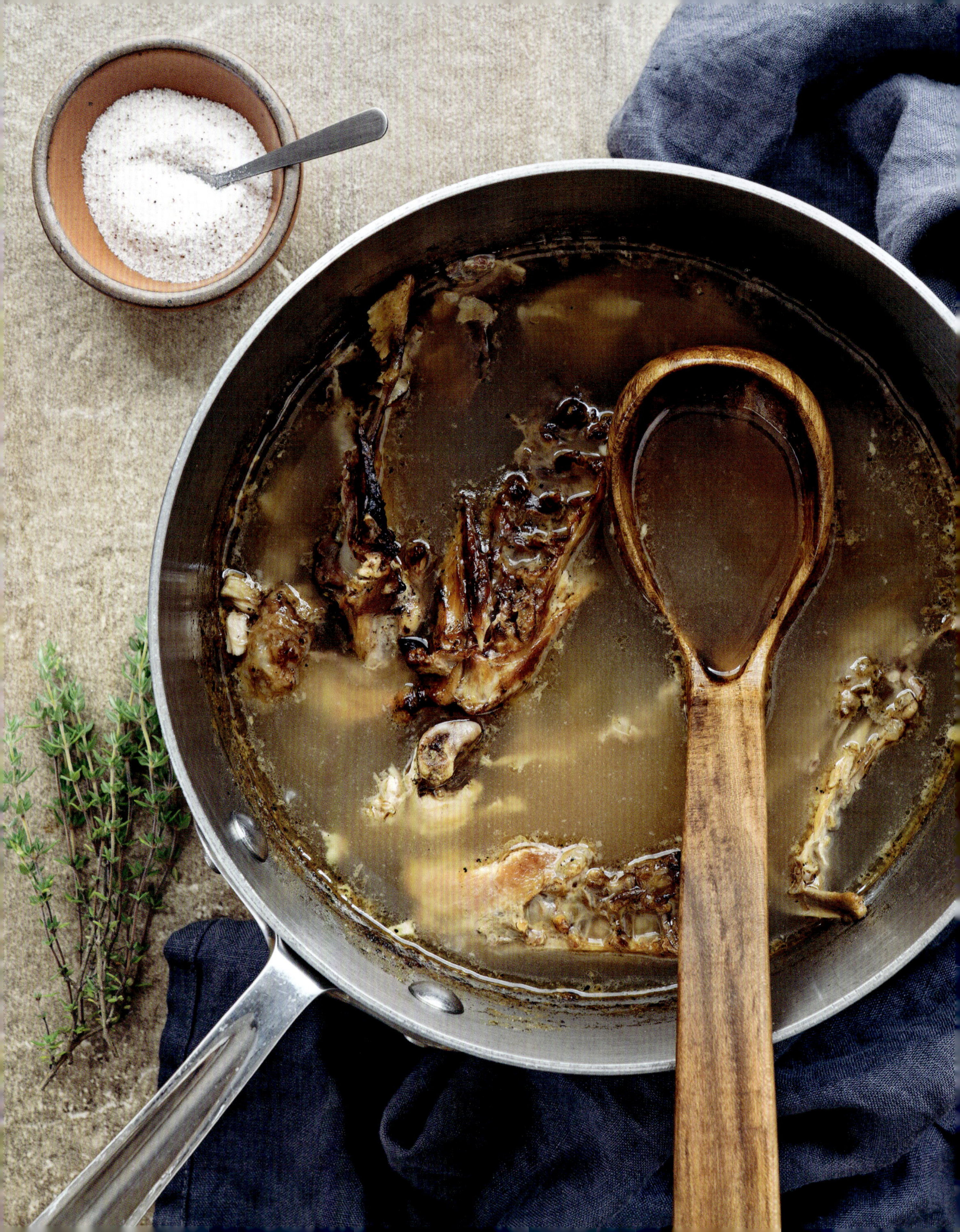

Healing Bone Broth

2 HOURS (PRESSURE COOKER) TO 24 HOURS (STOVETOP)

MAKES 3 TO 4 QUARTS

4 quarts water

2 or more pounds bones (see Sourcing Note)

2 tablespoons apple cider vinegar

1 bay leaf

SOURCING NOTE: *Bones should not be expensive or difficult to find. The best source is from a farmer you trust, maybe at a farmers' market or through a CSA. If you don't have those sources available to you, a lot of stores sell bones—be sure to ask the butcher. Also, you can start a bag in your freezer for storing any bones from the meat you consume—just toss them into the bag and freeze to make broth later. Feel free to use any type of bones, even if they have been previously cooked, to make broth—beef, lamb, chicken, and turkey all work well.*

STOVETOP

1. Place all the ingredients in a large stockpot and bring to a boil. Reduce the heat so the water is barely simmering.

2. Occasionally skim the surface for any scum that may appear during cooking. This is especially important in the first half hour or so of simmering. When there is no more scum rising to the surface, cover the pot, leaving the lid slightly ajar if your lowest setting still cooks too hot.

3. Cook for at least 8 and up to 24 hours, checking periodically to ensure the broth is still at only a bare simmer. If you notice the liquid cooking off too quickly, replace any loss with additional water. The longer you cook your bones, the richer and more nutritious the broth will be.

PRESSURE COOKER

1. Place all the ingredients in a pressure cooker, making sure not to exceed the fill line. Lock the lid and cook on high pressure for 90 minutes.

2. When the broth is finished (using either method):

3. Let the broth cool, then strain and portion it into containers for storage. Store in the refrigerator for up to 1 week, or in the freezer for a few months. I like to use wide-mouth canning jars and leakproof lids for freezing (if you are using glass jars, be careful to not use jars with shoulders, to not exceed the fill line, and to allow the broth to chill to refrigerator temperature before placing in the freezer).

4. After the liquid is strained, pick through any bones that are still intact and save them to add to the next batch, tossing those that fell apart. (You can usually get a few batches out of larger beef knuckle bones, while chicken bones last for only 1 or 2 batches.) You can refreeze used bones if you are not ready to make another batch of broth immediately.

Basic Sauerkraut

20 MINUTES, PLUS 2 TO 3 WEEKS FOR FERMENTATION

MAKES 2 QUARTS

4 to 5 pounds cabbage (about 2 medium heads)

2 tablespoons sea salt

YOU ALSO NEED

2 (1-quart) glass jars with airlocks

Clean fermenting weights or stones

Tamper (optional)

VARIATIONS: *The possibilities for varying your fermented vegetables are endless—you can use different types of cabbage, carrots, beets, garlic, ginger, and many other vegetables in different combinations to make a rich array of tasty probiotic foods.*

1. Finely shred the cabbage, either using a sharp knife or a food processor. Place the shredded cabbage in a bowl in batches, sprinkling each batch with a layer of salt. When you are finished, use your hands to massage the cabbage well until it breaks down and becomes soft, about 10 minutes. Let the massaged cabbage sit for 10 minutes to allow it to release its juices.

2. Pack the cabbage very tightly into jars, pushing all of it down until it is completely submerged by its own juices (a tamper is helpful here). Leave about 1½ inches headspace and add some additional brine if there is not enough liquid to fully submerge the cabbage (dissolve 1 teaspoon sea salt in 1 cup of water). Place the fermenting stones on top to weigh down the cabbage, tighten the lid, and ensure the airlock is installed properly (refer to the instructions that came with your unit, as they can vary). It is possible to ferment without an airlock—just be sure all the cabbage is submerged and check it often to make sure it hasn't spoiled.

3. Let the cabbage ferment at room temperature for 2 to 3 weeks; during this time, the vegetables will bubble a little and intensify in flavor. If any scum appears, remove it with a spoon. Taste it starting at 2 weeks, and when the taste is to your liking, you can remove the airlock, put a regular lid on the jars, and store in the refrigerator. Basic Sauerkraut will keep for a few months.

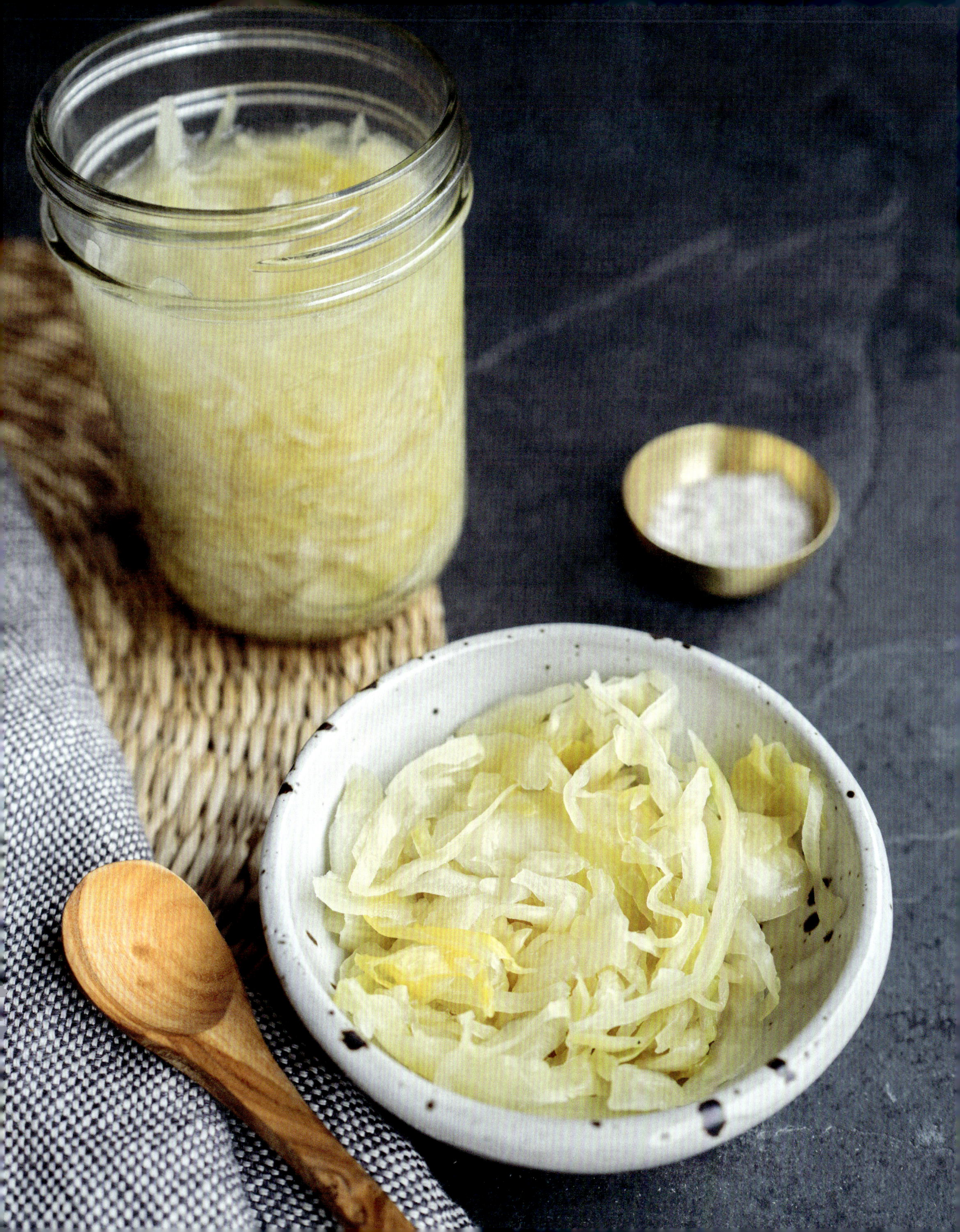

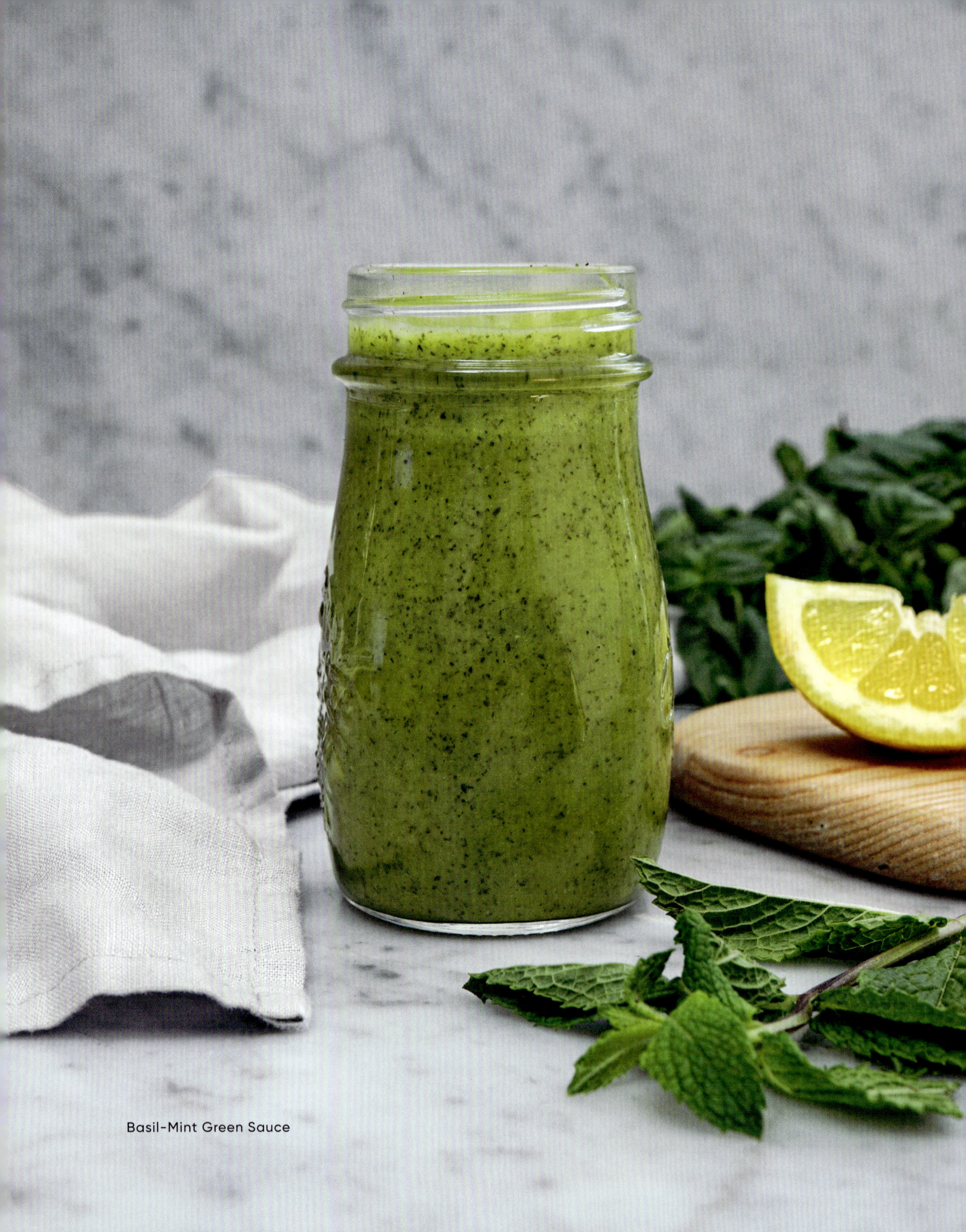
Basil-Mint Green Sauce

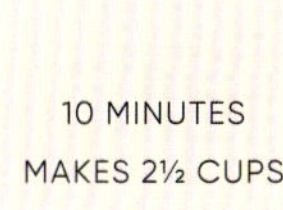

10 MINUTES
MAKES 2½ CUPS

Tangy Green Sauce

1¾ cups plain unsweetened coconut yogurt (check ingredients)

½ cup olive oil

½ cup water, plus more if needed

3 tablespoons lemon juice (about 1 lemon)

1 bunch cilantro, bottom stems removed

1 teaspoon sea salt

1. Place all the ingredients in a food processor or blender and process until just combined. If the mixture is too thick, add an additional tablespoon of water.

2. Use the sauce to drizzle over meats or vegetables, or as a salad dressing. If not using immediately, transfer to a storage container and keep in the refrigerator for up to 3 days.

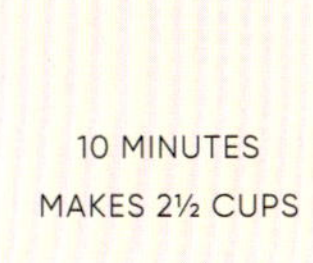

10 MINUTES
MAKES 2½ CUPS

Basil-Mint Green Sauce

2 medium avocados

¾ cup olive oil

¾ cup water, plus more if needed

3 tablespoons lemon juice (about 1 lemon)

¼ cup packed fresh mint leaves

½ cup packed fresh basil leaves

1 garlic clove

1 teaspoon sea salt

1. Cut the avocados in half and scoop out the flesh; you should have about 1½ cups.

2. Place the avocado flesh in a food processor or blender, add the rest of the ingredients, and process until just combined. If the mixture is too thick, add an additional tablespoon of water.

3. Use the sauce to drizzle over meats or vegetables, or as a salad dressing. If not using immediately, transfer to a storage container and keep in the refrigerator for up to 3 days.

40 MINUTES

MAKES ABOUT 2 CUPS

Chicken Liver Pâté with Apple and Thyme

4 slices thick-cut uncured bacon (check ingredients)

1 onion, chopped

4 garlic cloves, minced

1 pound chicken liver, sliced

1 green apple, cored and diced

2 tablespoons fresh thyme leaves, minced

¼ cup olive oil

½ teaspoon sea salt

Carrot, cucumber, or apple slices and additional fresh thyme leaves, for serving

1. Cook the bacon slices in a large skillet over medium-low heat, flipping as needed, until they are crisp, about 10 minutes. Transfer to a paper towel–lined plate to cool, keeping the fat in the pan.

2. Add the onion to the same pan over medium heat and cook for 5 minutes. Add the garlic and cook for a minute more, or until fragrant. Clear a space in the center of the skillet by moving the onion and garlic to the outside of the pan, then add the liver slices to the center one by one, making sure they lie flat, and then arrange the apple pieces around the outsides of the pan. Sprinkle with the thyme. Cook for 2 to 5 minutes per side, until the liver is no longer pink in the center when sliced open. Set aside to cool for a few minutes.

3. Transfer the mixture to a high-powered blender or food processor. Add the oil and salt and blend until a thick paste forms. Put the pâté into a medium bowl. Chop the bacon and fold it in.

4. If you are going to serve this immediately, transfer some into a small serving bowl, garnish with thyme leaves, and serve the vegetable and/or apple slices alongside. If you are making it for later, transfer to a storage container and refrigerate for up to 1 week. It also freezes well for up to three months.

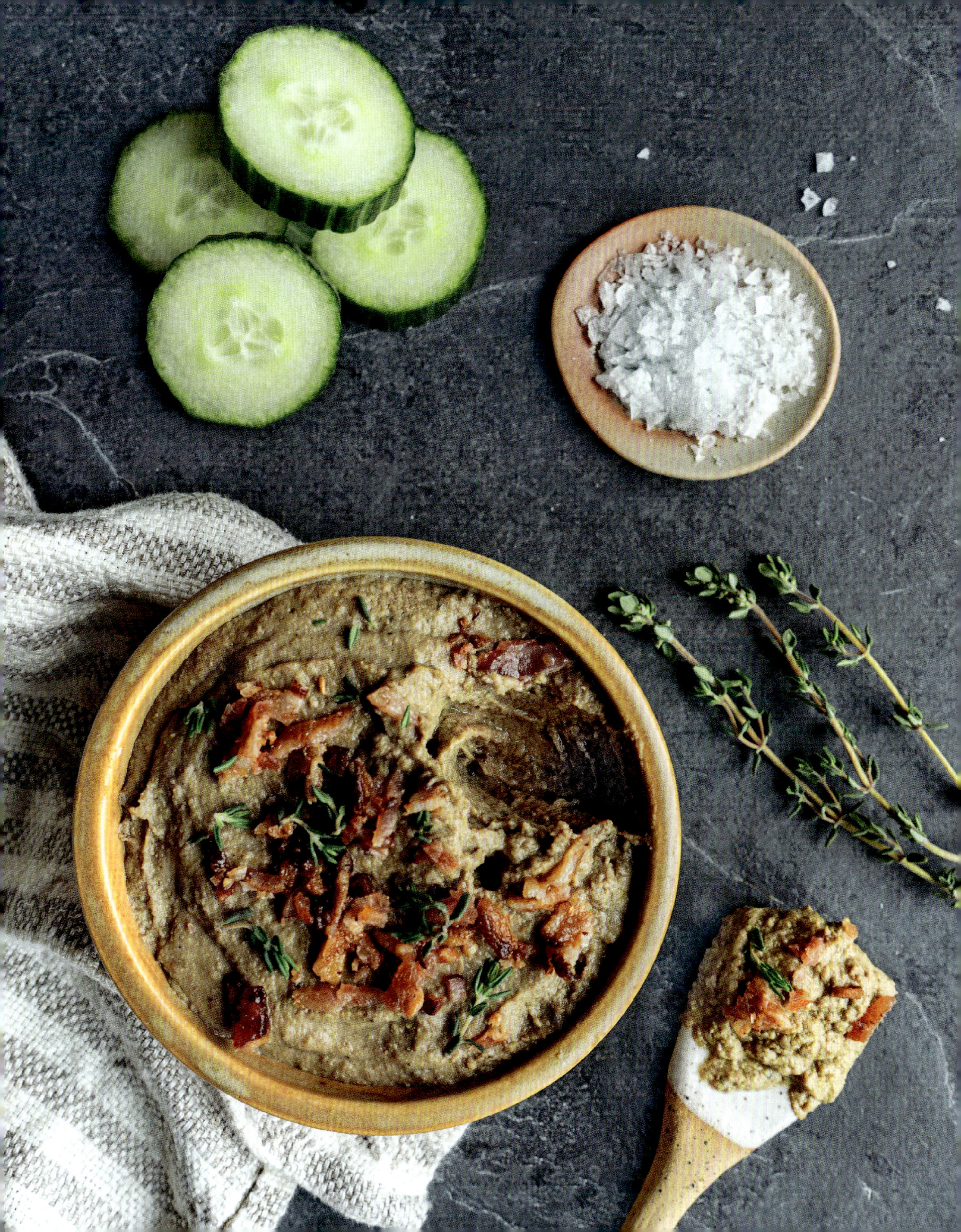

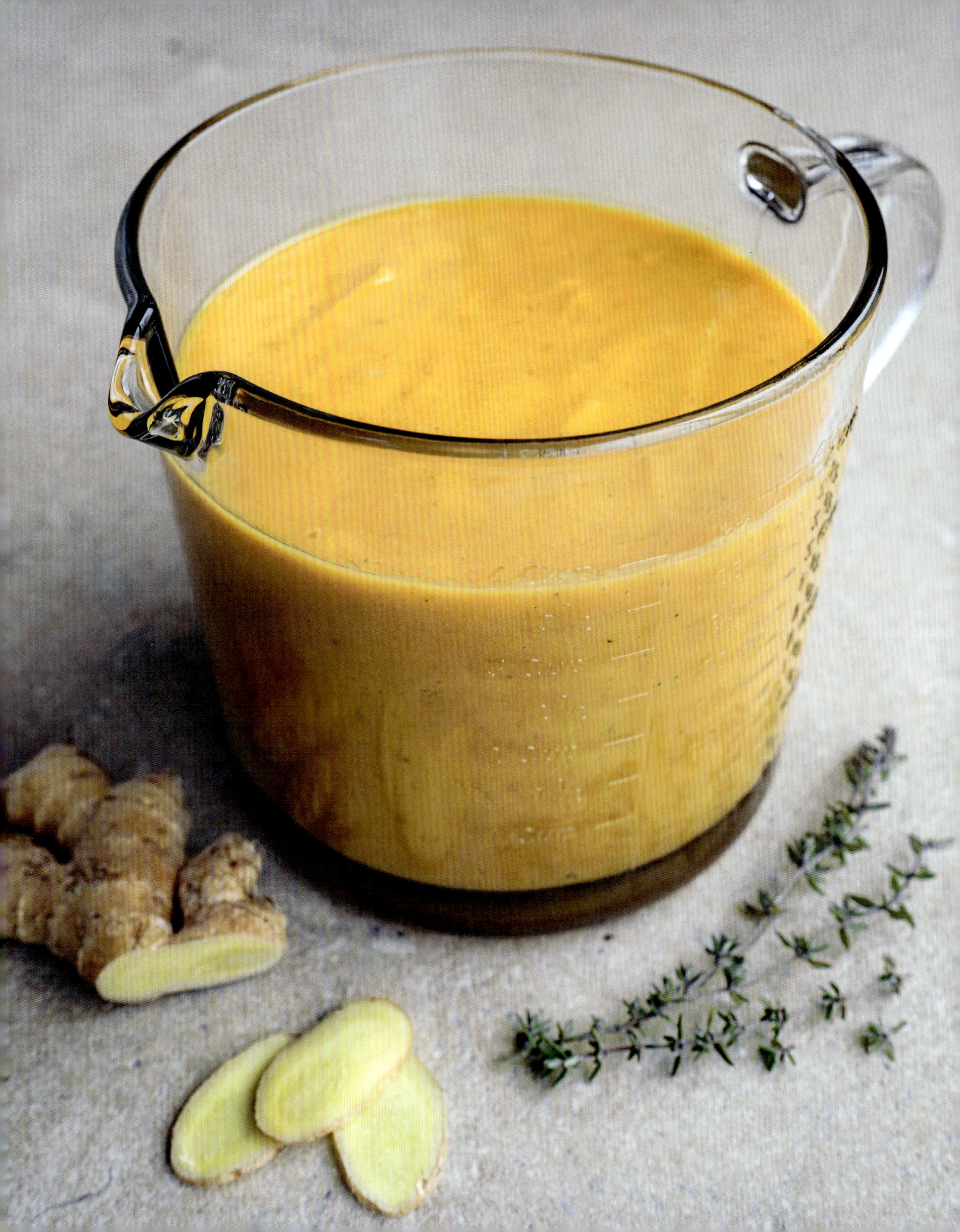

1 HOUR
15 MINUTES

MAKES
2 QUARTS

Earthy Roasted Roots Soup Base

2 large parsnips, chopped (about 4 cups)

3 tablespoons avocado or olive oil, divided

1 large sweet potato, peeled and chopped (about 4 cups)

1 onion, chopped

4 garlic cloves, minced

1 (1-inch) piece fresh ginger, minced (about 1 tablespoon)

2 cups water

2 tablespoons fresh thyme leaves, minced

1 teaspoon sea salt

½ teaspoon ground turmeric

⅛ teaspoon ground cinnamon

1 tablespoon apple cider vinegar

6 cups bone broth, homemade (page 119) or store-bought

Olive oil and thyme leaves, for serving (optional)

1. Preheat the oven to 425°F.

2. Place the parsnips in a large bowl and coat with 1 tablespoon of the oil. Transfer to a large rimmed baking sheet, place in the oven, and roast for 20 minutes.

3. Meanwhile, add the sweet potatoes to the bowl used for the parsnips and coat with another 1 tablespoon of the oil. When the parsnips have been in the oven for 20 minutes, remove from the oven, add the sweet potatoes to the sheet, and toss to combine. Place back in the oven and roast for 20 to 25 minutes, until the vegetables are fork-tender.

4. Meanwhile, heat the remaining 1 tablespoon oil in a soup pot over medium heat. When the pan is hot, add the onion and cook, stirring, until lightly browned, about 7 minutes. Add the garlic and ginger and cook for another 30 seconds, or until fragrant. Take off the heat and add the water to cool the mixture. Transfer to a blender along with the thyme, salt, turmeric, cinnamon, and vinegar and blend on high speed until fully combined. Pour the mixture back into the soup pot and set aside while the vegetables finish cooking.

5. When the vegetables are finished, blend them in two batches with the bone broth, then add the blended mixture to the pot with the onion mixture. Stir to combine. Drizzle in oil and top with thyme leaves, if desired.

6. Use as a handy base for adding shredded meat, like leftover chicken or beef, tender greens, and/or fermented vegetables for a quick meal or snack. It keeps in the refrigerator for up to 1 week; it also freezes well.

40 MINUTES
MAKES 4 CUPS

Golden Curry Sauce

2 tablespoons coconut or avocado oil

1 onion, roughly chopped

1 (2-inch) piece fresh ginger, minced (about 2 tablespoons)

3 garlic cloves, minced

1 cup bone broth, homemade (page 119) or store-bought

1 light-fleshed sweet potato, peeled and cut into 1-inch pieces (about 2 cups)

2 teaspoons tamarind paste

1 tablespoon ground turmeric

½ teaspoon ground ginger

¼ teaspoon ground cinnamon

1½ teaspoons sea salt

1 (14-ounce) can coconut milk (check ingredients)

1½ tablespoons lemon juice (about ½ lemon)

1. Heat the oil in a medium saucepan over medium heat. When the pan is hot, add the onion and cook, stirring, for 5 minutes, or until lightly browned and translucent. Add the minced ginger and garlic and cook, stirring, for another minute, or until fragrant.

2. Add the bone broth, sweet potato, tamarind paste, turmeric, ground ginger, cinnamon, and salt to the pot and mix. Bring to a boil, then cover and reduce the heat to maintain a simmer. Cook for 10 to 12 minutes, or until the sweet potatoes are soft. Add the coconut milk and lemon juice and let the mixture cool for 5 minutes.

3. When cool enough, carefully pour the mixture into a blender and secure the lid tightly. Place a kitchen towel on the lid to protect your hand, then blend for 30 seconds on high speed, or until fully combined and smooth.

4. Use the sauce to drizzle over meats or vegetables, or for reimagining leftovers. If not using immediately, transfer to a storage container and keep in the refrigerator for up to 1 week; it also freezes well.

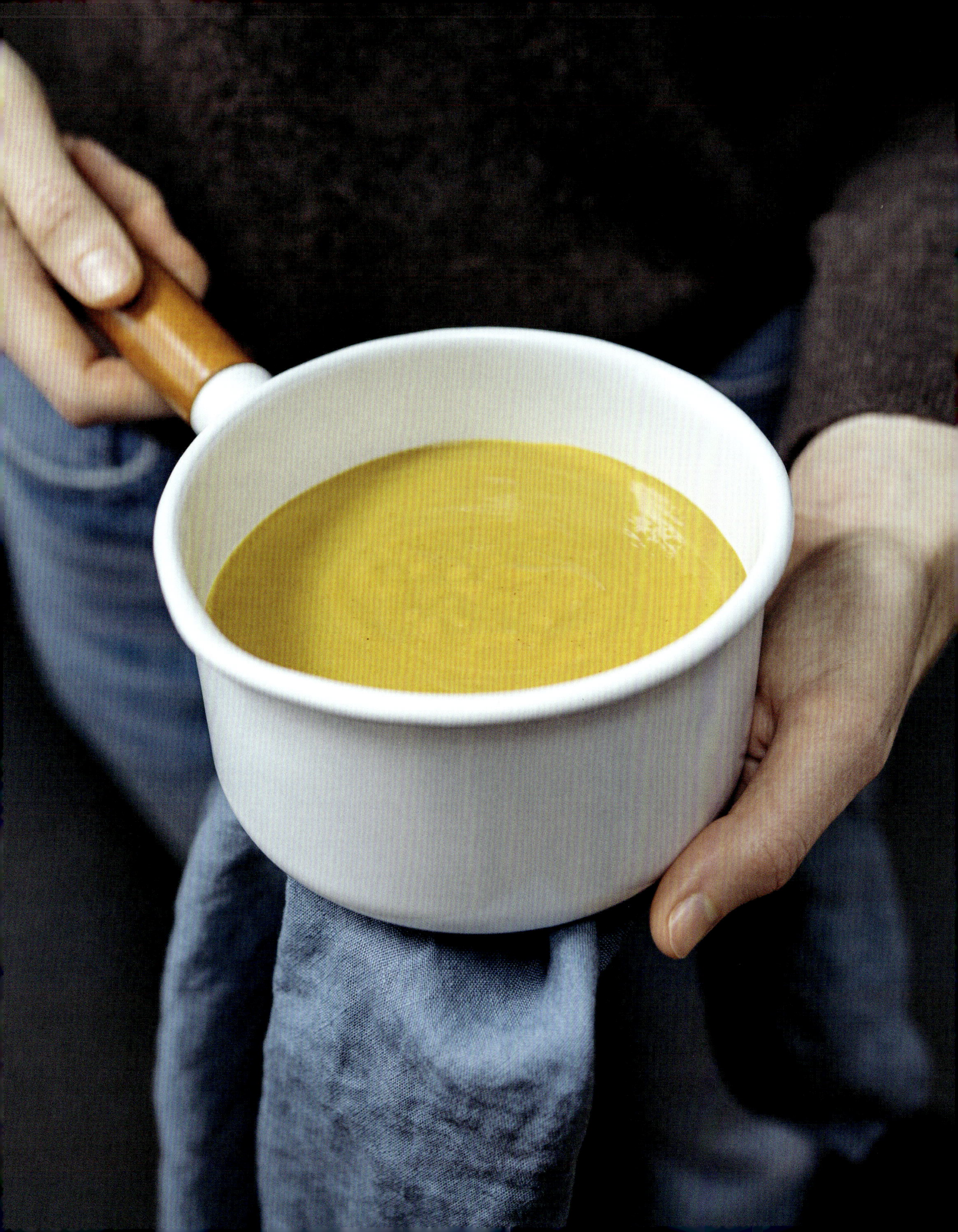

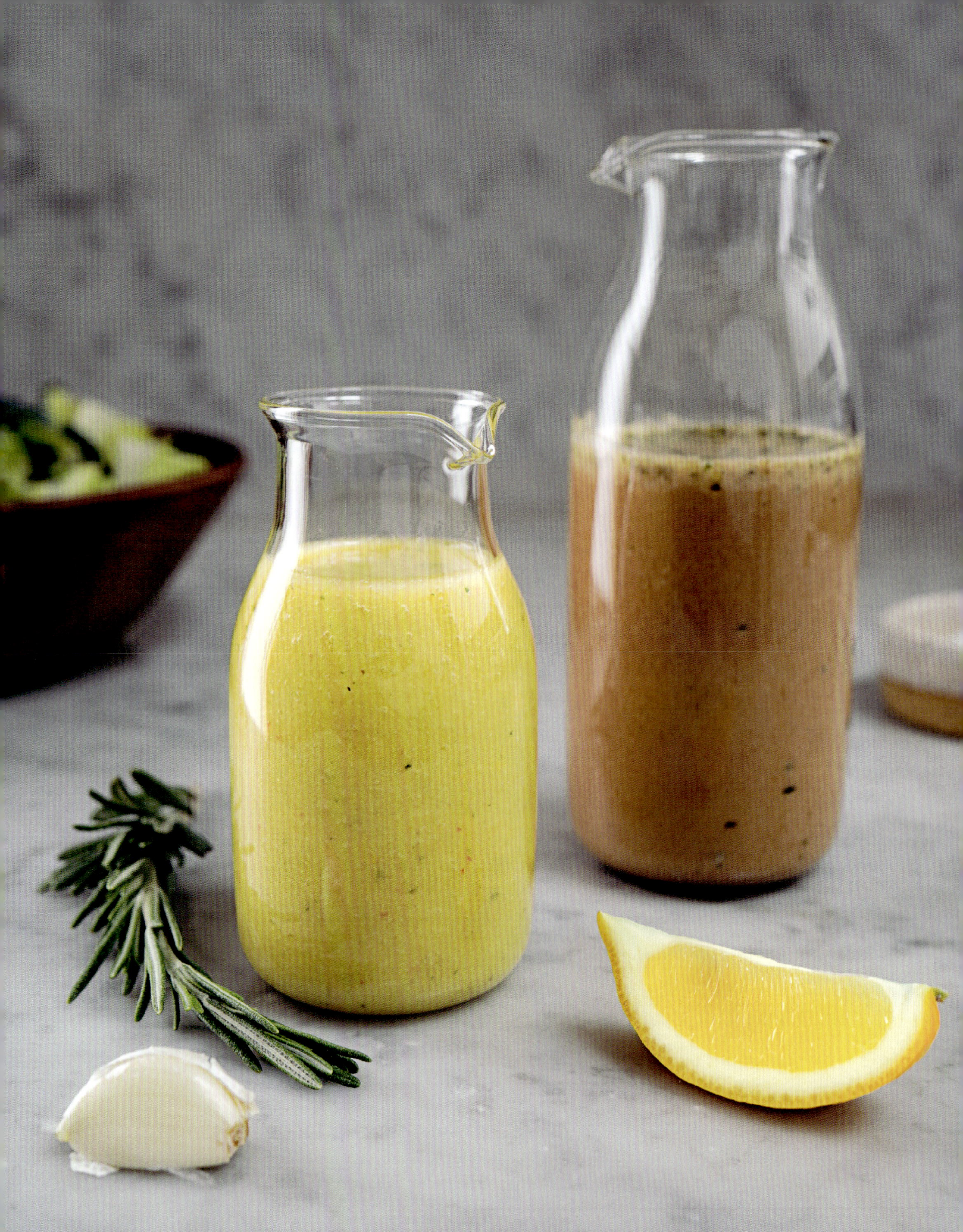

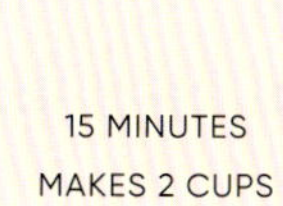

Meyer Lemon Dressing

1 cup olive oil

½ teaspoon Meyer lemon zest

½ cup fresh Meyer lemon juice (2 to 3 lemons)

1 teaspoon fresh thyme leaves

½ teaspoon minced garlic

½ teaspoon honey

½ teaspoon sea salt

SOURCING NOTE: *If you have trouble finding Meyer lemons, you can substitute half orange juice and half lemon juice for the Meyer lemon in this recipe.*

1. Place the oil, lemon zest and juice, the thyme, garlic, honey, and salt in a blender and blend until smooth. (Alternatively, you can use a bowl and whisk. If doing so, combine all the ingredients except the oil and whisk to combine, then slowly drizzle in the oil, whisking constantly to emulsify the dressing.)

2. Serve or transfer to a storage container. The dressing will keep for up to 1 week in the refrigerator.

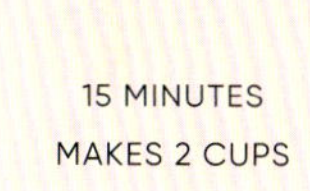

Maple Wine Vinaigrette

1 cup olive oil

½ cup red wine vinegar

1 tablespoon maple syrup

1 teaspoon minced fresh rosemary

½ teaspoon sea salt

1. Place the oil, vinegar, maple syrup, rosemary, and salt in a blender and blend until smooth. (Alternatively, you can use a bowl and whisk. If doing so, combine all the ingredients except the oil and whisk to combine, then slowly drizzle in the oil, whisking constantly to emulsify the dressing.)

2. Serve or transfer to a storage container. The vinaigrette will keep for up to 1 week in the refrigerator.

1 HOUR

MAKES 3 CUPS

Cranberry BBQ Sauce

2 tablespoons avocado oil

1 onion, chopped

6 garlic cloves, minced

3 cups cranberries, fresh or frozen (about 10 ounces)

¼ cup apple cider vinegar

¼ cup honey

½ cup pumpkin puree

2 teaspoons molasses

1 teaspoon smoked sea salt

½ cup water, plus more if needed

VARIATION: *You can substitute fresh or frozen cherries for the cranberries in this recipe—just cut the honey by half, as cherries are naturally sweeter.*

1. Heat the oil in a medium saucepan over medium heat. When the pan is hot, add the onion and cook, stirring, for 5 minutes. Add two-thirds of the garlic and cook for another minute, or until fragrant, reserving the remaining garlic for adding raw at the end of the recipe.

2. Add the cranberries, vinegar, honey, pumpkin, molasses, and salt. Cover and simmer for 10 minutes, or until the cranberries have popped and softened. Turn off the heat, add the water, and allow to cool for about 15 minutes.

3. Carefully transfer the mixture along with the remaining raw garlic to a blender and blend on high speed until smooth. If your mixture is too thick, add water 1 tablespoon at a time until the desired consistency is reached.

4. Serve right away or transfer to a storage container. The sauce will keep for up to 1 week in the refrigerator; it also freezes well.

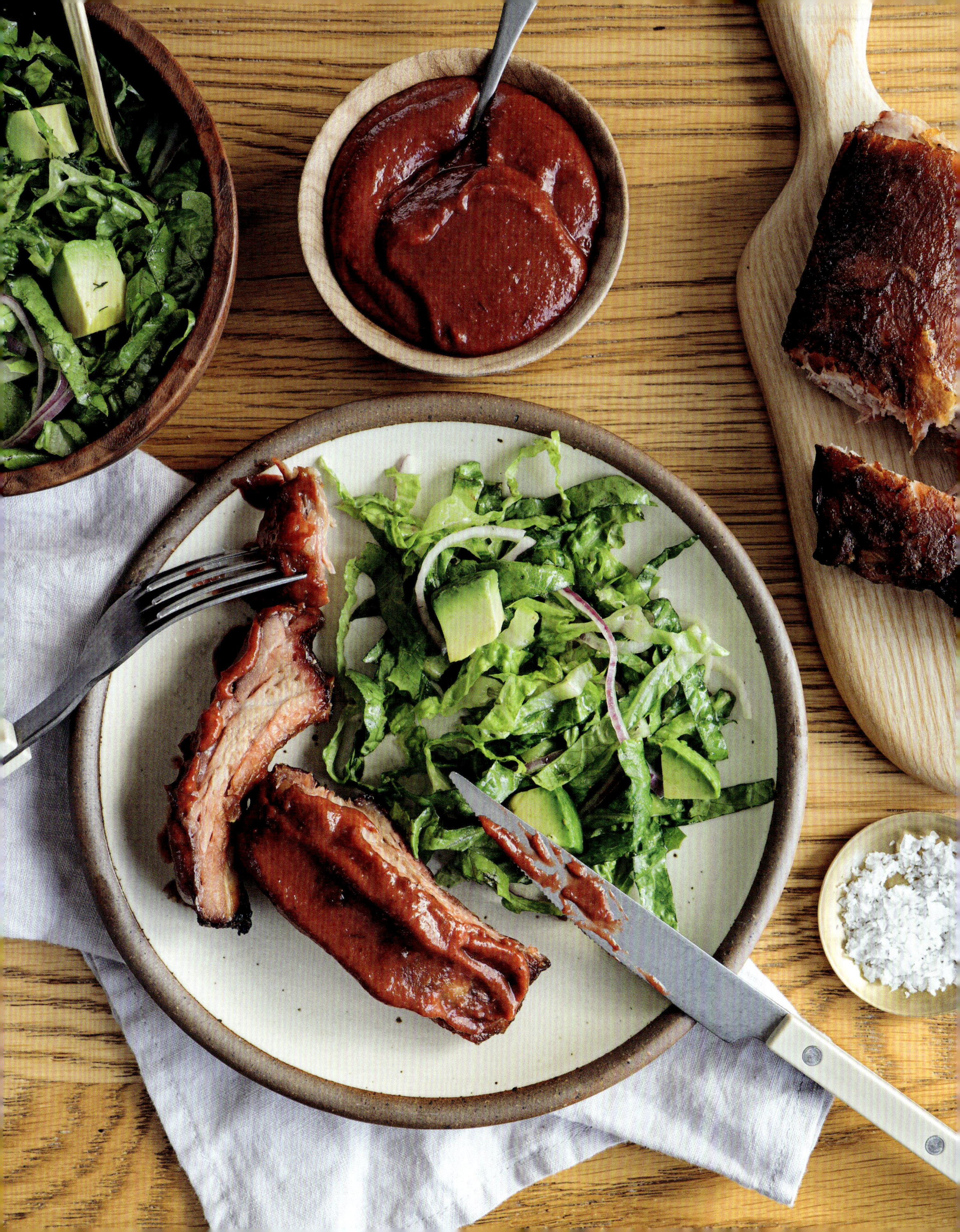

CHAPTER 8

Core Breakfasts

15 MINUTES

MAKES
2 SERVINGS

Salmon and Apple Breakfast Bowl

2 (6-ounce) cans boneless, skinless salmon

½ cup plain unsweetened coconut yogurt (check ingredients)

2 tablespoons olive oil

1 green apple, cored and diced

2 celery ribs, diced

2 green onions, white and green parts, ends removed and thinly sliced

1 tablespoon minced fresh dill

1½ tablespoons lemon juice (about ½ lemon)

½ teaspoon sea salt

1 avocado, sliced, for serving

1. Drain and discard the liquid from the canned salmon, then place the salmon in a medium bowl. Add the yogurt and oil and use a spoon to combine thoroughly.

2. Add the apple, celery, green onions, dill, lemon juice, and salt to the bowl and stir to combine. Serve topped with avocado slices. It will keep in the refrigerator for up to 3 days.

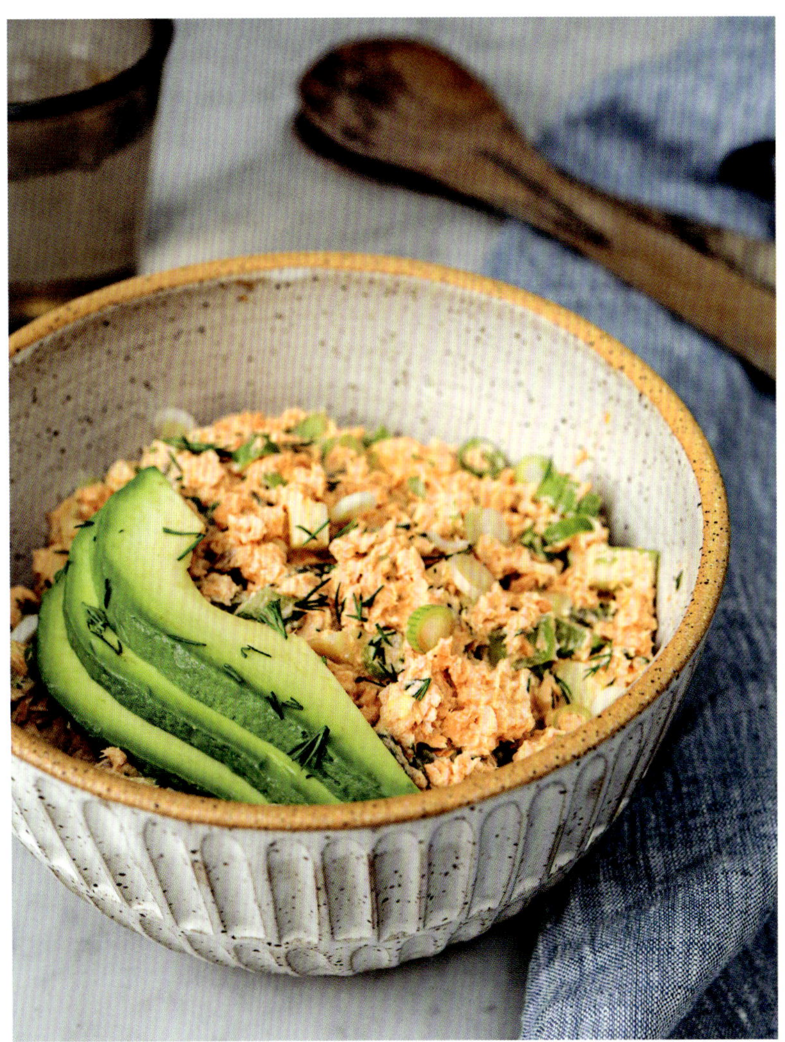

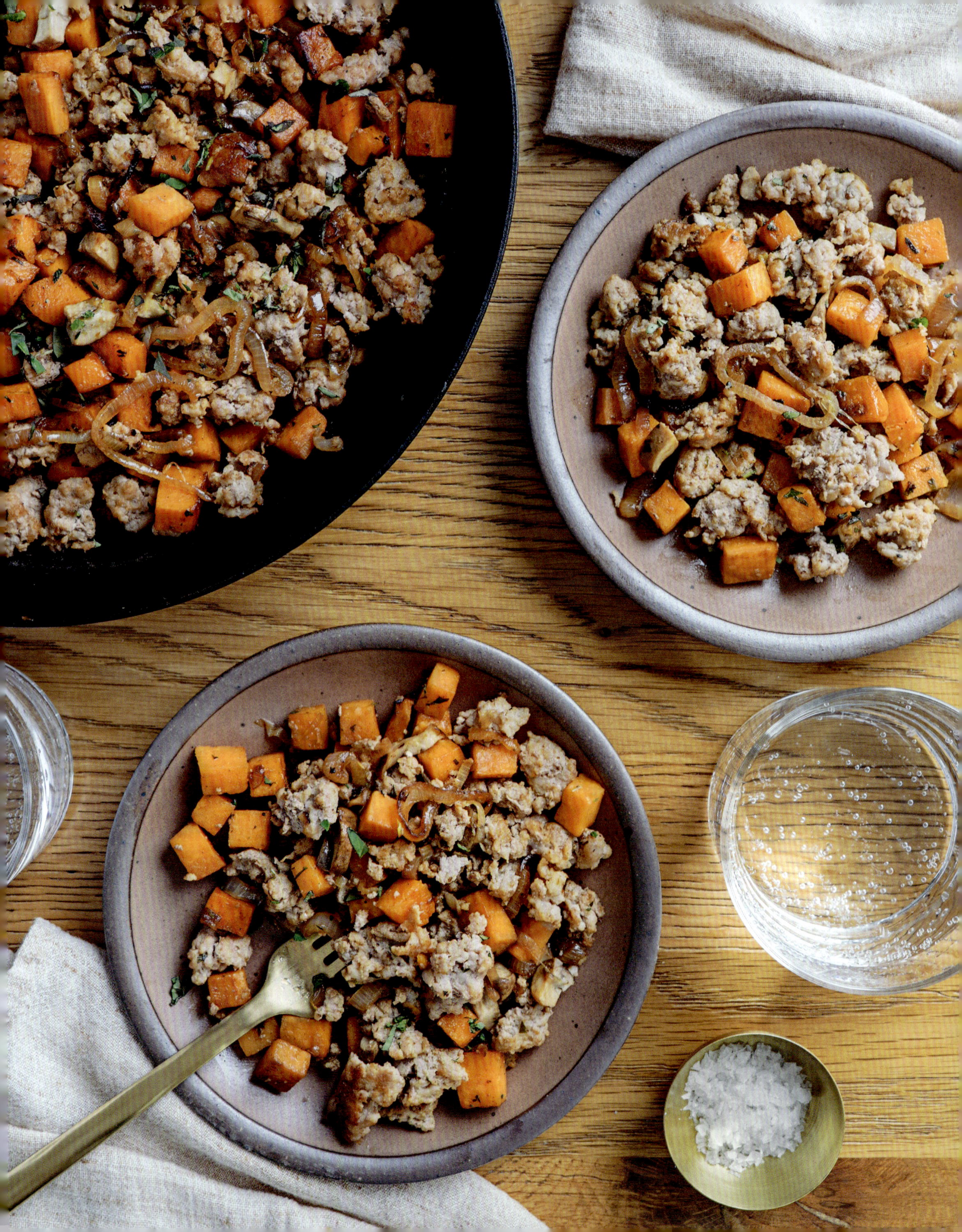

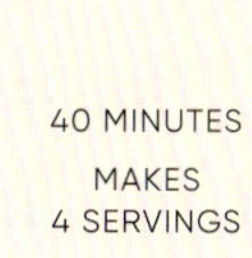

40 MINUTES

MAKES
4 SERVINGS

Pork Breakfast Skillet with Shallots and Marjoram

1 pound ground pork

3 shallots, thinly sliced

1 sweet potato, peeled and cut into ½-inch cubes (about 3 cups)

1 cup chopped mushrooms

2 tablespoons water

2 tablespoons apple cider vinegar

1 tablespoon coconut aminos

1 tablespoon fresh marjoram leaves, minced (or substitute oregano)

1 teaspoon sea salt

1. Place the pork in a large, cold skillet over medium heat. As it begins to cook, break up the meat into small bits. Cook, stirring and breaking it up occasionally, until most of the liquid is reabsorbed, the meat is lightly browned, and there is no pink left in any of the pieces, about 10 minutes. Transfer to a bowl and set aside, reserving any of the fat left over in the pan.

2. Turn the heat under the same skillet with the leftover fat back to medium. (If there is no reserved fat, add 2 tablespoons of avocado oil or another cooking oil.) Add the shallots and cook, stirring occasionally, until lightly browned, about 3 minutes. Add the sweet potatoes and cook, stirring, for 5 minutes.

3. Add the mushrooms, water, vinegar, coconut aminos, marjoram, and salt and stir to combine. Cook for 5 to 7 minutes, until the sweet potatoes are fork-tender.

4. Add the pork to the vegetable mixture, stir to combine and reheat the pork, and serve or portion into storage containers. It keeps in the refrigerator for up to 5 days.

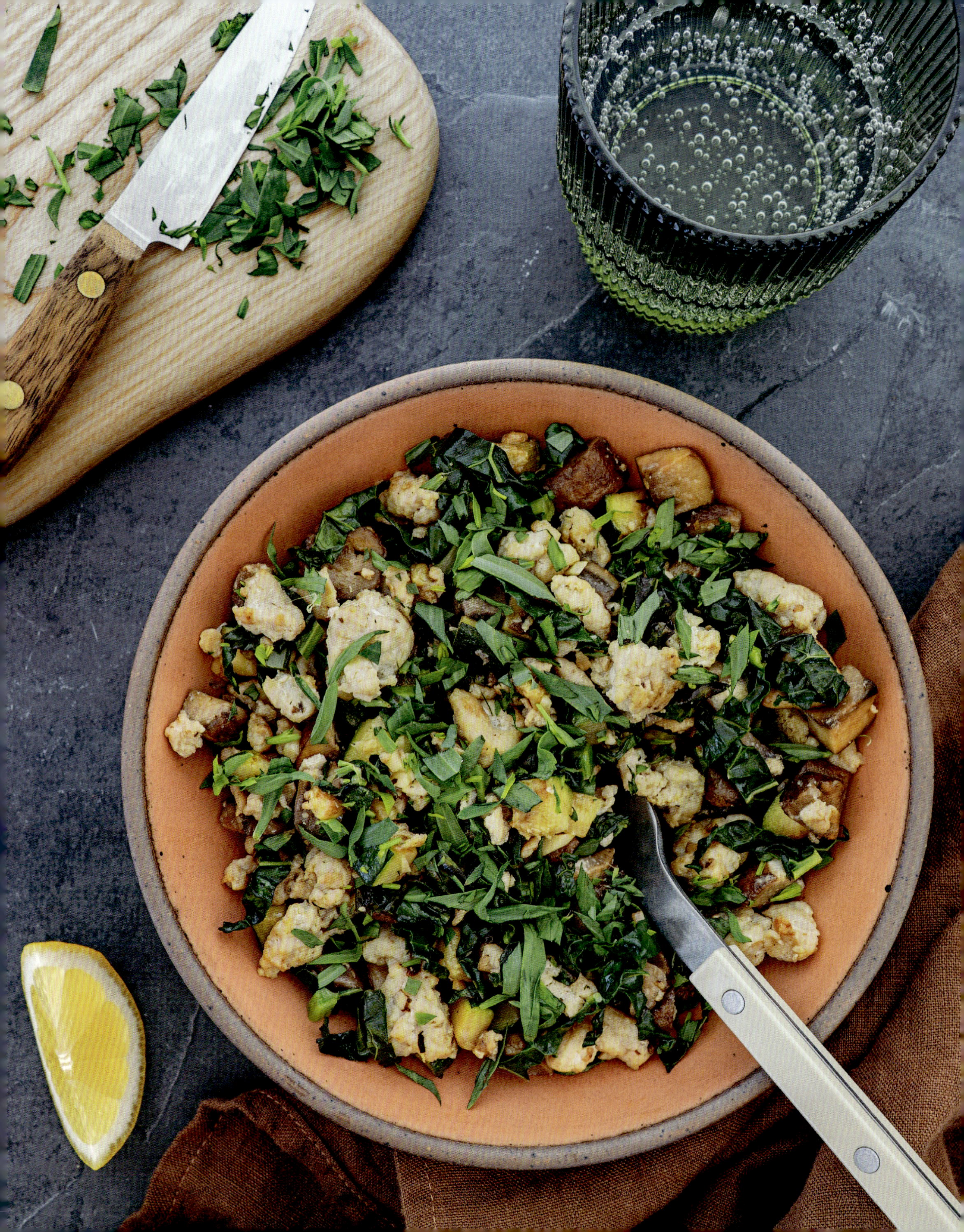

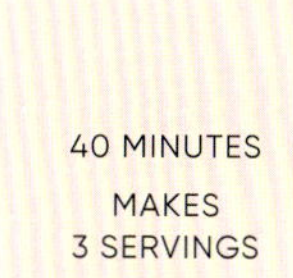

40 MINUTES

MAKES
3 SERVINGS

Lemon Tarragon Turkey Skillet

1 pound ground turkey

½ teaspoon baking soda

¼ cup olive oil, divided

1 large or 2 small zucchinis, diced

1 bunch Tuscan kale, stems removed and cut into ribbons

3 garlic cloves, minced

½ teaspoon sea salt

8 ounces mushrooms, diced

¼ cup tarragon leaves, minced

1½ tablespoons lemon juice (about ½ lemon)

1. Place the turkey in a medium bowl, sprinkle with the baking soda, and mix thoroughly. This treatment will ensure the meat browns evenly. Set aside for 15 minutes while you cook the vegetables.

2. Heat 2 tablespoons of the oil in a large skillet over medium-high heat. When the pan is hot, add the zucchini and cook, stirring, for 3 minutes. Add the kale and cook for 5 minutes, or until the kale cooks down and the zucchini is soft. Add the garlic and salt and cook for 1 minute more, or until the garlic is fragrant. Turn off the heat and transfer the vegetables to a bowl, then return the skillet to the stove.

3. Lower the heat to medium and add the remaining 2 tablespoons oil to the skillet. When the pan is hot again, add the mushrooms and cook for 2 minutes, or until they are beginning to brown. Break the turkey into pieces, then add to the pan to cook with the mushrooms. Cook for 7 to 8 minutes, continuing to break up and stir, until the turkey is cooked throughout. Turn off the heat.

4. Add the vegetables back to the skillet along with the tarragon and lemon juice and stir to combine. It keeps in the refrigerator for up to 5 days.

1 HOUR

MAKES
6 SERVINGS

Sausage and Veggie Bake

1 butternut squash, peeled and cut into 1-inch cubes

1 pound brussels sprouts, halved and thinly sliced

1 red onion, quartered and thinly sliced

2 tablespoons olive oil

2 teaspoons sea salt, divided

2 pounds ground beef, lamb, or pork

1 teaspoon ground ginger

1 teaspoon garlic powder

¼ teaspoon ground cinnamon

12 ounces sauerkraut or other fermented vegetable, homemade (page 120) or store-bought (check ingredients), for serving

1. Preheat the oven to 400°F.

2. Divide the squash, brussels sprouts, and onion evenly into two large rimmed baking dishes. Split the oil and ½ teaspoon of the salt between them and stir to combine thoroughly, then arrange evenly on the bottom of each dish. Set aside.

3. Put the meat, remaining 1½ teaspoons of salt, ginger, garlic powder, and cinnamon in a medium bowl. Use your hands to combine thoroughly, forming the mixture into about 20 large meatballs. Nest the meatballs evenly among the vegetables in the two baking dishes. Bake for 20 to 25 minutes, until the internal temperature of the meatballs reaches 165°F and the squash is fork-tender.

4. Serve each portion with a heaping portion of sauerkraut. The vegetables and meatballs will keep for up to 5 days in the refrigerator.

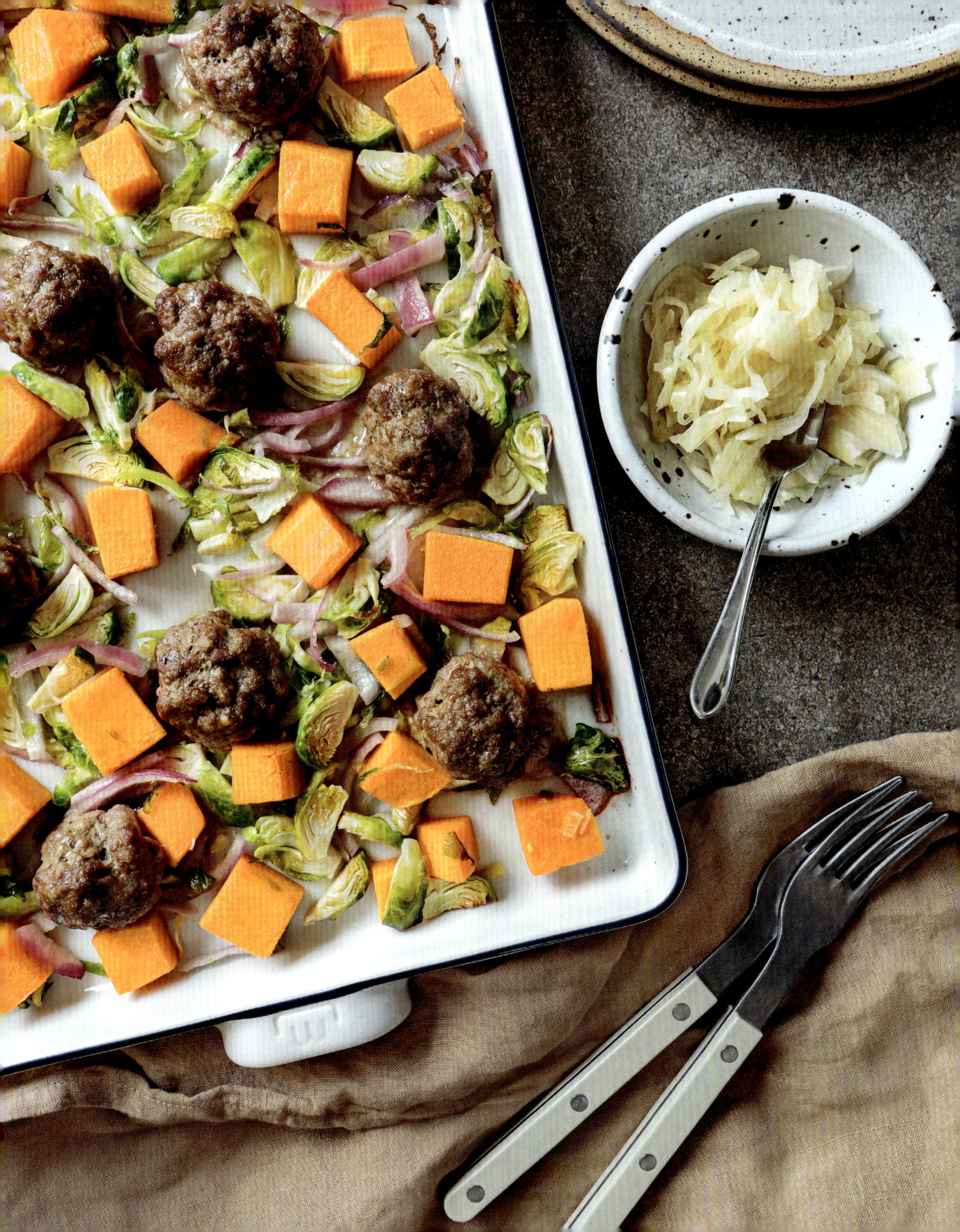

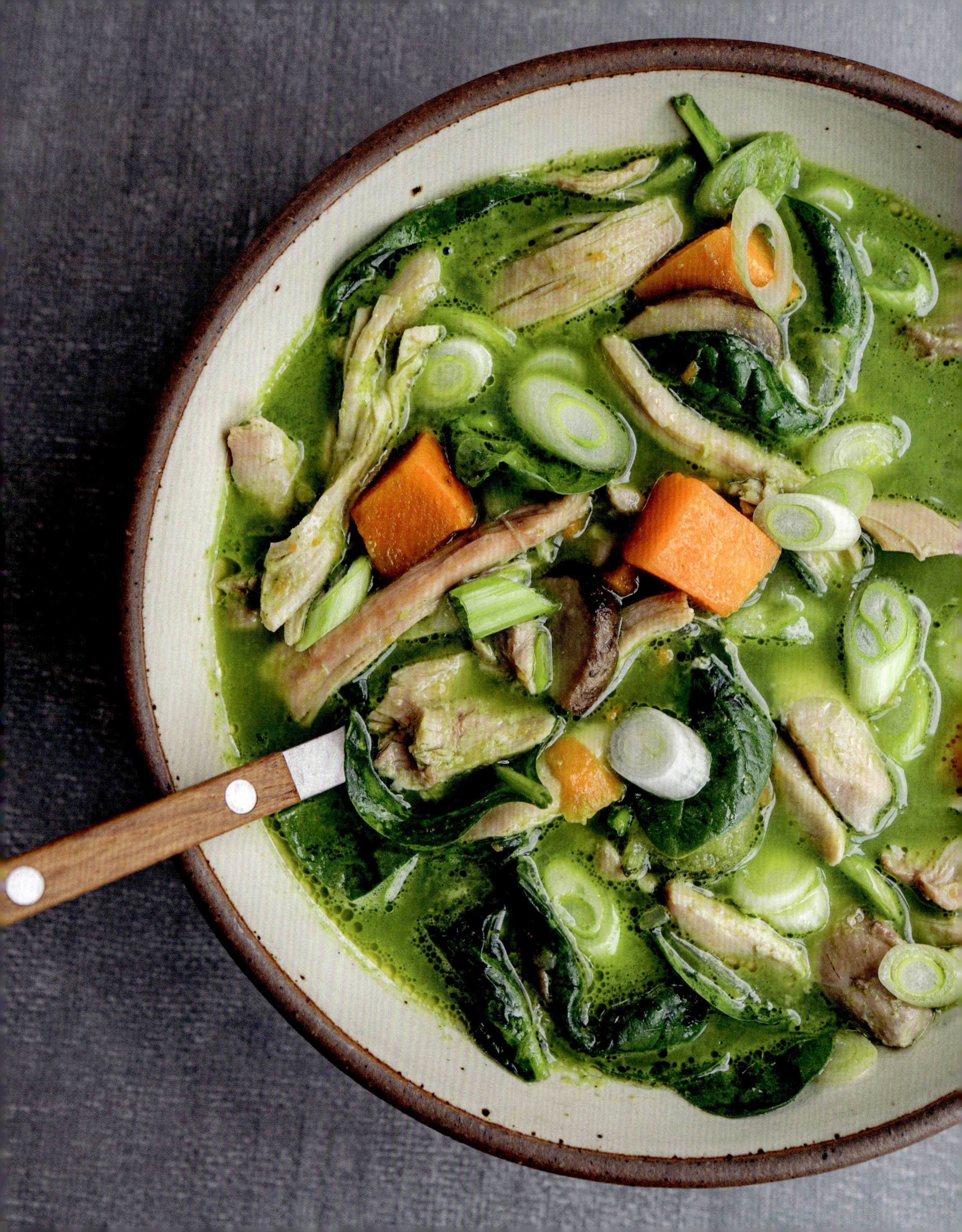

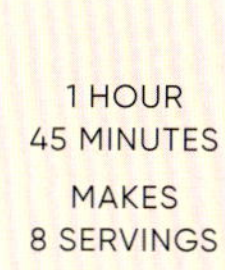

1 HOUR
45 MINUTES

MAKES
8 SERVINGS

Lemongrass Ginger Breakfast Soup

¼ cup olive oil

1 onion, chopped

12 ounces button mushrooms, thinly sliced (about 4 cups)

1 (3-inch) piece fresh ginger, minced (about ⅓ cup)

4 garlic cloves, minced

3 lemongrass stalks, ends removed and left whole

2 quarts water

3 pounds bone-in, skin-on chicken thighs

1 tablespoon sea salt

1 bay leaf

1 tablespoon apple cider vinegar

2 large sweet potatoes, peeled and chopped into 1½-inch pieces (about 6 cups)

2 large zucchinis, chopped into 1½-inch pieces (about 2 cups)

5 ounces spinach, divided

1 bunch green onions, white and green parts, ends removed and thinly sliced

1 lemon, cut into wedges (optional)

1. Heat the oil in a large, heavy-bottomed soup pot over medium heat. When the pan is hot, add the onion and cook, stirring, for 3 minutes. Add the mushrooms and cook, stirring occasionally, for 3 minutes. Add the ginger, garlic, and lemongrass and cook until fragrant, about 1 minute.

2. Add the water, chicken, salt, bay leaf, and vinegar to the pot. Bring to a gentle boil, then lower the heat to a bare simmer. Cook, covered, until the meat is tender and falling off the bone, 45 minutes to 1 hour—a low simmer ensures your chicken will come out perfectly tender.

3. Use tongs to remove the chicken from the pot and set aside to cool. Remove the bay leaf and lemongrass stalks and discard. Ladle 2 cups of the cooking liquid into a bowl or heatproof receptacle and set aside to cool. Add the sweet potatoes to the soup and simmer for 5 minutes, then add the zucchini and simmer for another 10 minutes, or until all the vegetables are just tender. Stir in half of the spinach and turn off the heat.

4. Meanwhile, when the chicken has cooled enough to handle, use your hands to remove the meat off the bone, discarding the skin and saving the bones for future batches of bone broth (see page 119).

5. Add the cooled cooking liquid to a blender with the remaining half of the spinach. Add this blended liquid to the soup pot with the shredded chicken. Serve each bowl garnished with green onions and a squeeze of lemon, if using. It keeps for up to 1 week in the refrigerator; it also freezes well.

45 MINUTES

MAKES 6 SERVINGS

Nutrivore Breakfast Batch Cook

SWEET POTATOES

3 pounds sweet potatoes, peeled and cut into 1-inch pieces

2 tablespoons avocado or olive oil

½ teaspoon sea salt

½ teaspoon garlic powder

¼ teaspoon ground cinnamon

PATTIES

1 pound ground beef

1 pound ground pork

1 teaspoon sea salt

1 teaspoon garlic powder

1 teaspoon onion powder

½ teaspoon ground ginger

1 tablespoon fresh herb leaves (oregano, rosemary, or thyme), minced

GREENS

2 tablespoons olive or avocado oil, divided

2 or 3 bunches kale, stemmed and cut into thin ribbons

½ teaspoon sea salt

1½ cups sauerkraut or other fermented vegetable, homemade (page 120) or store-bought (check ingredients)

3 ripe avocados, pitted and cubed

1. Arrange oven racks to accommodate three layers and preheat to 425°F.

2. Divide the sweet potatoes evenly between two large roasting dishes (giving them space to be spread out without touching enables them to crisp nicely; if you only have one large dish, it will do). Divide the 2 tablespoons of oil, ½ teaspoon of salt, ½ teaspoon of garlic powder, and ¼ teaspoon of cinnamon between them, and stir to combine thoroughly, then arrange evenly on the bottom of each dish. Set aside.

3. In a medium bowl, combine the meat, salt, the garlic powder, onion powder, ground ginger, and fresh herbs. Use your hands to combine thoroughly and form into about 6 large patties that are about ½ inch thick, slightly thinner in the center (this will ensure they stay flat and cook evenly). Place on a large rimmed baking sheet. When the oven is hot, add both dishes of sweet potatoes and the patties.

4. Cook the patties for 14 minutes, or until a thermometer inserted into the center of one reads 155°F. At the same time, cook the sweet potatoes for 20 to 25 minutes, stirring once, until they are just tender when probed with a fork.

5. While the patties and vegetables are in the oven, make the greens. Heat 1 tablespoon of oil in a large skillet over medium heat. When the pan is hot, add half of the greens. Cook, stirring, for 3 to 4 minutes, until the greens cook down. Transfer to a bowl and repeat with the remaining batch of oil and greens. Sprinkle the cooked greens with the salt and set aside (don't salt until after cooking, otherwise they might go soggy).

6. Serve each patty with a portion of sweet potatoes and greens, a heaping spoonful of fermented vegetables, and half an avocado. The vegetables and patties will keep for up to 5 days in the refrigerator.

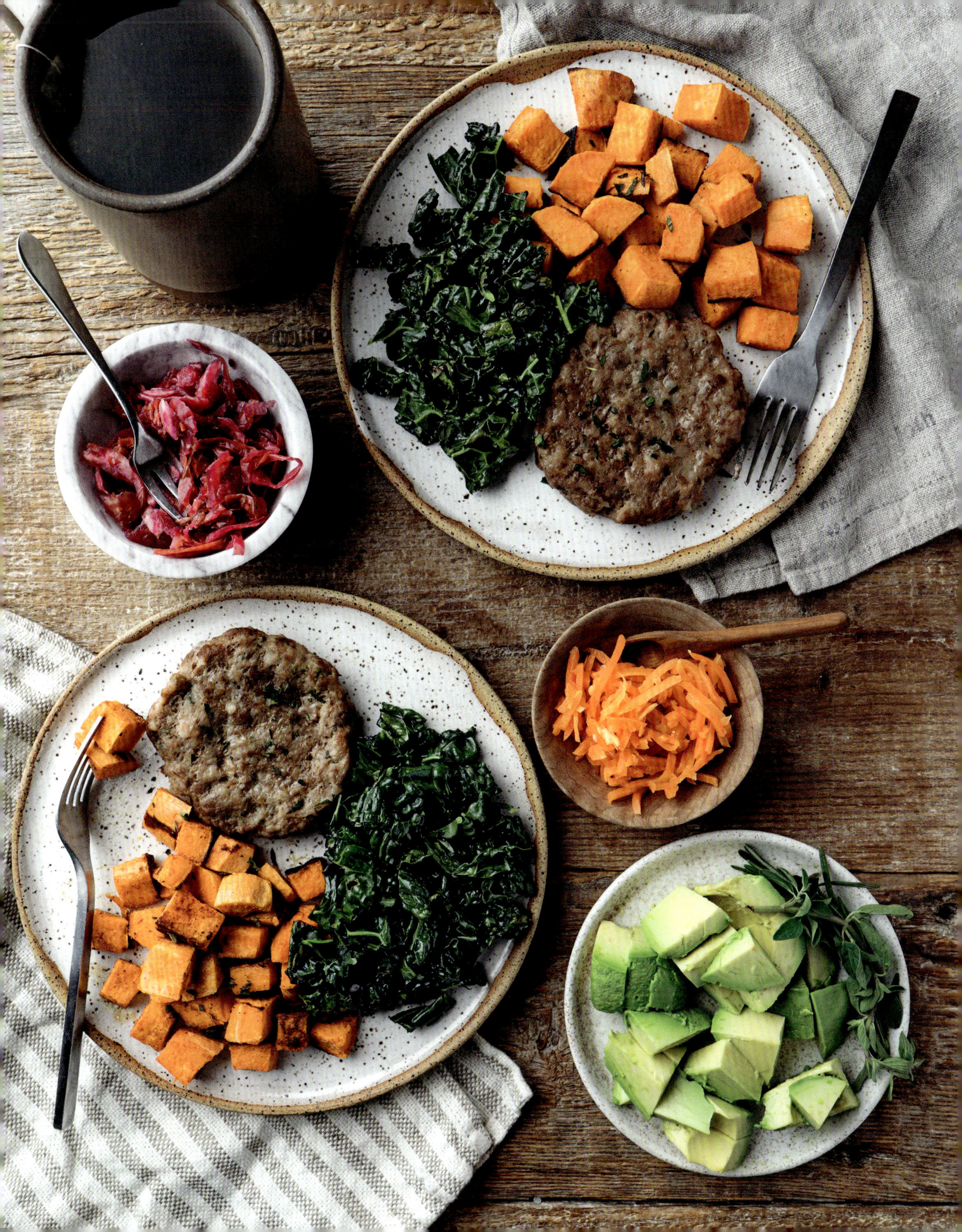

CHAPTER 9

Core Soups, Stews, and Salads

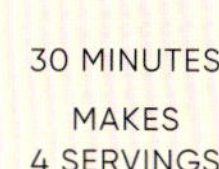

30 MINUTES

MAKES
4 SERVINGS

Superfood Sardine Salad

1½ pounds broccoli crowns, finely chopped

3 celery ribs, thinly sliced

4 radishes, halved and thinly sliced

2 cups microgreens

1 bunch cilantro, bottom stems removed, minced

½ cup thinly sliced red onion

1 green apple, cored and diced

12 ounces grapes, halved

1 cup plain unsweetened coconut yogurt (check ingredients)

¼ cup olive oil (or substitute avocado oil)

1½ tablespoons lemon juice (about ½ lemon)

¾ teaspoon sea salt

4 (4-ounce) cans sardines or mackerel packed in olive oil, drained (check ingredients)

PREP NOTE: *If batch-cooking this meal ahead, store the salad and dressing separately; toss fresh and serve with a can of fish.*

1. In a large bowl, combine the broccoli, celery, radishes, microgreens, cilantro, onion, apple, and grapes and stir to combine. Set aside.

2. In a medium bowl, combine the yogurt, oil, lemon juice, and salt and whisk until thoroughly combined. Add to the salad and toss until all the vegetables are completely coated. Set aside for 10 minutes to allow the flavors to combine before serving.

3. Serve each portion of salad with a can of sardines or mackerel. The dressed salad keeps for up to 2 days in the refrigerator.

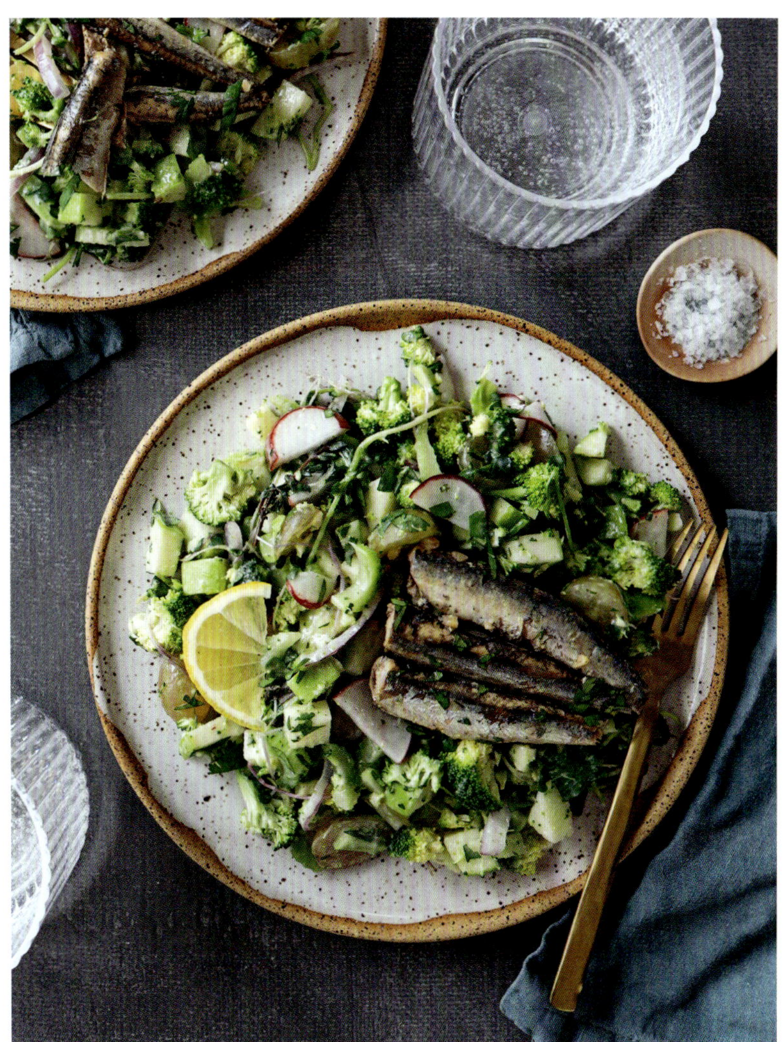

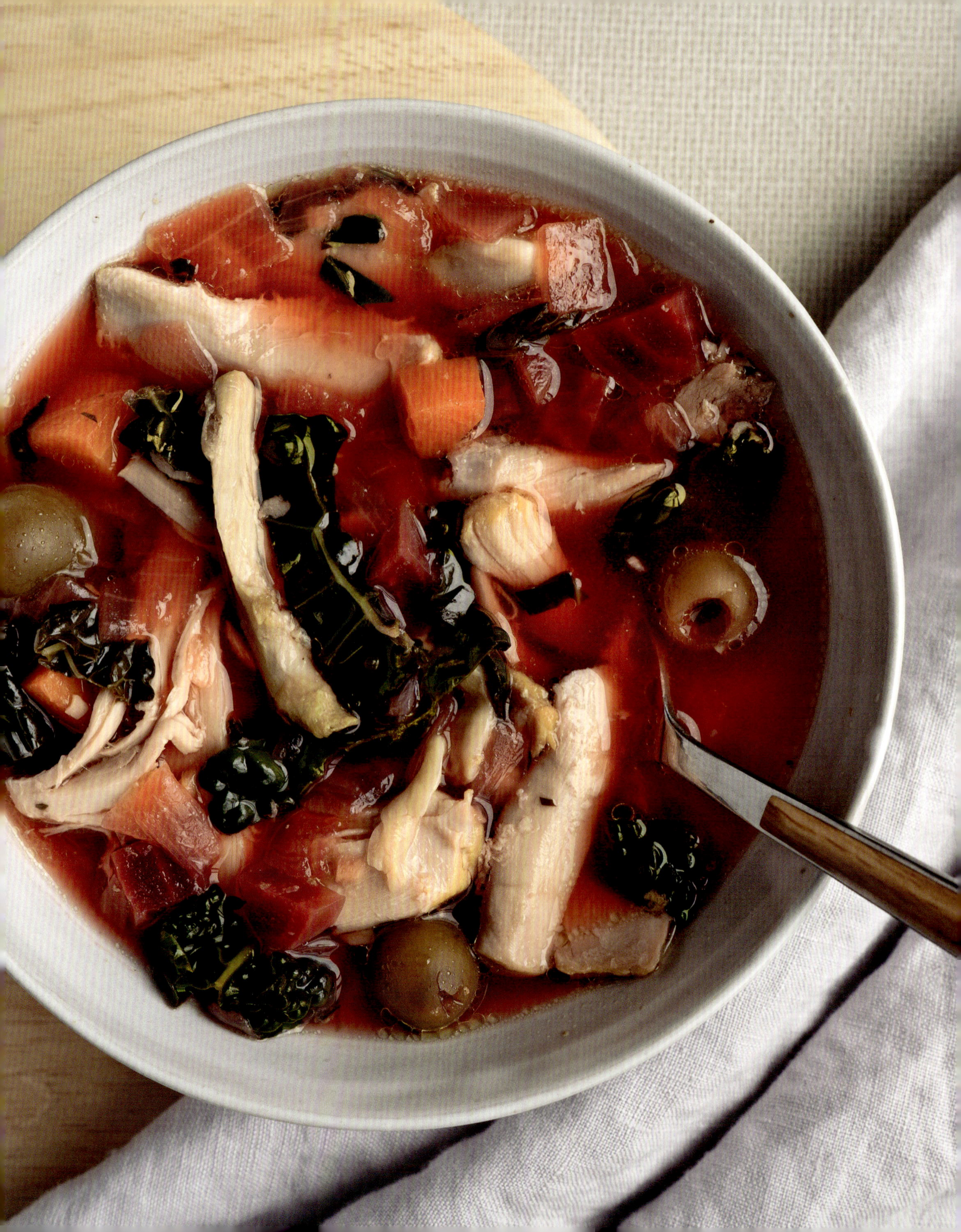

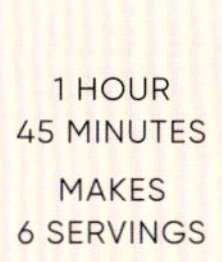

Rustic Chicken and Kale Stew

¼ cup olive oil

1 onion, chopped

4 garlic cloves, minced

2 quarts water

3 pounds bone-in, skin-on chicken thighs

3 carrots, chopped (about 2 cups)

1 small beet, diced (about 1 cup)

½ cup pitted olives (check ingredients)

1 tablespoon sea salt (reduce if using salt-cured olives)

1 bay leaf

1 teaspoon fresh thyme leaves, minced

1 teaspoon fresh oregano leaves, minced

1 bunch kale, stemmed and cut into ribbons

1½ tablespoons lemon juice (about ½ lemon)

1. Heat the oil in a large, heavy-bottomed soup pot over medium heat. When the pan is hot, add the onion and cook, stirring, for 5 minutes, or until starting to brown. Add the garlic and cook until fragrant, about 1 minute.

2. Add the water, chicken, carrots, beet, olives, salt, bay leaf, thyme, and oregano to the pot. Bring to a gentle boil, then cover tightly and lower the heat to maintain a bare simmer. Cook until the meat is tender and falling off the bone, 45 minutes to 1 hour—a low simmer ensures your chicken will come out perfectly tender.

3. Use tongs to remove the chicken from the pot and set aside to cool. Remove the bay leaf and discard. Add the kale and lemon juice to the soup and simmer for 5 minutes.

4. When the chicken has cooled enough to handle, use your hands to remove the meat off the bones and add it back to the soup, discarding the skin and saving the bones for future batches of bone broth (see page 119). It keeps for up to a week in the refrigerator; it also freezes well.

1 HOUR

MAKES
6 SERVINGS

Nourishing Core Chili

4 slices thick-cut uncured bacon (check ingredients)

1 pound ground beef

1 pound ground pork

1 onion, diced

4 celery ribs, diced

3 large carrots, diced (about 4 cups)

5 garlic cloves, minced

2 cups bone broth, homemade (page 119) or store-bought

2 cups water

1 beet, grated (or diced)

¼ cup fresh oregano leaves, minced

2 teaspoons onion powder

2 teaspoons garlic powder

1 teaspoon sea salt

1 (14-ounce) can pumpkin puree

2 tablespoons apple cider vinegar

1 teaspoon fish sauce

1. Place the bacon in a cold, heavy-bottomed soup pot. I like to cut the slices in half so that they more easily cover the bottom surface of the pot. Turn the heat to medium-low and cook, turning occasionally, until browned and slightly crisp, about 10 minutes. Transfer to a paper towel–lined plate to cool, leaving the rendered fat in the pot.

2. While the bacon is cooking, place the beef and pork in a large, cold skillet. Use a utensil to break the meat into smaller pieces, then turn the heat to medium. Cook, stirring and continuing to break up the pieces, until the meat is cooked and the liquid is reabsorbed, about 10 minutes. Set aside.

3. Turn the heat under the soup pot with the rendered fat to medium and, when hot, add the onion. Cook, stirring occasionally, for 3 minutes, or until starting to brown. Add the celery and carrots and cook for another 3 minutes. Add the garlic and cook for 1 minute, or until fragrant. Meanwhile, roughly chop the cooked bacon and set aside.

4. Add the broth, water, beet, oregano, onion powder, garlic powder, salt, and bacon to the pot and simmer uncovered for 20 minutes. Add the pumpkin and meat to the pot and simmer, covered, for 10 minutes. Add the vinegar and fish sauce, stir to combine, and serve. It keeps for up to 1 week in the refrigerator; it also freezes well.

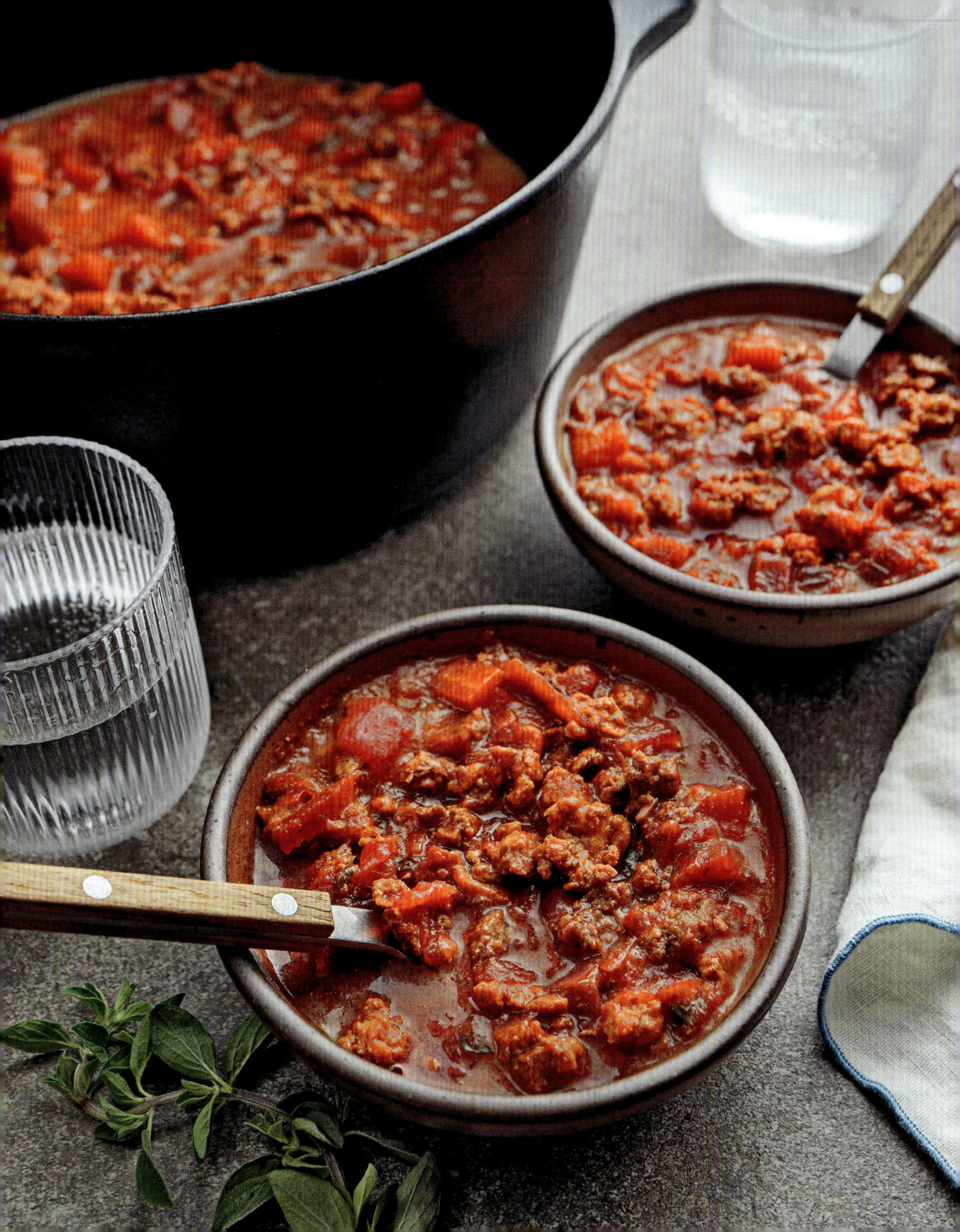

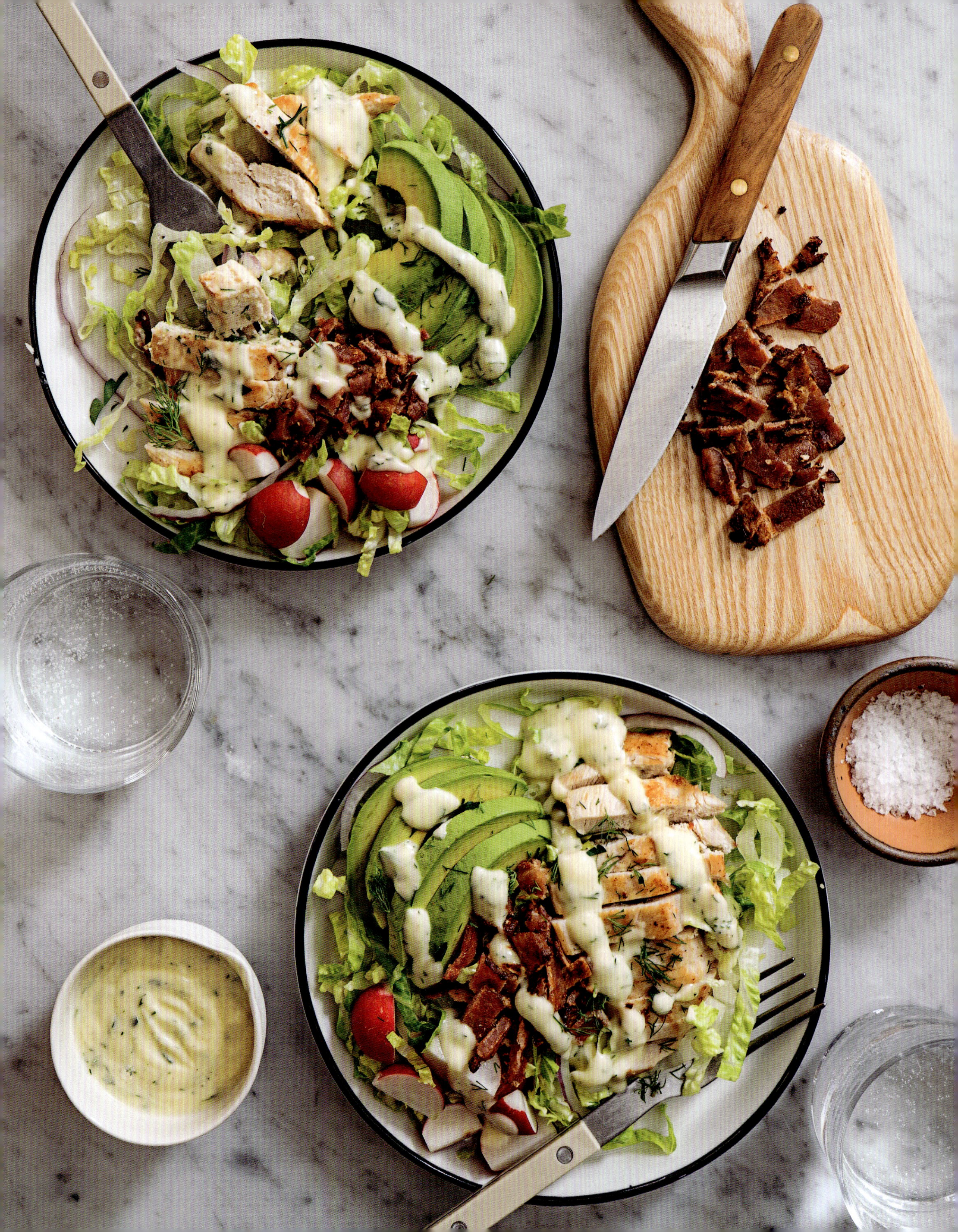

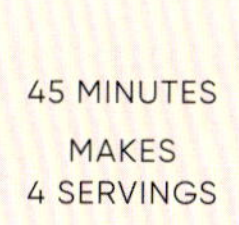

45 MINUTES

MAKES
4 SERVINGS

Bacon Chicken Ranch Salad

4 slices thick-cut uncured bacon (check ingredients)

2 large chicken breasts (about 1½ pounds), butterflied and lightly salted

½ cup bone broth, homemade (page 119) or store-bought

½ cup olive oil (or substitute avocado oil)

½ cup plain unsweetened coconut yogurt (check ingredients)

¼ cup water

1½ tablespoons lemon juice (about ½ lemon)

½ teaspoon sea salt

½ teaspoon garlic powder

½ teaspoon onion powder

1 teaspoon minced fresh dill

½ teaspoon minced fresh thyme

½ teaspoon minced fresh parsley

1 large head romaine lettuce, chopped

1 bunch radishes, trimmed and quartered

¼ cup thinly sliced red onion

2 avocados, pitted and thinly sliced

1. First, make the bacon. Place the slices in a large, cold skillet and turn the heat to medium-low. Cook, turning occasionally, until browned and slightly crisp, about 10 minutes. Transfer to a paper towel–lined plate to cool.

2. Use the same skillet for the chicken (if there are more than 2 tablespoons of bacon fat left over, transfer it to a container for another use). Heat the pan over medium heat, and when it is hot, add the chicken. Cook for 5 minutes, or until the bottom has started to brown. Flip, add the broth, cover, and cook for another 7 minutes, or until the chicken reaches an internal temperature of 165°F. (If your skillet won't fit both breasts, you'll need to do this in two batches using half of the broth and leftover bacon grease.) Rest the chicken while you make the salad.

3. To make the ranch dressing, combine the oil, yogurt, water, lemon juice, salt, garlic powder, and onion powder in a blender and blend on high speed for 30 seconds. Add the dill, thyme, and parsley and pulse to combine (don't overblend, or your dressing will be green). Set aside while you make the salad.

4. When the chicken is cool, slice it. Assemble each bowl with lettuce, radishes, onion, bacon, avocado, and chicken. Drizzle with the ranch dressing and serve. The chicken keeps for up to 5 days in the refrigerator.

PREP NOTE: *If batch-cooking this meal ahead, store the greens and dressing separately and toss fresh for each portion.*

35 MINUTES

MAKES
6 SERVINGS

Salmon and Mushroom Chowder with Tarragon and Dill

2 tablespoons coconut oil (or substitute olive oil)

6 shallots, halved and thinly sliced

3 celery ribs, thinly sliced

3 cups bone broth, homemade (page 119) or store-bought

1 cup water

1 teaspoon sea salt

2 large parsnips, cut into 1-inch pieces (about 4 cups)

12 ounces button mushrooms, halved and thinly sliced

1 (14-ounce) can coconut milk (check ingredients)

2 tablespoons minced fresh tarragon

2 tablespoons minced fresh dill

14 ounces salmon, skin removed and cut into 2-inch pieces

1½ tablespoons lemon juice (about ½ lemon)

NOTE: *If you need to reheat this stew, do so on low, stirring often, to avoid overcooking the salmon.*

1. Heat the oil in a soup pot over medium heat. When it has melted and the pan is hot, add the shallots and cook, stirring occasionally, for 3 minutes, or until starting to brown. Add the celery and cook for another 2 minutes.

2. Add the broth, water, salt, and parsnips to the pot and bring to a simmer. Cook, covered, for 8 minutes, then add the mushrooms and cook for another 2 minutes. The pot may seem low on liquid, but it will eventually release from the vegetables as they cook.

3. Add the coconut milk, tarragon, and dill and bring back to a simmer. Turn off the heat, add the salmon and lemon juice, and stir. Cover and leave for 1 to 2 minutes, with the heat off, to gently cook the salmon. Serve immediately. It keeps in the refrigerator for up to 3 days.

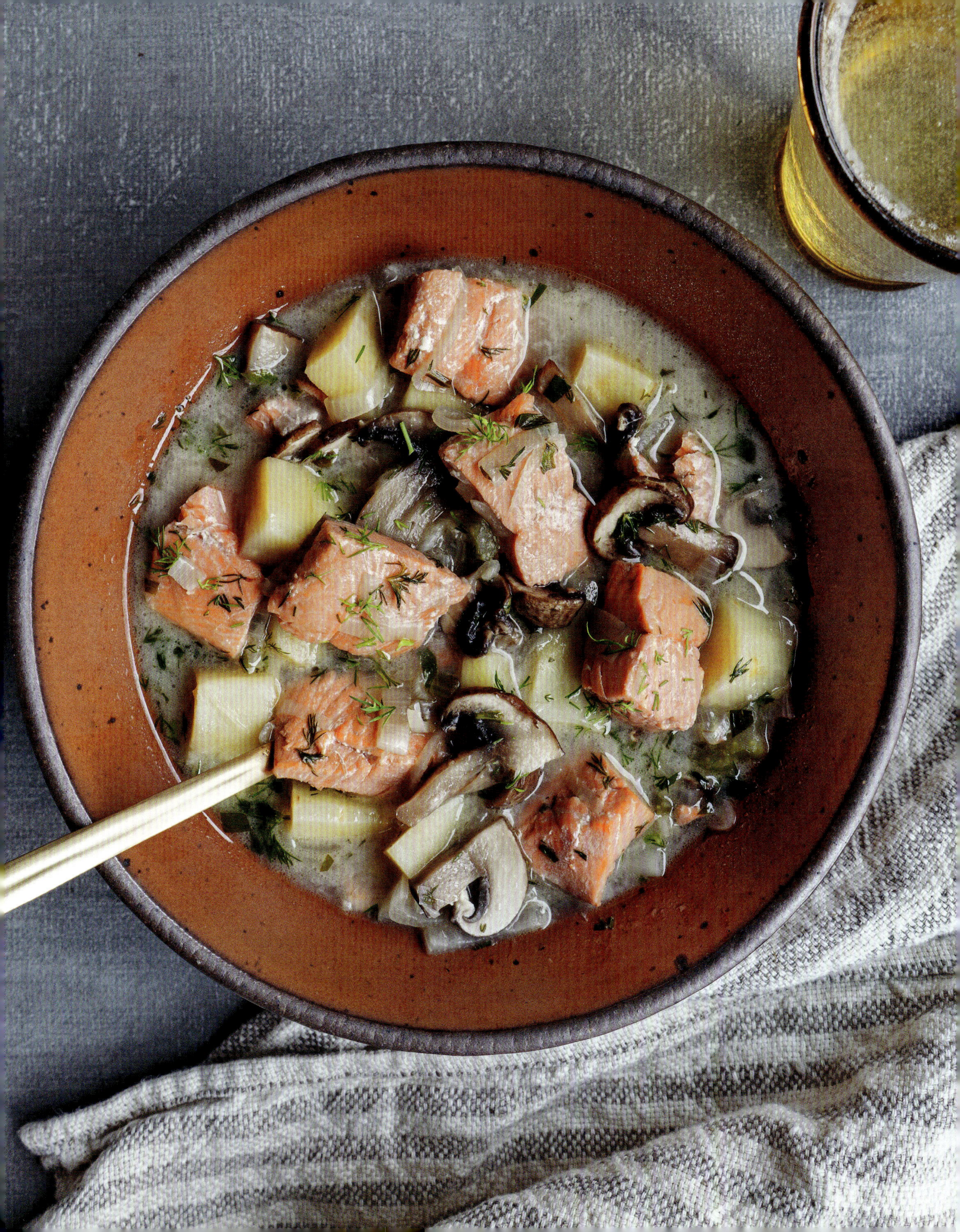

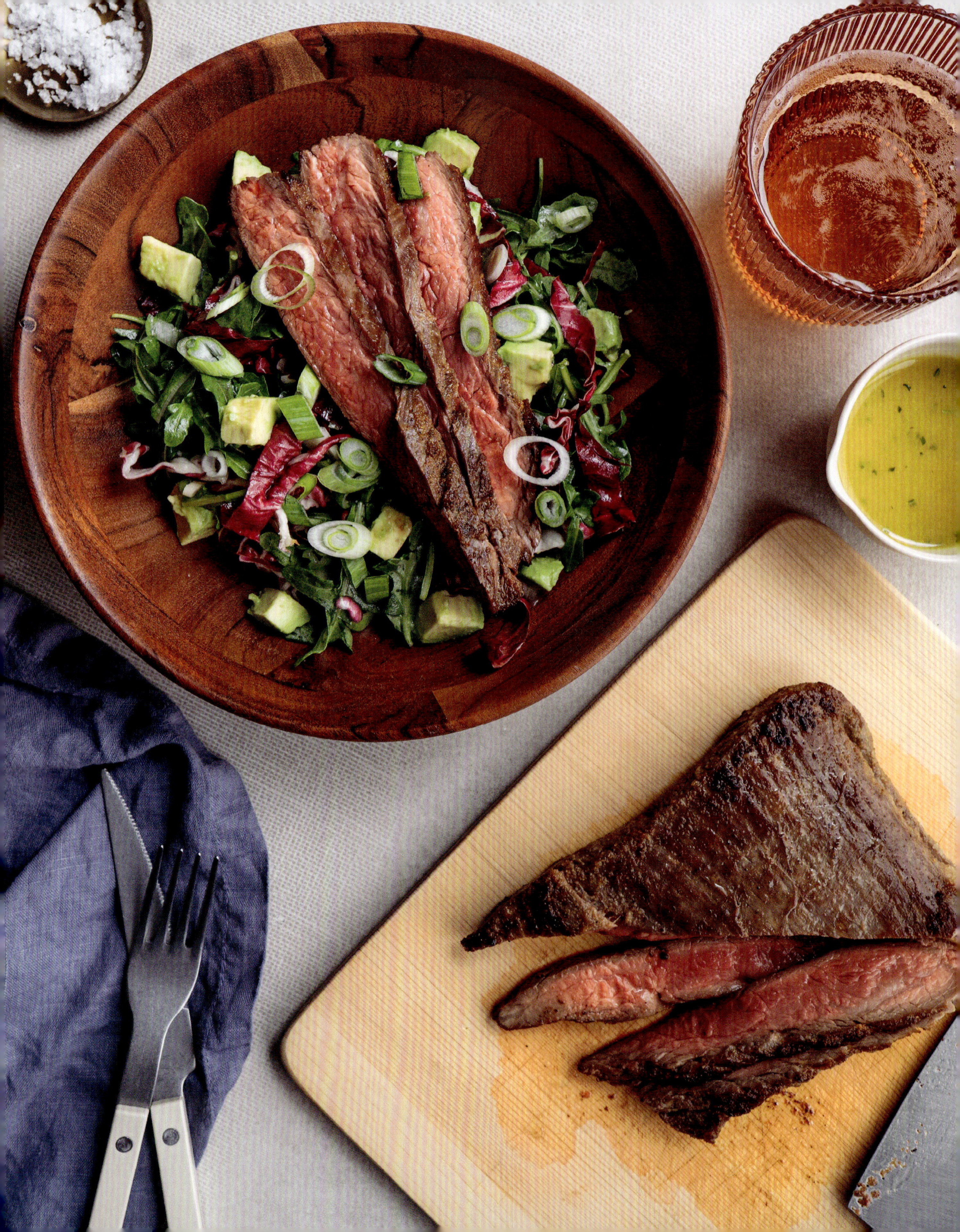

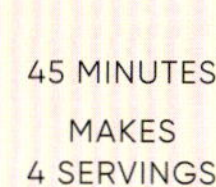

45 MINUTES

MAKES
4 SERVINGS

Maple Lime Steak and Radicchio Salad

1 head radicchio, chopped

2 quarts cold water

1½ pounds 1-inch-thick flank steak

¾ teaspoon plus ½ teaspoon sea salt

½ teaspoon garlic powder

½ teaspoon onion powder

¼ cup plus 2 tablespoons olive oil (or substitute avocado oil)

2 tablespoons lime juice (about 1 juicy lime)

1 tablespoon maple syrup

½ teaspoon sea salt

¼ teaspoon minced fresh rosemary

5 ounces arugula

2 avocados, pitted and cubed

1 bunch green onions, white and green parts, ends removed and thinly sliced

PREP NOTE: *If batch-cooking this meal ahead, store the greens and dressing separately and toss fresh for each portion.*

1. Place the radicchio in a large bowl with the cold water. (This helps reduce the bitter flavor.) Set aside. Sprinkle both sides of the steak with ¾ teaspoon of the salt, garlic powder, and onion powder, using your hands to rub it in and coat evenly. Allow the radicchio and steak to sit for at least 20 minutes.

2. Meanwhile, make the dressing. Combine ¼ cup of the oil, lime juice, maple syrup, the remaining ½ teaspoon salt, and rosemary in a blender and blend until smooth. (Alternatively, you can use a bowl and whisk. If doing so, combine all the ingredients except the oil and whisk to combine, then drizzle in the oil slowly, whisking constantly to emulsify the dressing.) Set aside.

3. When the radicchio has finished soaking, place it in a strainer and drain the water, then use a salad spinner or a kitchen towel to dry it. Place in a large bowl along with the arugula and set aside.

4. To cook the steak, heat the remaining 2 tablespoons of oil in a large skillet over medium-high heat. When the pan is hot, add the steak and cook for 5 minutes, or until a nice brown crust has developed on the first side. Flip and cook for another 3 minutes, then turn down the heat to medium and cover with a lid. Cook for another 3 minutes, or until the internal temperature reaches 125°F (for medium-rare), or longer if your steak is more than 1 inch thick. When finished, place on a cutting board, cover with a piece of foil, and let rest for 5 minutes.

5. While the steak is resting, add the dressing to the salad and toss to combine. Slice the steak thinly against the grain. Serve each plate of dressed salad with steak slices, avocado, and green onions. The steak keeps for up to 5 days in the refrigerator.

1 HOUR

MAKES
6 SERVINGS

Hearty Pork and Cabbage Stew

2 pounds ground pork

1 onion, chopped

½ medium green cabbage, cored and shredded (about 4 cups)

3 garlic cloves, minced

3 cups bone broth, homemade (page 119) or store-bought

3 cups water

2 large carrots, chopped (about 3 cups)

2 large parsnips, chopped (about 4 cups)

1 teaspoon sea salt

1 bay leaf

2 tablespoons minced fresh dill

1 cup sauerkraut, homemade (page 120) or store-bought (check ingredients)

1. Place the ground pork in a heavy-bottomed soup pot over medium heat. Use a utensil to break up the meat; cook, stirring occasionally, until browned and the juices are mostly reabsorbed, 10 to 12 minutes. Use a slotted spoon to transfer the pork to a bowl and set it aside, leaving any fat remaining in the pot.

2. Keeping the heat at medium, add the onion and cook, stirring occasionally, for 3 minutes, or until starting to soften. Add the cabbage and cook for an additional 5 minutes, or until beginning to soften. Add the garlic and cook until fragrant, about 1 minute. Add the broth, water, carrots, parsnips, salt, and bay leaf. Bring to a boil, then turn down the heat to maintain a simmer. Cover and cook for 20 minutes. (If your stovetop can't manage a covered simmer on the lowest setting, you can set the lid ajar to allow some heat to escape.)

3. Add the pork, cover again, and cook for 10 more minutes, or until the vegetables are just fork-tender. Remove the bay leaf, stir in the dill and sauerkraut, and serve. It keeps for up to 5 days in the refrigerator; it also freezes well.

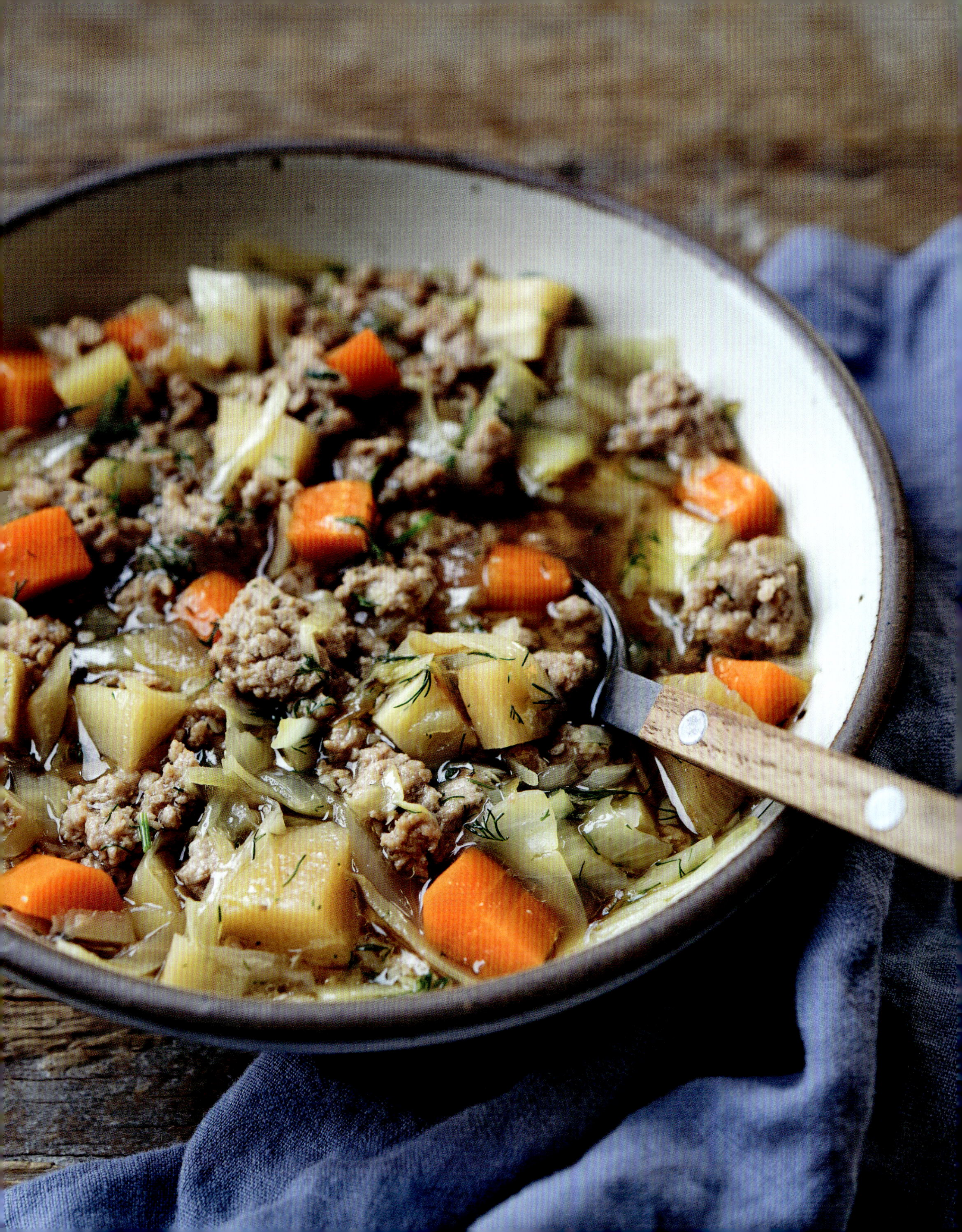

45 MINUTES

MAKES
6 SERVINGS

Beef Taco Salad Bowl with Pickled Onions

QUICK-PICKLED ONIONS

½ cup water

½ cup apple cider vinegar

1 teaspoon sea salt

1 teaspoon coconut sugar (or substitute date sugar)

1 cup thinly sliced red onion

TACO BEEF

2 tablespoons avocado oil

1 onion, diced

6 ounces button mushrooms, diced

4 garlic cloves, minced

¾ cup bone broth, homemade (page 119) or store-bought

2 teaspoons garlic powder

2 teaspoons onion powder

1 teaspoon fresh thyme leaves

1 teaspoon sea salt

2 pounds ground beef

SALAD

10 ounces mixed greens

¼ cup avocado oil

2 tablespoons lime juice (about 1 juicy lime)

¼ teaspoon sea salt

1 bunch cilantro, bottom stems removed, chopped

2 avocados, pitted and sliced

10 ounces plantain or cassava chips

1. First, make the quick-pickled onions. Combine the water, vinegar, salt, and sugar in a small saucepan over medium heat. Bring to a boil, then turn off the heat, stirring until the salt and sugar are dissolved. Place the onion in a glass jar and add the vinegar mixture. Set aside to marinate while you make the rest of the meal.

2. Next, make the beef. Heat the oil in a large skillet over medium heat. When the pan is hot, add the onion and mushrooms and cook, stirring, for 5 minutes. Add the garlic and cook until fragrant, about 1 minute. Add the broth, garlic powder, onion powder, thyme, and salt and stir to combine, then add the beef, breaking it into pieces as you add it to the pan. Cook for 10 to 15 minutes, stirring occasionally to break up the meat as it cooks, until the liquid is absorbed. Turn off the heat and allow to cool while you assemble the bowls.

3. Place the greens in a large bowl, add the oil, lime juice, and salt, and toss to combine well. Strain the onions, discarding the brine. Serve each bowl of dressed greens with a serving of taco meat, cilantro, pickled onions, avocado slices, and chips. The taco meat keeps in the refrigerator for up to 1 week.

PREP NOTE: *If batch-cooking this meal ahead, make the pickled onions and the taco meat for storage (the onions may be stored in their pickling liquid). Before serving, toss a portion of greens with dressing and add the reheated meat, pickled onions, avocado, and chips.*

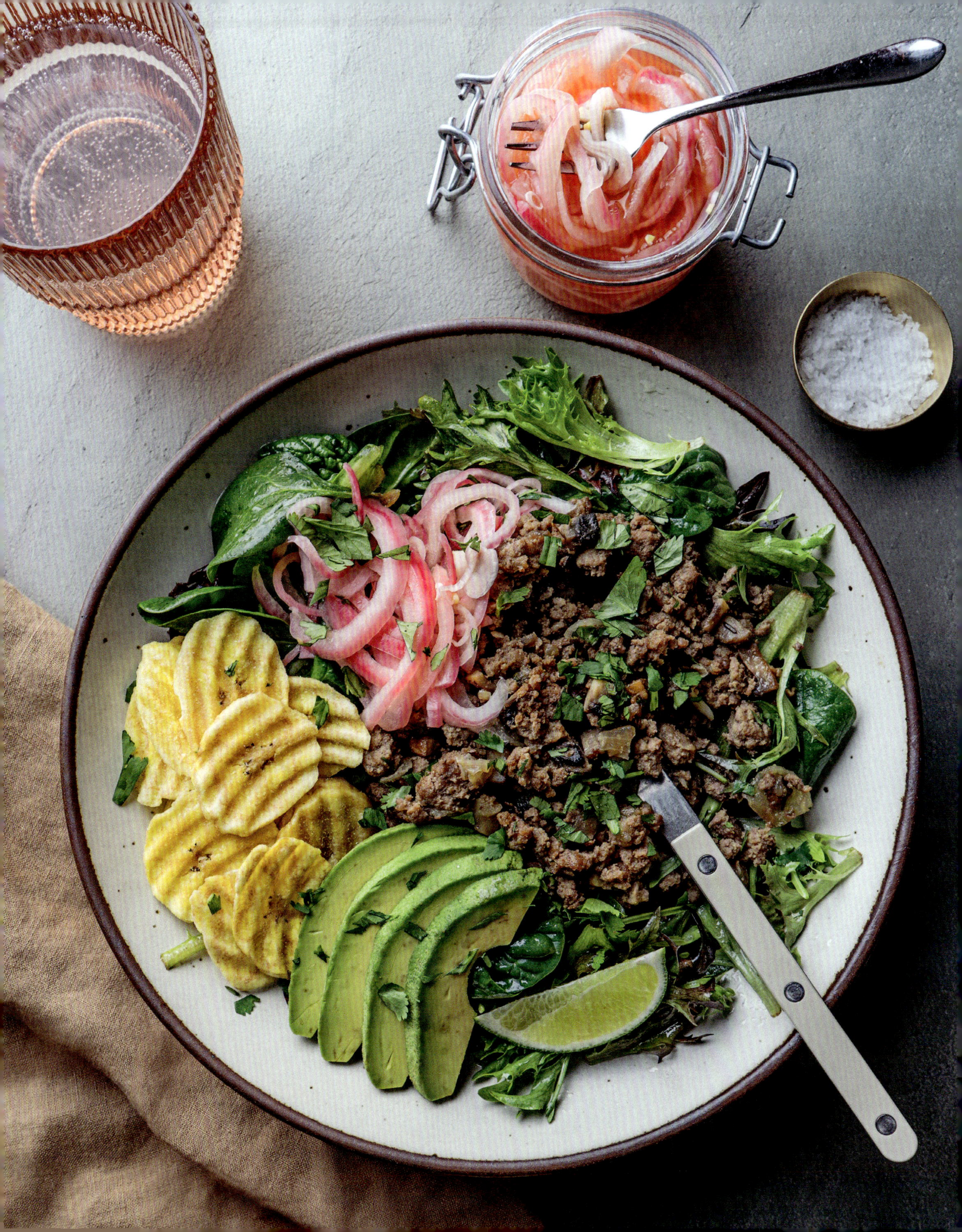

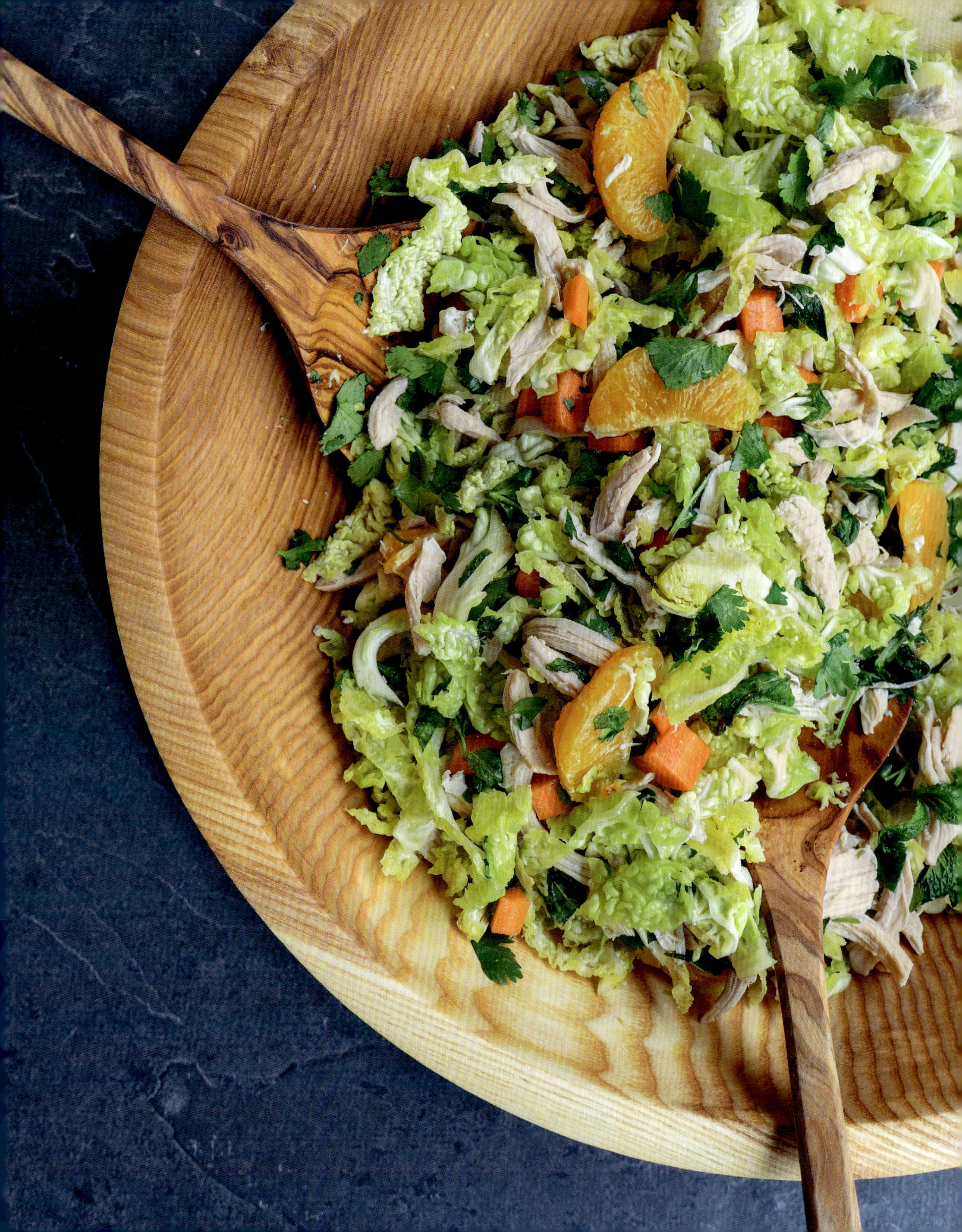

45 MINUTES

MAKES
4 SERVINGS

Massaged Cabbage and Mandarin Chicken Salad

1 head Savoy cabbage, shredded (or substitute napa cabbage)

4 tablespoons avocado oil, divided

1 teaspoon sea salt, divided

1½ pounds chicken breast

½ cup water

1 carrot, diced (about 1 cup)

3 tangerines, peeled and sectioned

½ cup fresh mint leaves, chopped

½ cup fresh cilantro leaves, chopped

2 tablespoons lime juice (about 1 juicy lime)

1 tablespoon coconut aminos

½ teaspoon fish sauce

1. Place the cabbage in a large bowl, drizzle with 3 tablespoons of the oil, and sprinkle with ½ teaspoon of the salt. Massage the cabbage gently with your hands for 5 minutes, or until the tough fibers of the cabbage break down and soften somewhat. Set aside.

2. Sprinkle the chicken breasts with the remaining ½ teaspoon salt. Heat the remaining 1 tablespoon oil in a large skillet over medium heat. When the pan is hot, place the chicken top-side down and cook for 5 to 7 minutes, until browned. Flip the chicken, add the water, cover, and lower the heat to maintain a simmer. Cook for about 15 minutes, until the internal temperature of the chicken reaches 165°F, adding additional water if necessary if the pan goes dry. Set the chicken aside to cool for 10 to 15 minutes, then shred it.

3. Add the shredded chicken, carrot, tangerines, mint, cilantro, lime juice, coconut aminos, and fish sauce to the bowl with the cabbage and toss to combine. Serve immediately.

PREP NOTE: *If batch-cooking this ahead, store the massaged cabbage separately from the rest of the dry salad ingredients and dressing. Before serving, toss the massaged cabbage portion with the herbs, tangerines, chicken, and dressing. It keeps for up to 3 days in the refrigerator.*

45 MINUTES

MAKES
4 SERVINGS

Coastal Harvest Stew

⅓ cup olive oil

2 leeks, ends removed and whites thinly sliced

10 ounces trumpet mushrooms, diced (or substitute button mushrooms)

8 garlic cloves, minced

2 cups bone broth, homemade (page 119) or store-bought

2 cups water

1 large parsnip, diced (about 2 cups)

2 carrots, diced (about 2 cups)

1 small beet, diced (about 1 cup)

½ cup canned pumpkin puree

1 bay leaf

½ teaspoon sea salt

1 tablespoon coconut aminos

1 teaspoon fish sauce

6 ounces cod, skin and bones removed, cut into 1½-inch pieces

6 ounces scallops

8 ounces shrimp, peeled and deveined

3 tablespoons lemon juice (about 1 lemon)

½ cup fresh dill, minced

NOTE: *If you need to reheat this stew, do so gently over low heat, while stirring, to avoid overcooking the seafood.*

1. Heat the oil in a large soup pot over medium heat. When hot, add the leeks and mushrooms and cook, stirring occasionally, for 5 minutes, or until beginning to brown. Add the garlic and cook until fragrant, about 1 minute.

2. Add the broth, water, parsnips, carrots, beet, pumpkin, bay leaf, salt, coconut aminos, and fish sauce and bring to a boil. Turn down the heat to maintain a simmer and cook, covered, for 20 minutes (if your stovetop can't manage a simmer on the lowest setting, adjust the lid so that a little steam can escape and produce a simmer).

3. Add the cod, scallops, shrimp, lemon juice, and dill and cook for 3 minutes, or until the seafood is no longer translucent and the fish flakes easily. Take off the heat and either serve immediately or transfer directly to a container for storage (leaving the stew in the hot pot may cause the seafood to overcook). It keeps in the refrigerator for up to 3 days.

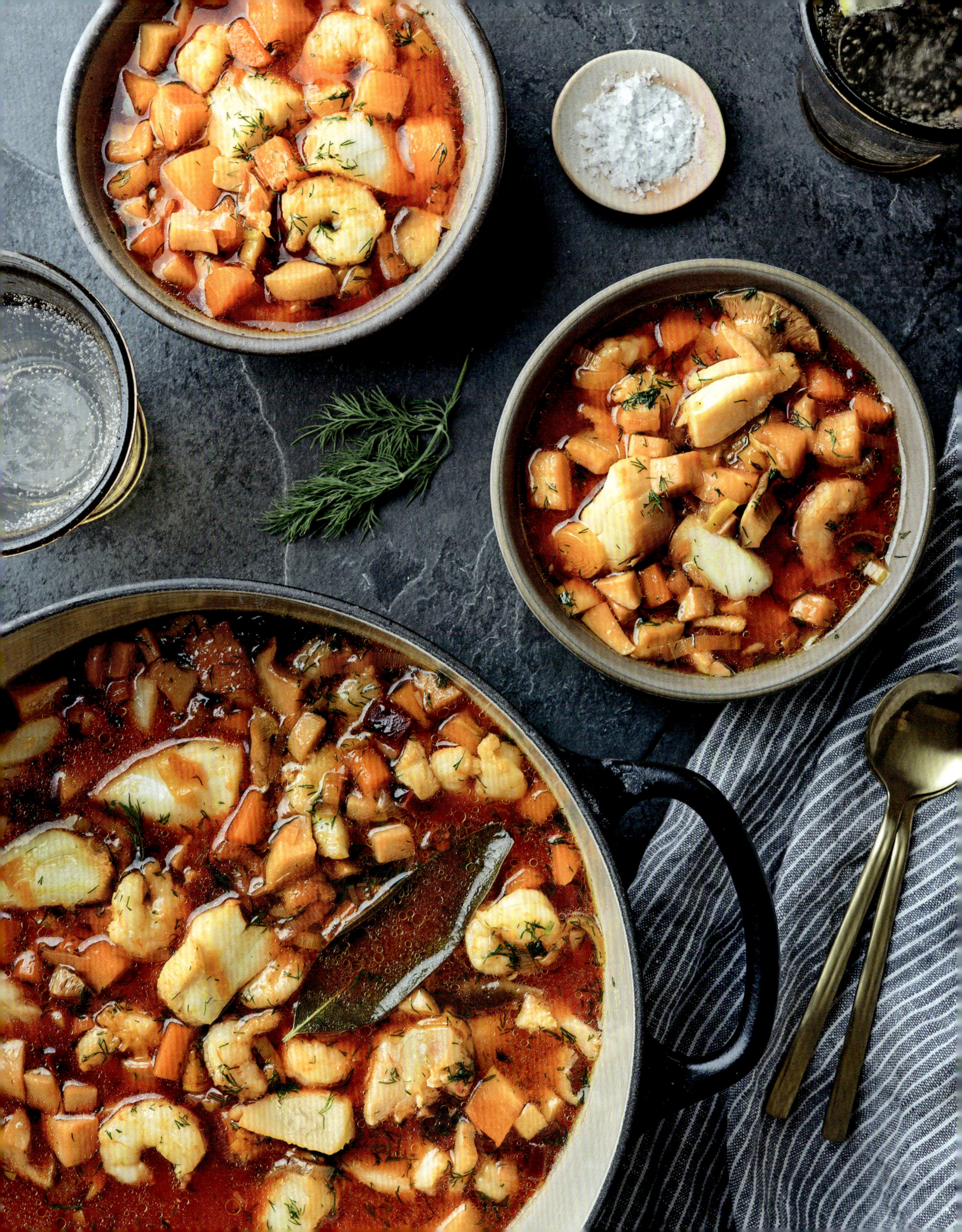

CHAPTER 10

Core Main Meals

40 MINUTES

MAKES 3 SERVINGS

Cauli-Shrimp Stir-Fry

4 tablespoons avocado oil, divided

14 ounces frozen riced cauliflower*

½ teaspoon sea salt, plus more if needed

½ white onion, diced

3 garlic cloves, minced

1 (1-inch) piece fresh ginger, minced

6 ounces shiitake mushrooms, thinly sliced (or substitute button mushrooms)

¼ cup coconut aminos

1 tablespoon apple cider vinegar

1 pound medium shrimp, peeled, deveined, and without tails

Green onions and fresh cilantro, for garnish

**Many grocers sell frozen cauliflower processed into rice-sized granules, but if you can't source it at your local store, you can use a food processor to process half a head of cauliflower for this recipe.*

1. First, make the cauliflower base. Heat 2 tablespoons of the oil in a large skillet over medium-high heat. When the pan is hot, add the frozen riced cauliflower. Cook, stirring occasionally, for 7 to 10 minutes, until all the granules are fully defrosted and begin to lightly brown. Add the salt and transfer to a large bowl while you make the rest of the meal.

2. In the same skillet, heat the remaining 2 tablespoons oil over medium-high heat. When the pan is hot, add the onion and cook, stirring, for about 3 minutes, until just starting to brown. Add the garlic, ginger, and mushrooms and cook until the garlic is fragrant, about 30 seconds.

3. Add the coconut aminos and vinegar and cook until the liquid thickens, about 2 minutes. Add the shrimp and cook, stirring, until they are cooked throughout, 1 to 2 minutes. Turn off the heat, taste, and add salt if necessary.

4. Serve each bowl of cauliflower rice topped with the shrimp stir-fry and garnished with green onions and cilantro. It keeps for up to 3 days in the refrigerator.

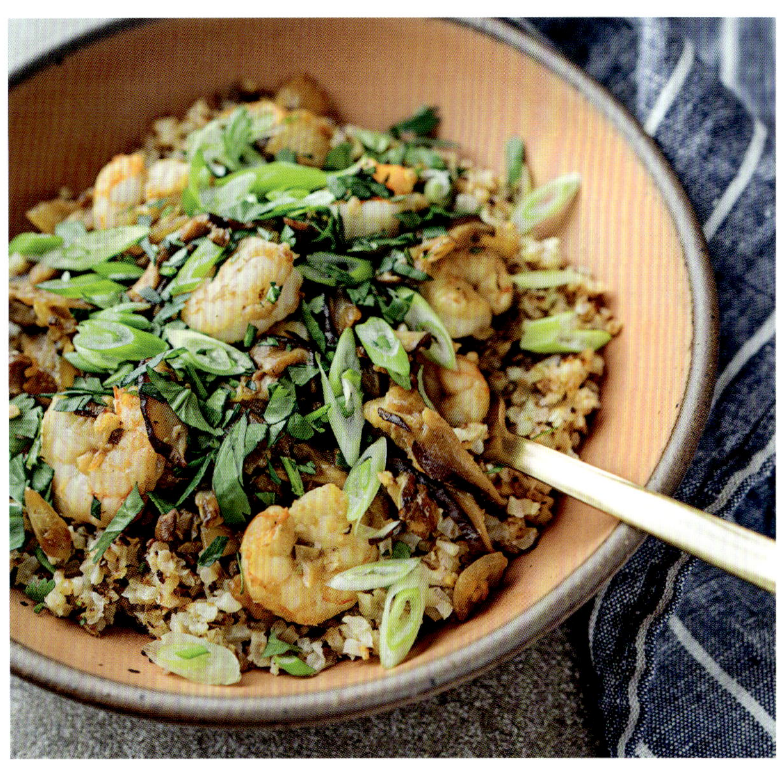

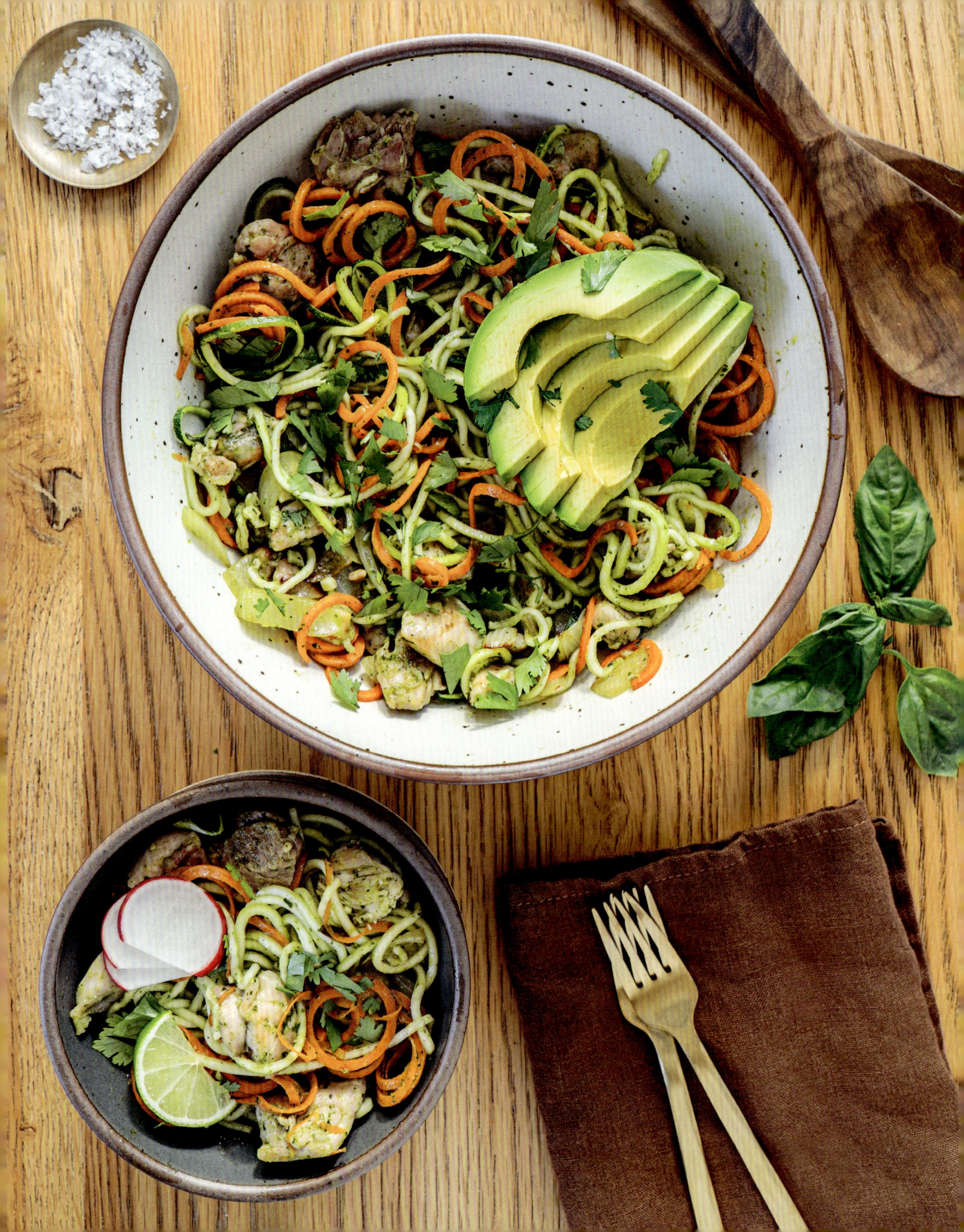

30 MINUTES
MAKES
4 SERVINGS

Chicken Noodle Pesto Bowl

SAUCE

½ cup packed fresh cilantro (or substitute basil)

½ cup olive oil

2 tablespoons lime juice (about 1 juicy lime)

¼ teaspoon sea salt

1 garlic clove

CHICKEN

1½ pounds boneless, skinless chicken thighs, cut into 1½-inch pieces

½ teaspoon sea salt

2 tablespoons olive oil

½ onion, diced

3 garlic cloves, minced

2 zucchinis, spiralized into noodles*

2 carrots, spiralized into noodles*

Cilantro (or basil) leaves, thinly sliced radishes, lime wedges, and avocado, for serving (optional)

**Spiralizing tools come in both handheld and countertop varieties and make this task incredibly easy. And some grocers sell pre-spiralized vegetables that you can use for this recipe.*

1. Preheat the oven to 425°F.

2. First, to make the sauce, place all the ingredients in a blender and blend until thoroughly combined. Set aside.

3. Season the chicken with the salt. Heat the oil in an ovenproof skillet over medium heat. When the pan is hot, add the onion and cook, stirring occasionally, for 5 minutes, or until lightly browned. Add the garlic and cook for another 30 seconds, or until fragrant.

4. Turn the heat to high. Add the chicken to the pan and spread it out so that the pieces are in a thin layer. Cook for 1 to 2 minutes without stirring, to allow the bottom of the chicken pieces to brown. Give them a good stir, then place in the oven and cook for 10 to 12 minutes, until the internal temperature reaches 165°F.

5. While the chicken is cooking, place the spiralized zucchini and carrots in a large bowl and toss with the dressing. Set aside.

6. When the chicken is finished cooking, allow to cool for a few minutes, then toss your desired portion with the vegetables and dressing. Serve garnished with additional cilantro leaves, radish slices, a lime wedge, and avocado slices, if desired. The chicken keeps for up to 3 days in the refrigerator.

PREP NOTE: *If batch-cooking this ahead, store the spiralized vegetables, dressing, and cooked chicken separately; toss each portion fresh and serve with the accompaniments, if including.*

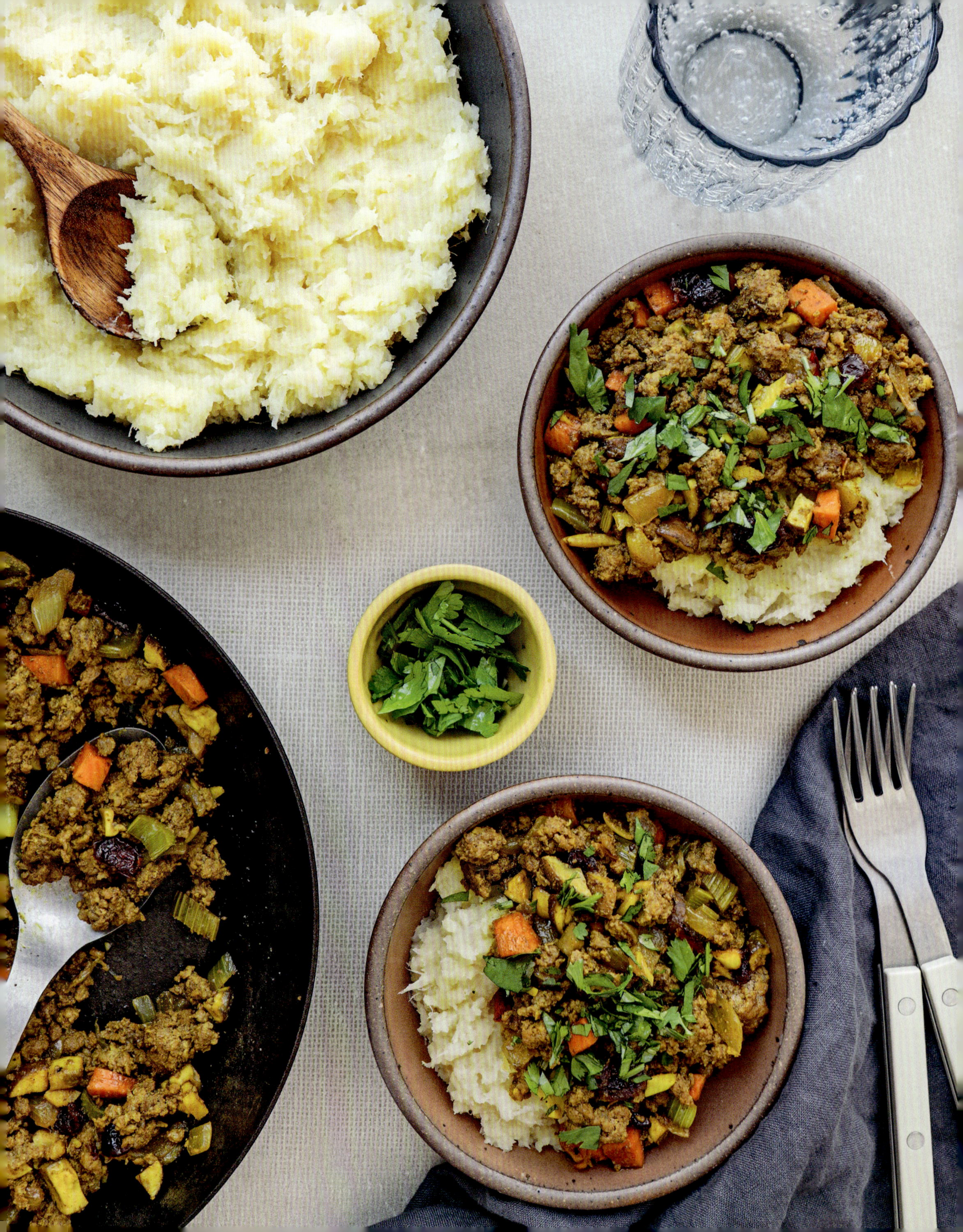

1 HOUR

MAKES
8 SERVINGS

Curried Beef Vegetable Pie

2 pounds parsnips, cut into large pieces

2 pounds light-fleshed sweet potatoes, peeled and cut into large pieces

2 pounds ground beef

1 onion, diced

3 celery ribs, diced

1 large carrot, diced (about 1 cup)

6 garlic cloves, minced

1 (1-inch) piece ginger, minced

8 ounces mushrooms, diced

½ cup water

2 teaspoons ground turmeric

1 teaspoon tamarind paste

1 teaspoon garlic powder

1 teaspoon onion powder

Pinch ground cinnamon

2 teaspoons sea salt, divided

¼ cup unsweetened dried tart cherries or raisins, chopped (check ingredients)

¼ cup avocado oil

Fresh cilantro, for garnish

1. First, cook the root vegetables. Fill a large pot with water, bring to a boil, and add the parsnips and sweet potatoes. Cook for about 10 minutes, until fork-tender.

2. In the meantime, prepare the beef and vegetables. Place the beef in a large, cold skillet and break it into large pieces. Turn the heat to medium and cook, continuing to break up and turn the meat until browned and cooked throughout, about 10 minutes. Use a slotted spoon to transfer the meat to a bowl, reserving the fat and cooking juices in the pan. Set aside.

3. Add the onion to the same skillet over medium heat and cook, stirring, for 3 minutes, or until just starting to brown. Add the celery and carrots and cook for 5 minutes. Add the garlic, ginger, and mushrooms and cook, stirring, for another minute, or until aromatic.

4. Add the water, turmeric, tamarind paste, garlic powder, onion powder, cinnamon, and 1 teaspoon of the salt to the pan. Cook, stirring, for 1 to 2 minutes, until the water is absorbed and the spices are incorporated. Add the dried fruit and beef and cook until warmed. Turn off the heat and set aside.

5. When the root vegetables are finished cooking, drain and mash with the oil and remaining 1 teaspoon salt. If necessary, heat up the beef mixture for serving. Serve garnished with cilantro. It keeps in the refrigerator for up to 1 week; it also freezes well.

PREP NOTE: *This recipe is perfect for batch-cooking, as it keeps well in both the refrigerator and freezer. I like to portion each serving of meat topped with a serving of root mash into wide-mouth, pint-sized glass jars and store them in the freezer. To protect against breakage, just be sure not to use jars with shoulders or overfill your jars.*

1 HOUR

MAKES
4 SERVINGS

Pork Tenderloin with Cabbage and Honey-Cider Glaze

1½ pounds pork tenderloin

1½ teaspoons sea salt, divided

1 teaspoon honey, warmed if not liquid

1 teaspoon apple cider vinegar

½ teaspoon ground ginger

4 tablespoons avocado oil (or substitute olive oil), divided

1 small sweet potato, peeled and cut into 1-inch pieces

1 green apple, cored and cut into 1-inch pieces

1 teaspoon fresh thyme leaves

4 shallots, thinly sliced

½ head red cabbage (about 1½ pounds), shredded

1. Preheat the oven to 400°F.

2. Remove the silverskin membrane off the tenderloin. This is a tough, silvery-looking membrane on the surface of the meat. Use a sharp knife to slide under the silverskin and carefully pull it away as you cut the membrane away from you. Once you are finished, season the tenderloin with 1 teaspoon of the salt, using your hands to rub it in. Set aside.

3. In a small bowl or jar, combine the honey, vinegar, and ginger and whisk to combine. Set aside.

4. Heat 1 tablespoon of the oil in a large skillet over medium-high heat. When the pan is hot, brown the tenderloin on all sides, 2 to 3 minutes. Turn off the heat and set aside.

5. Place the sweet potato and apple in a roasting dish and toss with 1 tablespoon of the remaining oil and ¼ teaspoon of the remaining salt. Place the tenderloin in the center, arranging the potato and apple pieces around it, then spoon or brush with the honey mixture and sprinkle with the thyme. Cook in the oven for 20 to 25 minutes, stirring the sweet potato and apple pieces halfway, until the pork reaches 145°F as measured on an instant-read thermometer.

6. While the pork is cooking, heat the remaining 2 tablespoons oil in the large skillet over medium-high heat. When the pan is hot, add the shallots and cook, stirring, for 2 minutes, or until beginning to brown. Add the cabbage and cook for 5 to 7 minutes, until tender. Add the remaining ¼ teaspoon salt and set aside.

7. When the pork is finished cooking, allow to rest for 10 minutes, then slice and serve. It keeps for up to 5 days in the refrigerator.

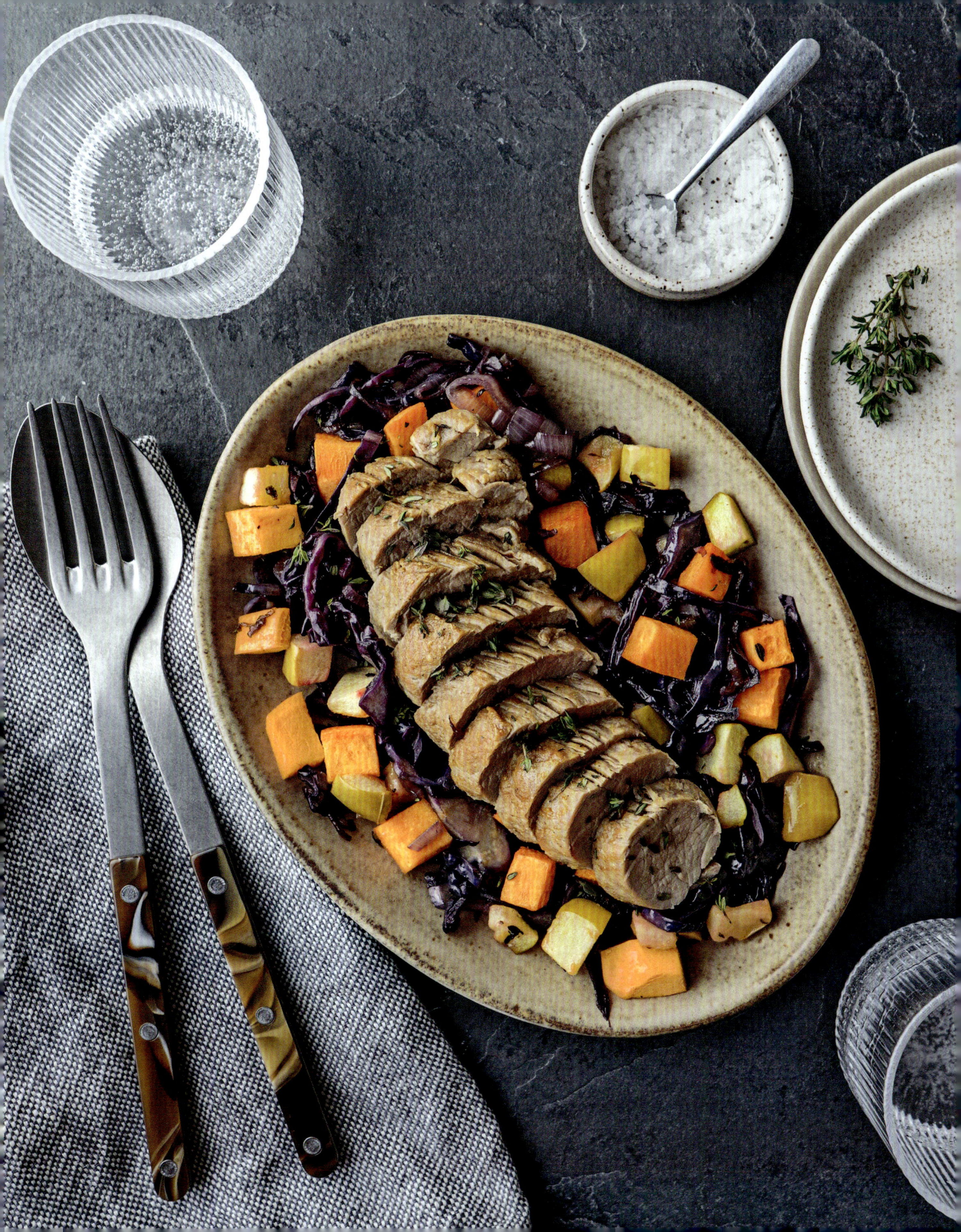

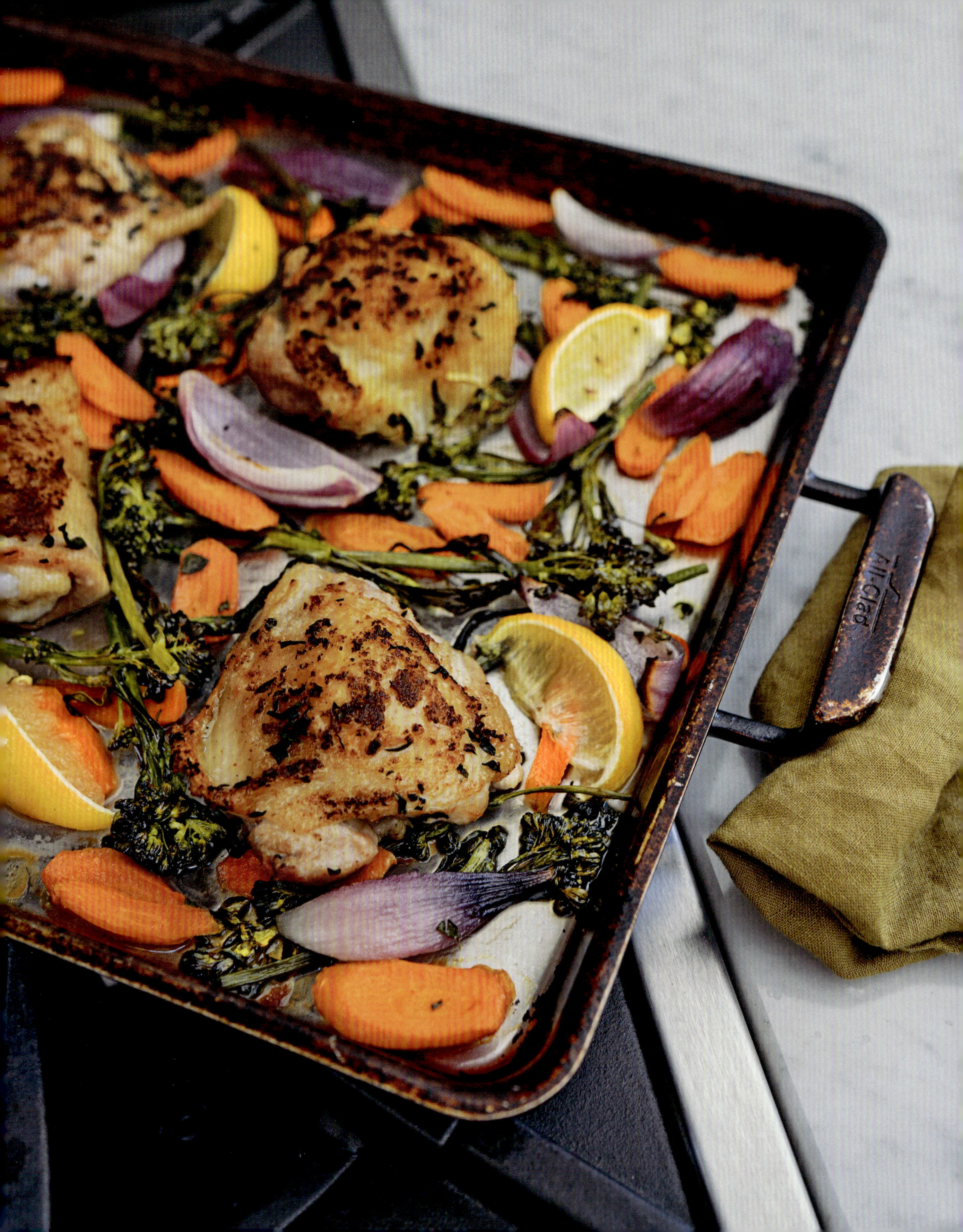
All-Clad

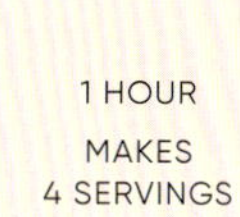
1 HOUR

MAKES
4 SERVINGS

One-Pan Roasted Chicken with Broccolini and Lemon

- 1½ teaspoons sea salt, divided
- ¾ teaspoon garlic powder
- ¾ teaspoon onion powder
- 3 pounds bone-in, skin-on chicken thighs
- 1 pound carrots, thinly sliced on the diagonal
- 1 pound Broccolini, roughly chopped
- 1 red onion, roughly chopped
- 1 lemon, cut lengthwise into 6 sections
- 3 tablespoons olive oil (or substitute avocado oil), divided
- 1 tablespoon minced fresh oregano

1. Preheat the oven to 425°F.

2. Combine 1 teaspoon of the salt, the garlic powder, and onion powder in a small bowl. Sprinkle all over the chicken and use your hands to rub it in thoroughly. Set aside.

3. Divide the carrots, Broccolini, onion, and lemon between two large rimmed baking sheets or roasting dishes. Add 1 tablespoon of the oil and ¼ teaspoon of the remaining salt to each dish and stir to coat evenly. Set aside.

4. Heat the remaining 1 tablespoon oil in a large skillet over medium-high heat. When the pan is hot, add half of the chicken thighs, skin-side down. Allow to cook, undisturbed, for about 2 minutes, until the skin is nice and brown. Transfer the browned batch of chicken to one of the trays or dishes, nestling them skin-side up among the vegetables. Set aside and repeat with the other half of the chicken.

5. Sprinkle both trays or dishes with the oregano, place in the oven, and cook for 20 to 25 minutes, until the chicken reaches 165°F as tested by an instant-read thermometer inserted into a thigh. Discard the lemon before serving. It keeps for up to 5 days in the refrigerator.

40 MINUTES

MAKES
4 SERVINGS

Coconut Curried Cod

3 tablespoons avocado oil, divided

1½ pounds frozen riced cauliflower*

1 teaspoon sea salt, divided

1 pound cod, skin and bones removed and cut into 1½-inch pieces

1 onion, diced

1 large carrot, diced (about 1 cup)

4 garlic cloves, minced

1 (1-inch) piece ginger, minced

1 (14-ounce) can coconut milk (check ingredients)

2 tablespoons coconut aminos

1 teaspoon tamarind paste

1 teaspoon ground turmeric

¼ teaspoon ground cinnamon

2 baby bok choy, ends removed and chopped

1 tablespoon lime juice (about ½ juicy lime)

Microgreens or fresh cilantro, for garnish (optional)

**Many grocers sell frozen cauliflower processed into rice-sized granules, but if you can't source this at your local store, you can use a food processor to process half a head of cauliflower for this recipe.*

1. Start by making the cauliflower base. Heat 1 tablespoon of the oil in a large skillet over medium-high heat, and when the pan is hot, add half of the frozen riced cauliflower. Cook, stirring occasionally, for 7 to 10 minutes, until all the granules are fully defrosted and they begin to lightly brown. Transfer to a bowl and repeat with the second half of the cauliflower. Add ½ teaspoon of the salt to the cooked cauliflower and set aside, keeping the skillet handy for reheating before serving.

2. Once the cauliflower is ready, sprinkle the remaining ½ teaspoon salt on the cod and set aside.

3. Heat the remaining 1 tablespoon oil in a large skillet over medium heat (it is helpful to use a separate skillet here). When the pan is hot, add the onion and cook for 2 minutes, or until starting to soften. Add the carrot and cook for 3 more minutes, or until beginning to brown. Add the garlic and ginger and cook, stirring, for 30 seconds, or until fragrant. Add the coconut milk, coconut aminos, tamarind paste, turmeric, and cinnamon and stir to combine. When the mixture begins to simmer, add the cod and bok choy. Cover and simmer for about 5 minutes, stirring occasionally, until the cod is flaky and the bok choy is wilted. Take off the heat and stir in the lime juice.

4. Serve portions of cauliflower rice topped with the curry and garnished with microgreens, if using. It keeps for up to 3 days in the refrigerator.

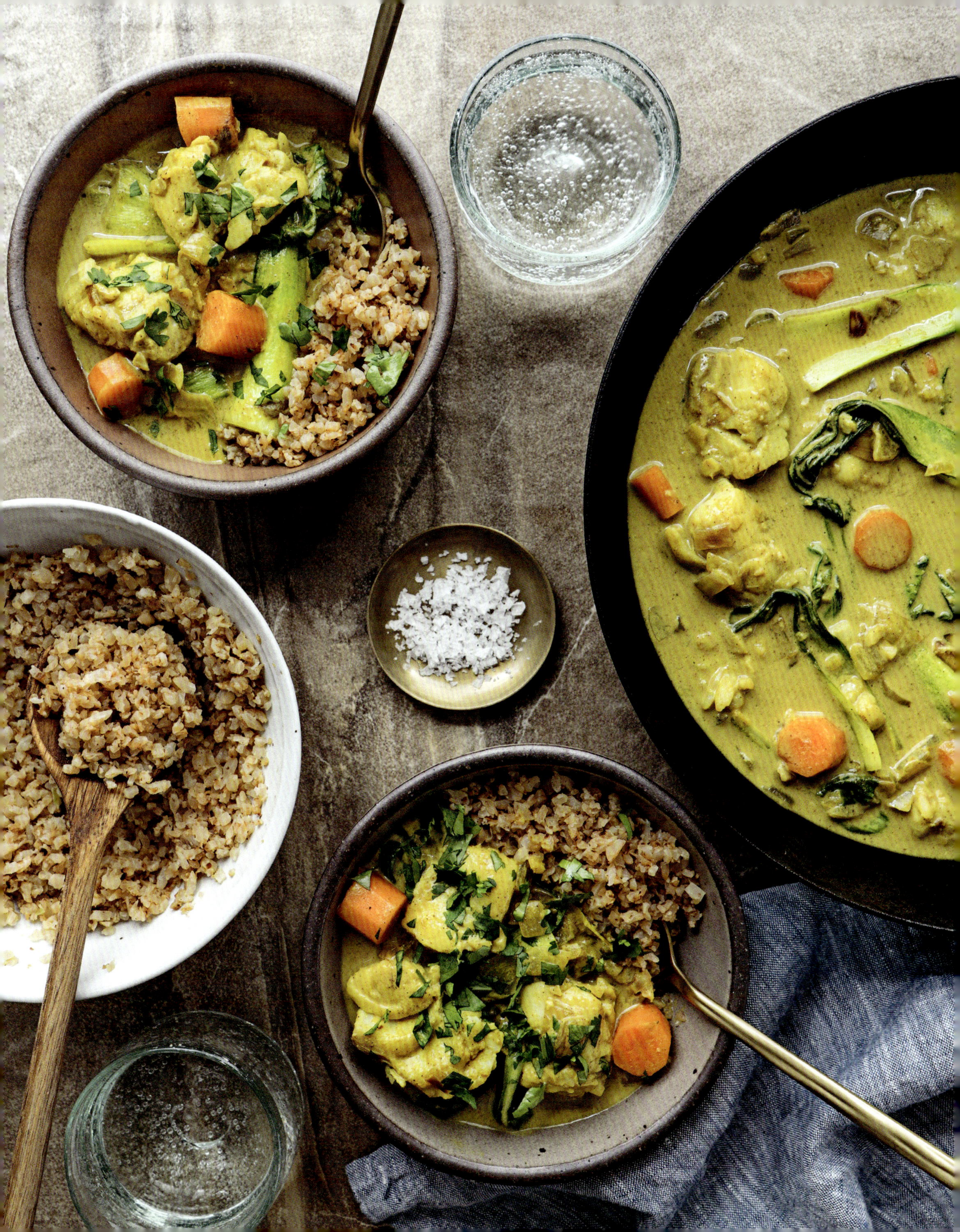

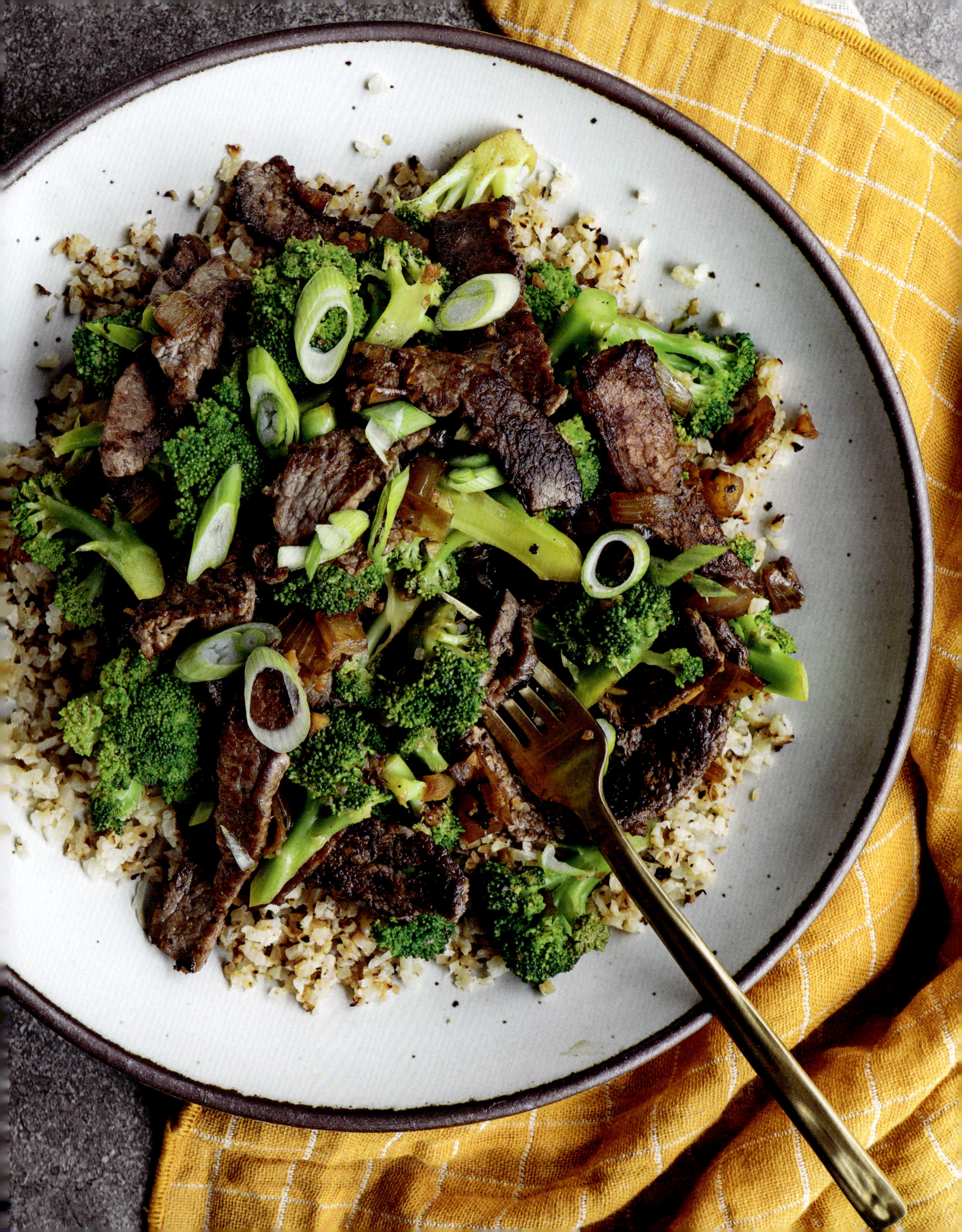

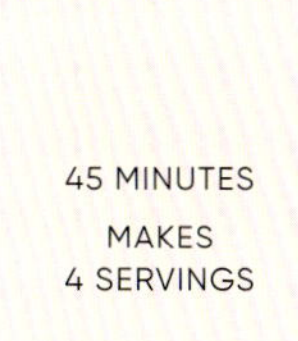

45 MINUTES

MAKES
4 SERVINGS

Zesty Orange Ginger Beef and Broccoli

3 tablespoons avocado oil, divided, plus more if needed

1½ pounds frozen riced cauliflower*

½ teaspoon sea salt

1 pound broccoli crowns, chopped

1½ pounds beef strips (flank, skirt, or sirloin cut for stir-fry)

½ onion, chopped

3 garlic cloves, minced

1 (2-inch) piece ginger, minced

¾ cup orange juice

¼ cup coconut aminos

1 teaspoon fish sauce

1 bunch green onions, white and green parts thinly sliced on the diagonal

**Many grocers sell frozen cauliflower processed into rice-sized granules, but if you can't source this at your local store, you can use a food processor to process half a head of cauliflower for this recipe.*

1. Start by making the cauliflower base. Heat 1 tablespoon of the oil in a large skillet over medium-high heat. When the pan is hot, add half of the frozen riced cauliflower. Cook, stirring occasionally, for 7 to 10 minutes, until all the granules are fully defrosted and begin to lightly brown. Transfer to a bowl and repeat with the second half of the riced cauliflower. Add the salt to the cooked cauliflower and set aside, keeping the skillet handy to reheat before serving.

2. While the cauliflower is cooking, steam the broccoli. Pour 2 cups of water into a pot with a steaming basket and heat over medium heat. When the water is boiling, add the broccoli and steam for 5 minutes, or until just tender but not fully cooked. Set aside, uncovered.

3. Once the cauliflower and broccoli are ready, make the beef and sauce. Heat 1 tablespoon of the remaining oil in a large skillet over medium-high heat (it is helpful to use a separate skillet here). Add half of the beef strips and cook for 4 to 5 minutes, stirring once or twice for even browning. Transfer to a bowl and repeat with the remaining 1 tablespoon of oil and beef strips, then add them to the bowl and set aside.

4. Once the beef is finished, turn down the heat to medium and add an additional tablespoon of oil if necessary. Add the onion and cook, stirring, for 3 minutes, or until just beginning to brown. Add the garlic and ginger and cook until fragrant, about 30 seconds. Add the orange juice, coconut aminos, and fish sauce to the pan and cook for 5 minutes, or until reduced to a thick sauce.

5. Add the steamed broccoli and beef and stir to combine. Cook for 1 to 2 more minutes to reheat, while you reheat the cauliflower if necessary. Serve warm garnished with green onions. It keeps for up to 5 days in the refrigerator.

45 MINUTES

MAKES 4 SERVINGS

Herb Roasted Salmon with Asparagus and Cauli Steaks

ROASTED SALMON AND VEGETABLES

1 head cauliflower, cut horizontally into ½-inch-thick "steaks"

3 tablespoons olive oil, divided

¾ teaspoon sea salt, divided

1½-pound salmon fillet, skin-on

1 bunch thin asparagus spears, ends removed and cut into thirds

HERB SAUCE

¼ cup minced fresh cilantro

2 tablespoons minced fresh parsley

2 tablespoons minced fresh mint

4 garlic cloves, minced

⅓ cup olive oil

1½ tablespoons lemon juice (about ½ lemon)

½ teaspoon sea salt

1. Preheat the oven to 400°F.

2. Brush each side of the cauliflower steaks with 1 tablespoon of the oil and sprinkle with ¼ teaspoon of the salt. Place in a roasting dish and cook for 20 minutes.

3. Meanwhile, place the salmon skin-side down on a large rimmed baking sheet, drizzle with 1 tablespoon of the remaining oil, and sprinkle with ¼ teaspoon of the remaining salt. Place the asparagus pieces in a medium bowl, add the remaining 1 tablespoon oil, toss, then sprinkle with the remaining ¼ teaspoon salt and arrange on the baking sheet around the salmon.

4. When the cauliflower has been in the oven for 20 minutes, add the sheet of salmon and asparagus and cook for 12 minutes, or until the salmon is just tender when probed with a fork. Both dishes should be finished at approximately the same time, but you may need to leave either the cauliflower or the salmon in for a minute or two longer, until they are both fully cooked.

5. While the salmon and vegetables are cooking, prepare the herb sauce. Combine the cilantro, parsley, mint, garlic, oil, lemon juice, and salt in a small bowl or jar and whisk or shake to combine. Serve each portion of salmon and vegetables topped with a generous serving of herb sauce spooned on top. It keeps for up to 3 days in the refrigerator.

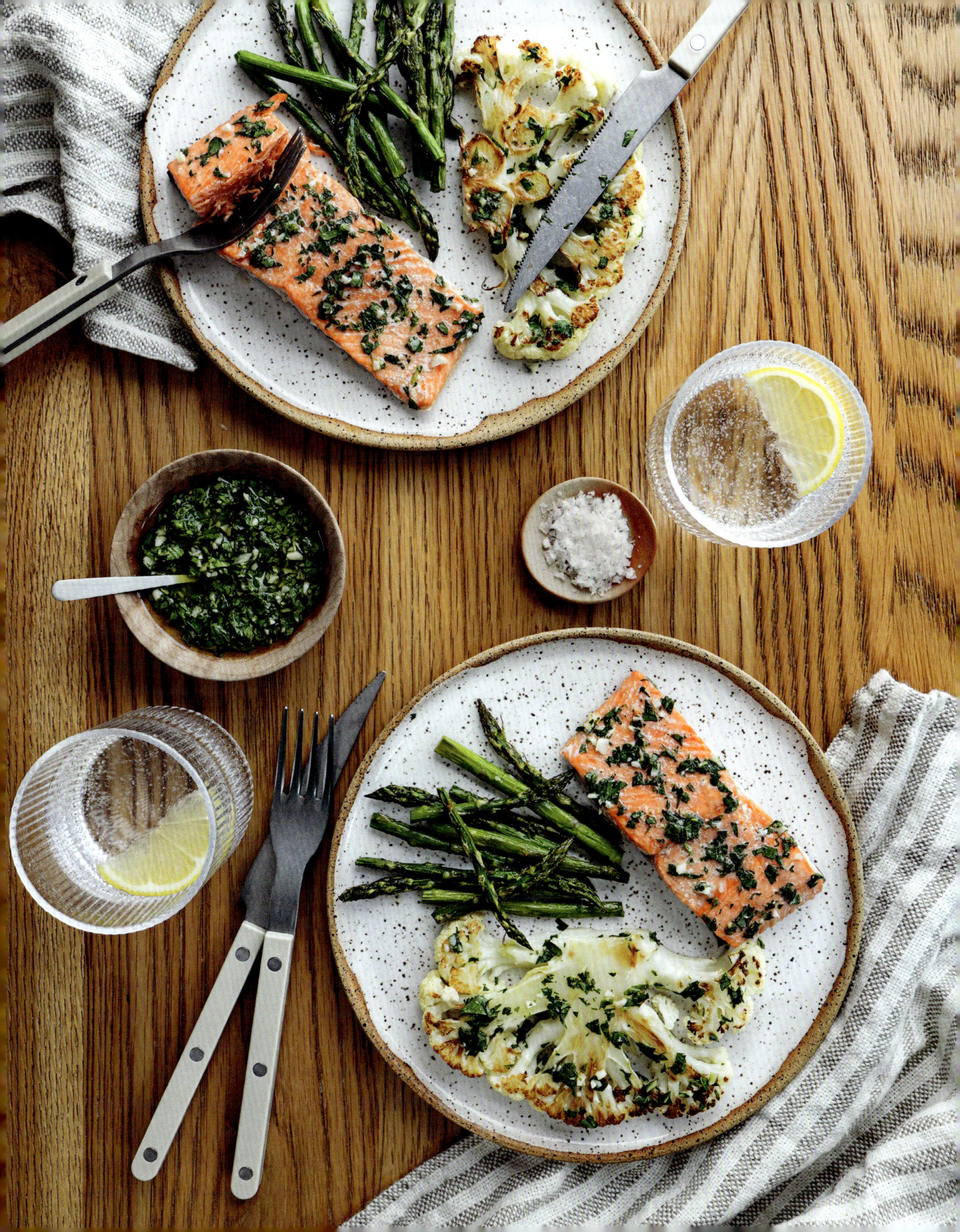

CHAPTER 11

Core Sweet Treats

Cosmic Fruit Tart, Two Ways

1 HOUR
30 MINUTES, PLUS
2 HOURS TO SET

MAKES
8 SERVINGS

CRUST

1 cup tightly packed pitted dates

⅔ cup sustainable palm shortening

1½ cups (216 grams) arrowroot powder, plus more if needed

¼ cup maple sugar

CRANBERRY VERSION

1½ pounds cranberries, fresh or frozen

1 cup orange juice, divided

¾ cup maple sugar

2½ teaspoons gelatin powder

½ cup sustainable palm shortening

CITRUS VERSION

1½ cups freshly squeezed Meyer lemon juice (8 to 10 lemons)

1 tablespoon gelatin powder

¼ teaspoon ground turmeric

½ cup sustainable palm shortening

½ cup maple sugar (or substitute date or coconut sugar)

½ cup freshly squeezed orange juice (about 2 oranges)

¼ cup (28 grams) arrowroot powder

1. Preheat the oven to 350°F.

2. To make the crust, place the dates in the bowl of a food processor and pulse until small granules form. Don't overmix or it will turn into a paste. Add the shortening, arrowroot, and maple sugar and pulse until combined into a crumbly mixture. If it is too sticky, add some arrowroot powder 1 tablespoon at a time.

3. Place the mixture in the bottom of a 9-inch tart pan. Use your hands to work the mixture evenly across the bottom and up the sides, pressing it into an even form. Bake for 15 minutes, or until lightly browned; the crust will be slightly soft but will develop a firmer texture as it cools. Set aside to cool to room temperature, about 1 hour.

CRANBERRY VERSION

1. Combine the cranberries, ½ cup of the orange juice, and the maple sugar in a large saucepan. Bring to a simmer over medium-low heat and simmer uncovered for 10 minutes, or until the cranberries have popped and softened. Set aside to cool for 5 to 10 minutes, then transfer to a high-speed blender or food processor and blend until completely smooth.

2. Pour the remaining ½ cup orange juice into a small bowl. Sprinkle the gelatin over the juice and set aside for 5 minutes to bloom. While you are waiting, wipe out the pot you used to cook the cranberries. Return the cranberry puree to the pot along with the orange juice/gelatin mixture and heat over low heat, stirring constantly with a whisk, for 5 to 10 minutes, until the mixture reaches 120°F (this is to mix in the gelatin, but be cautious not to heat it too quickly). Take off the heat and whisk in the shortening until completely smooth. Immediately pour into the tart crust.

3. Allow to cool for 5 to 10 minutes, then place in the refrigerator for at least 2 hours to set. Once set, the tart will keep at room temperature for 1 day and up to 3 in the refrigerator.

(Citrus version on next page)

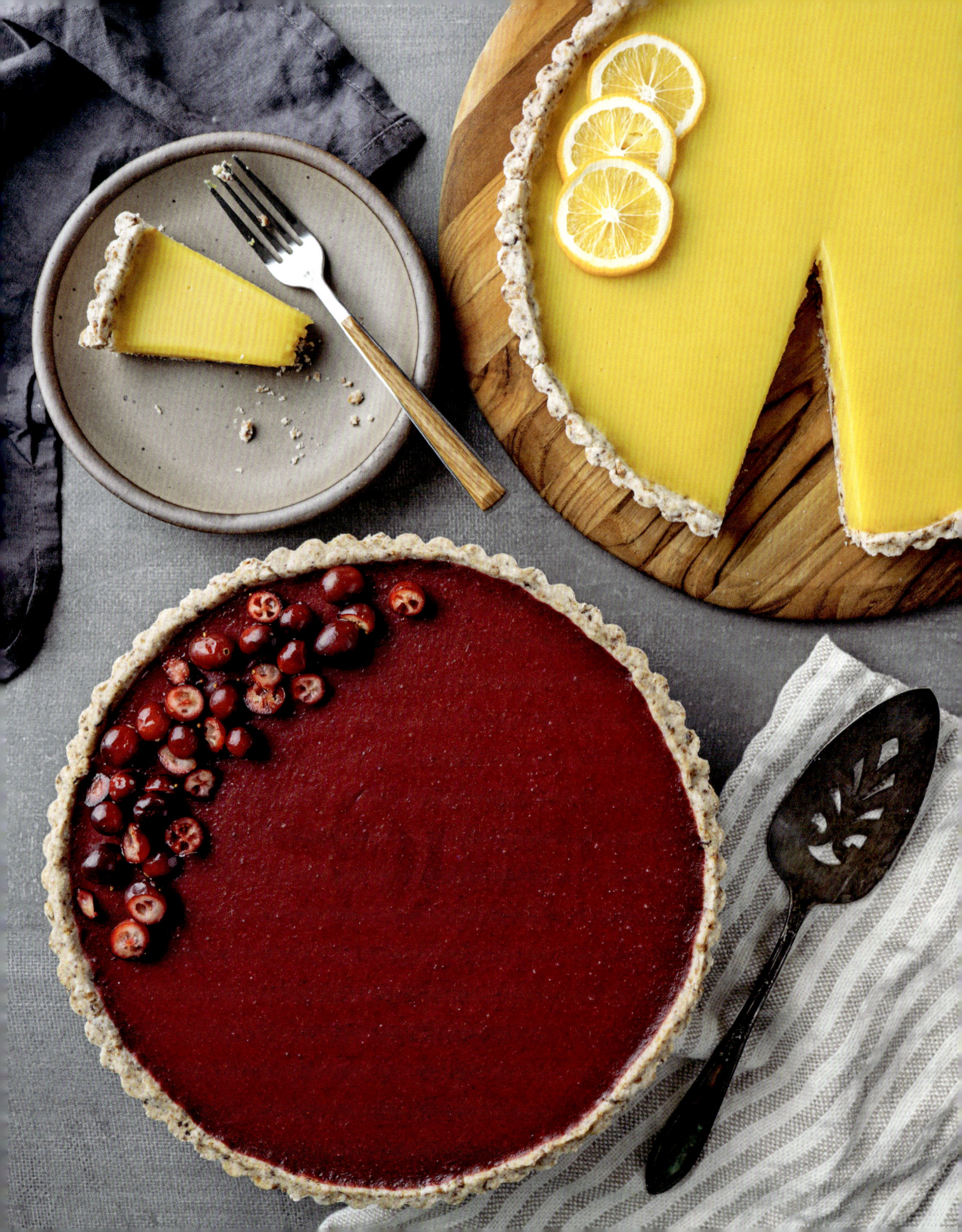

CITRUS VERSION

1. Pour the lemon juice into a small bowl. Sprinkle the gelatin and turmeric over the lemon juice and set aside for 5 minutes for the gelatin to bloom.

2. Combine the shortening and maple sugar in a medium saucepan and heat over low heat to melt and dissolve. Take off the heat and allow to cool a bit, then add the lemon juice, turmeric, and gelatin mixture. Stirring constantly with a whisk, heat on the lowest setting until the mixture is lukewarm and all of the fat, sugar, and gelatin are dissolved, or until the mixture reaches 120°F (this is to mix in the gelatin, but be cautious not to heat it too quickly). Take off the heat and set aside.

3. In a small bowl, whisk together the orange juice and arrowroot powder, then add to the pan with the lemon juice mixture. Place the pan over low heat and cook, stirring constantly with a whisk, until just thickened, about 5 minutes. You'll notice the texture of the mixture change from fully viscous to that of thin pancake batter. Do not overcook. When the mixture has thickened, immediately pour it into the tart crust.

4. Allow to cool for 5 to 10 minutes, then place in the refrigerator for at least 2 hours to set. Once set, the tart will keep at room temperature for 1 day and up to 3 in the refrigerator.

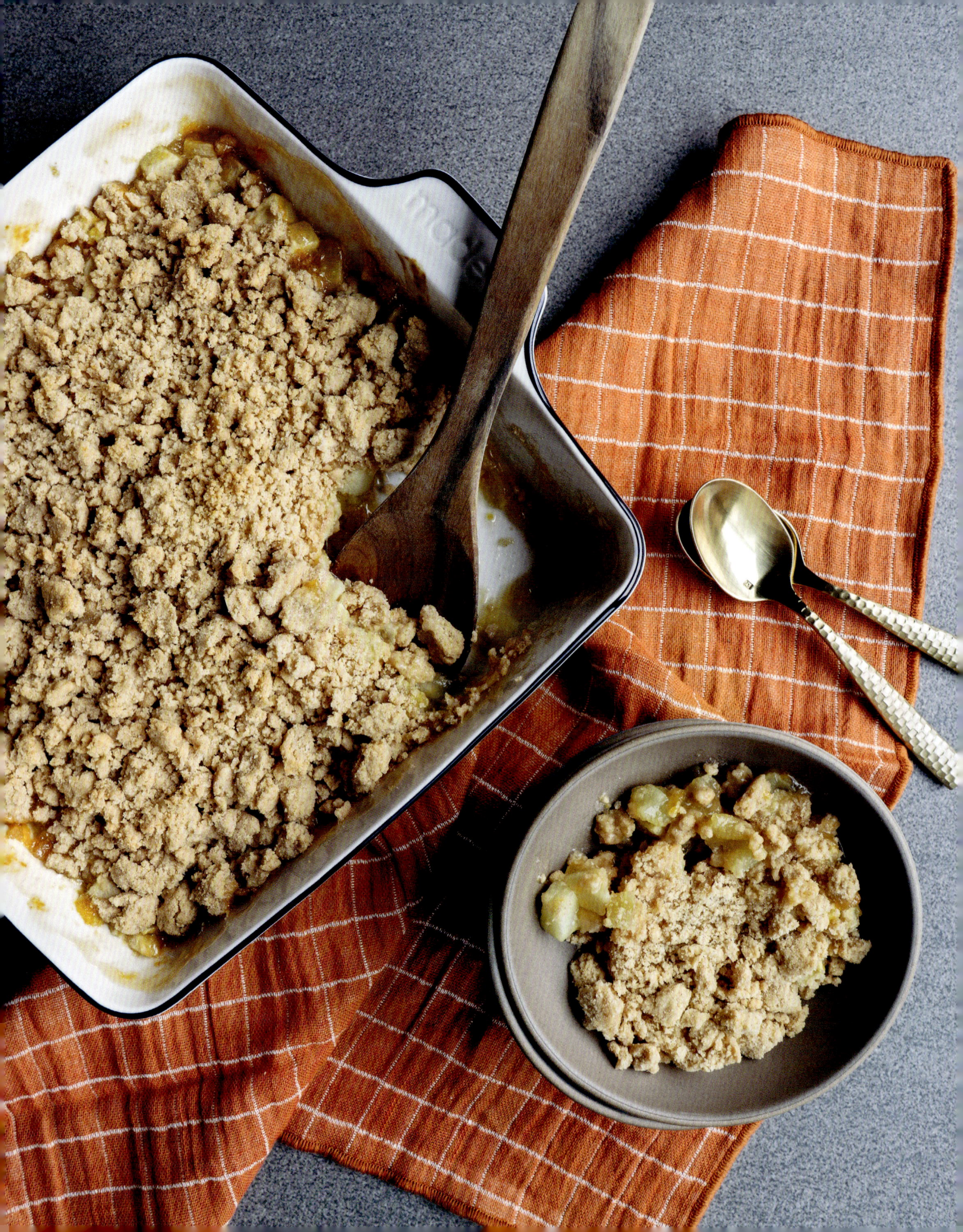

1 HOUR
30 MINUTES

MAKES
6 SERVINGS

Apricot and Apple Crumble

FILLING

6 tart apples, peeled, cored, and cut into 1-inch pieces

¾ cup apricot preserves

¼ cup (30 grams) tapioca flour (or substitute arrowroot flour)

2 tablespoons maple sugar (or substitute coconut or date sugar)

1 teaspoon lemon zest

2 tablespoons lemon juice (about ½ lemon)

¼ teaspoon sea salt

TOPPING

1 cup (150 grams) cassava flour

⅓ cup maple sugar (or substitute coconut or date sugar)

¼ cup tapioca flour

½ teaspoon ground cinnamon

½ teaspoon ground ginger

¼ teaspoon sea salt

½ cup sustainable palm shortening

1 teaspoon vanilla extract

NOTE: *If you are serving a crowd, double this recipe and bake it in a 9 by 13-inch baking dish.*

1. Preheat the oven to 350°F.

2. To make the filling, combine the apples, preserves, tapioca flour, maple sugar, the lemon zest and juice, and salt in a large bowl. Stir to combine thoroughly. Transfer to an 8-inch square baking pan and use a spatula to gently level it. Set aside.

3. To make the topping, combine the cassava flour, maple sugar, tapioca flour, cinnamon, ginger, and salt in a medium bowl. Add the shortening and vanilla and work it in with your hands to combine until pea-size granules form. You might have to work it until the dough comes together as a large ball and then crumble it into smaller granules.

4. Use your hands to distribute the topping evenly over the apple mixture, without disrupting the granules too much. Bake for 45 to 50 minutes, until the topping is just browned. Cool to room temperature before serving.

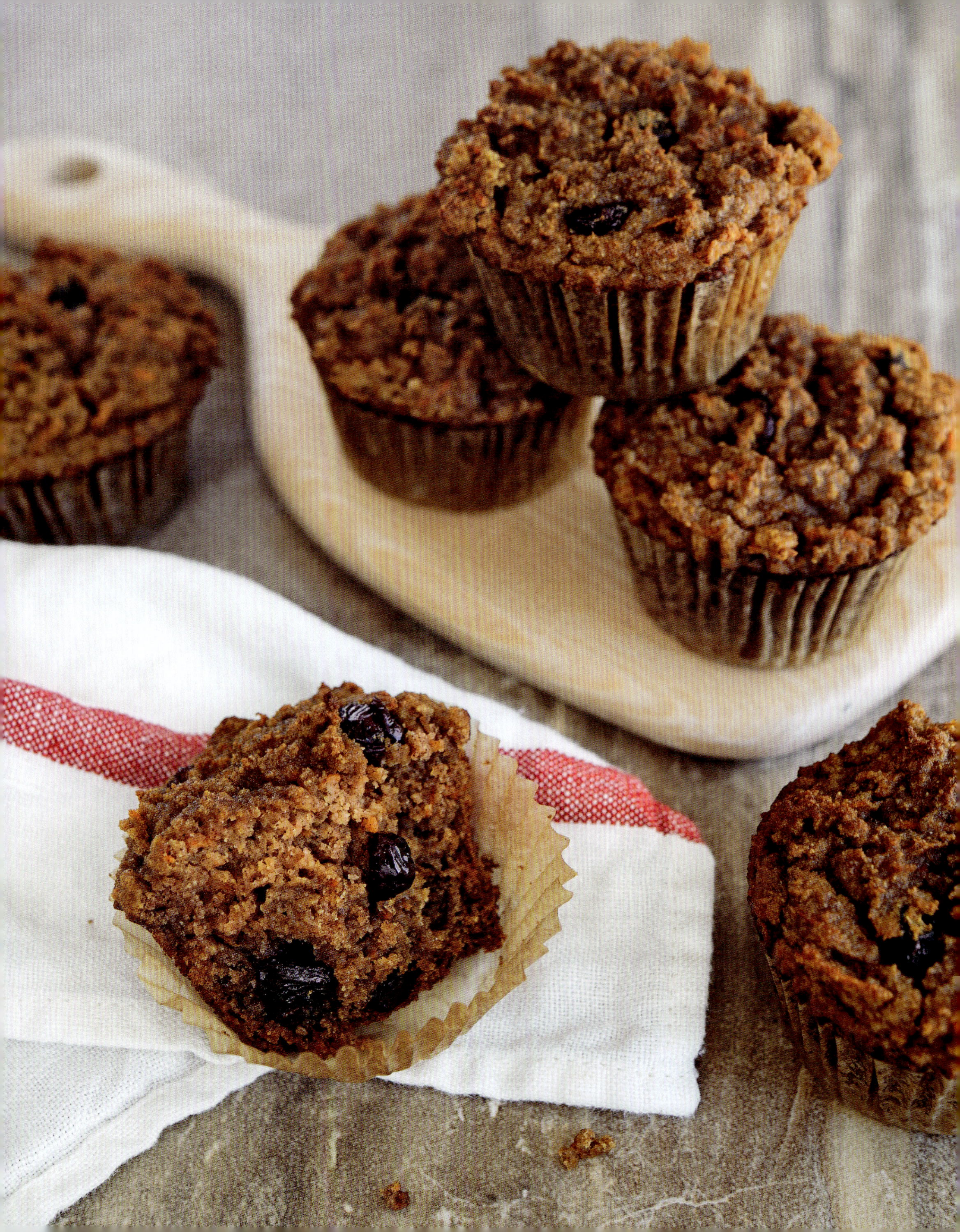

45 MINUTES, PLUS TIME TO COOL

MAKES 12 MUFFINS

Morning Glory Muffins

¾ cup water

½ cup unsweetened applesauce

2 tablespoons gelatin powder

1 cup (120 grams) tapioca flour

1¼ cups (140 grams) coconut flour

2 teaspoons baking soda

1 tablespoon ground cinnamon

2 teaspoons ground ginger

½ teaspoon sea salt

1 cup maple syrup

½ cup avocado oil

1 teaspoon vanilla extract

1 teaspoon apple cider vinegar

⅔ cup finely grated carrot

⅓ cup dried cherries or raisins (check ingredients)

1. Preheat the oven to 350°F and prepare a 12-hole muffin tray with paper liners.

2. Place the water in a small saucepan. Add the applesauce, stir, then sprinkle the gelatin on top of the mixture. Set aside for 5 minutes to allow the gelatin to absorb the liquid.

3. In a large bowl, combine the tapioca flour, coconut flour, baking soda, cinnamon, ginger, and salt and stir to combine. In a medium bowl, combine the maple syrup, oil, vanilla, and vinegar. Set both aside.

4. Place the saucepan with the gelatin mixture on the stovetop on the lowest heat setting. Heat gently as you whisk until the mixture thins and the gelatin has dissolved (the liquid should only be warm to the touch, or about 120°F when probed with a thermometer). Don't overheat. Once warm and thin, turn off the heat and add to the bowl with the other wet ingredients. Use a whisk or handheld electric mixer on low speed to combine the wet ingredients and gelatin mixture. Add to the bowl with the dry ingredients and mix again until just combined.

5. Add the carrot and dried fruit to the mix and stir until combined. You will have a mixture that is thicker than typical muffin batter—this is normal. Use two spoons to fill each muffin tin with a large scoop almost to the brim. Bake for 35 minutes, or until browned on top and you can no longer hear moisture cooking off when removed from the oven. Allow to cool fully to room temperature—this is essential for developing the correct texture with the gelatin eggs. If desired, the muffins may be reheated gently before enjoying. Store in an airtight container at room temperature for up to 3 days.

2 TO 3 HOURS

MAKES
6 SERVINGS

Citrus and Cherry Celebration Cake

¾ cup unsweetened applesauce

½ cup maple syrup

¼ cup water

2 tablespoons gelatin

¾ cup (84 grams) coconut flour

½ cup (60 grams) tapioca flour

1 teaspoon baking soda

¼ teaspoon sea salt

½ cup avocado oil

1 teaspoon lemon zest

1 tablespoon lemon juice (about ½ lemon)

1 teaspoon vanilla extract

1 recipe Maple-Yogurt Cream (page 192)

1 pound cherries, pitted and quartered

Lemon zest and mint leaves, for decorating

NOTE: *You can make this cake 1 to 2 days before frosting and serving. Because the cream is delicate, it doesn't transport or store well. If you need to bring it to an event, bring the wrapped cakes, cream, cherries, and garnishes with you and take a few minutes to assemble just before serving.*

1. Preheat the oven to 325°F and line two 6-inch cake pans with parchment paper (see the Lining Cake Pans tutorial on page 287).

2. In a small saucepan, combine the applesauce, maple syrup, and water and whisk to combine. Sprinkle with the gelatin and set aside for 5 minutes so the gelatin can absorb the liquid.

3. Meanwhile, in a large bowl, combine the coconut flour, tapioca flour, baking soda, and salt. Stir to combine and set aside. In a medium bowl, combine the oil, lemon zest and juice, and vanilla. Whisk to combine and set aside.

4. Place the saucepan with the gelatin mixture on the stovetop on the lowest heat setting. Whisk as it warms and take off the heat when the gelatin has dissolved (around 120°F—do not overheat). Add the warm gelatin mixture to the bowl with the oil and whisk or use a handheld electric mixer on low speed to combine thoroughly, then add to the bowl with the flours and continue to mix until fully combined. Your mixture will be thicker than usual cake batter—this is normal.

5. Divide the mixture evenly between the two prepared cake pans and use a spatula to level the surfaces (the mixture will be too thick to naturally even out). Bake for 1 hour, or until golden brown and just firm to the touch. Place the pans on a wire rack to cool completely, allowing the cakes to remain in the pans. Once fully cooled, wrap in plastic wrap and place in the refrigerator to chill until ready to decorate—at least 1 hour to allow the gelatin to set properly.

6. When you are ready to assemble the cake, place one of the cake layers on a flat surface. Add about half of the cream to the center, using a spatula to work it evenly to ½ inch from the edges. Add a single layer of quartered cherries on top of the frosting, being careful not to place them too close to the edges. Add the second cake layer and gently press down to level (be careful your frosting and cherries don't get squished out between the layers). Add the remaining cream to the top, again using a spatula to work it evenly to about ½ inch from the edges. Top with the remaining cherries and decorate with lemon zest and mint leaves.

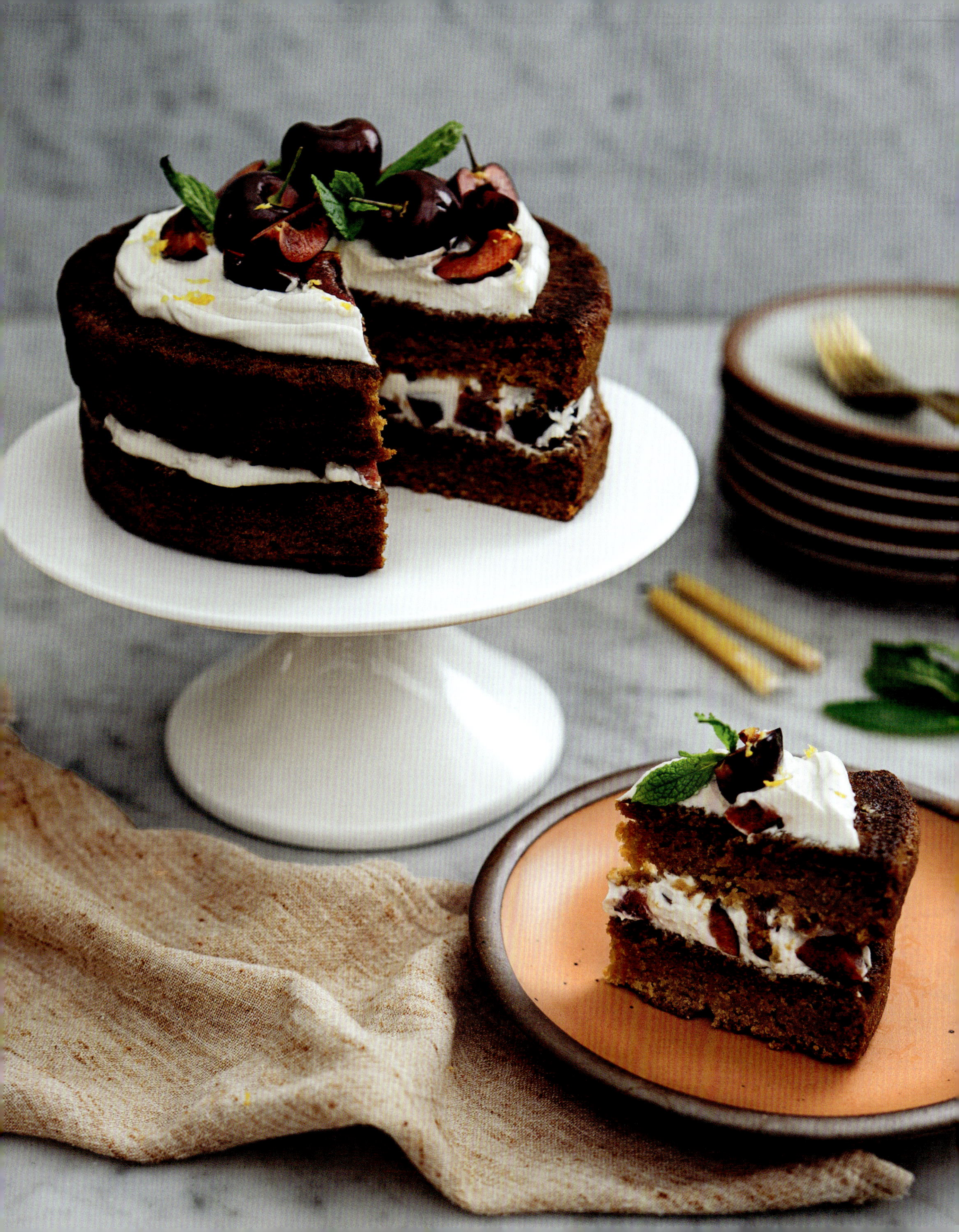

15 MINUTES
MAKES 1 CUP

Maple-Yogurt Cream

¾ cup plain unsweetened coconut yogurt (check ingredients)*

⅓ cup maple sugar

¾ teaspoon vanilla extract

**This recipe works best with a thick coconut yogurt. Look for brands that market their coconut yogurt as extra-thick or Greek-style for best results.*

1. Combine the yogurt, maple sugar, and vanilla in a large bowl and use an electric mixer or whisk to combine thoroughly. Use fresh or store in an airtight container in the refrigerator for up to 3 days.

2. Use this cream on Citrus and Cherry Celebration Cake (page 190) or Morning Glory Muffins (page 189) to turn them into cupcakes, or on a bowl of fresh fruit.

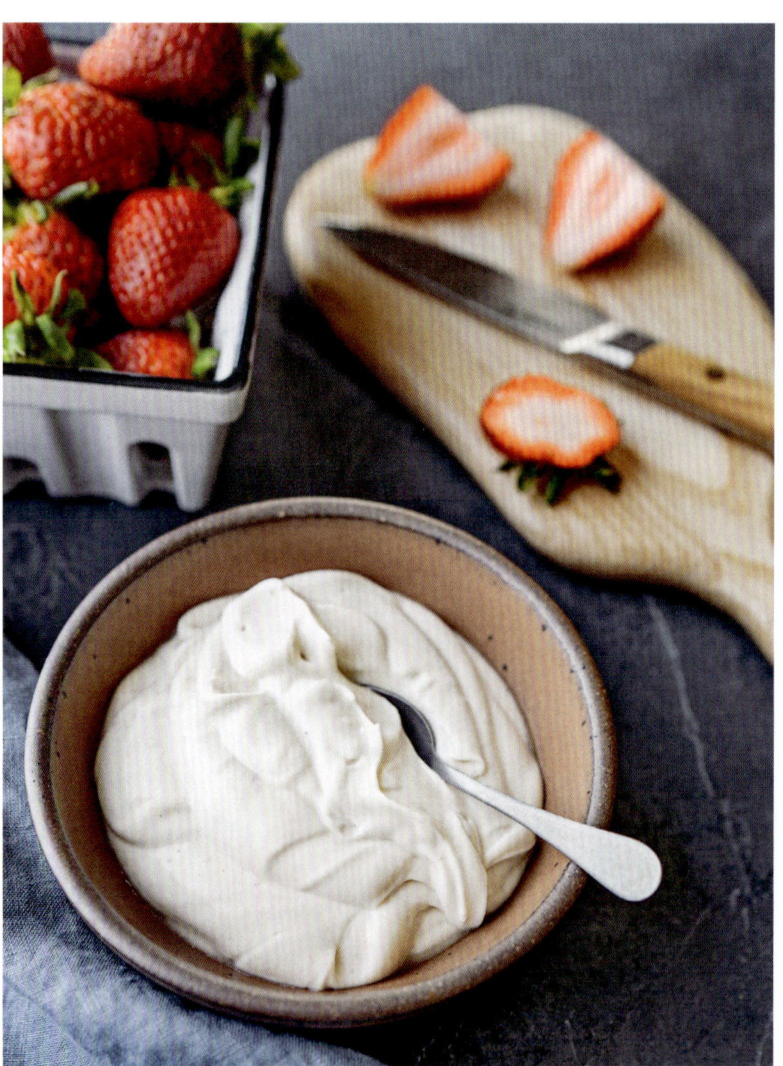

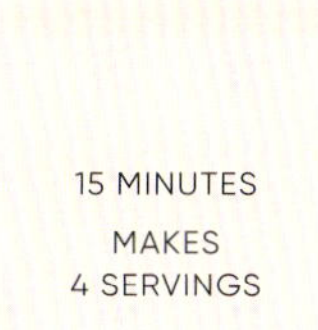

15 MINUTES

MAKES
4 SERVINGS

Avocado Blackberry Mousse

2 cups mashed avocado (2 to 3 medium avocados)

1½ cups blackberries (fresh or frozen)

⅓ cup honey

¼ cup blueberry, cranberry, or pomegranate juice

1 teaspoon vanilla extract

¼ teaspoon sea salt

Plain unsweetened coconut yogurt (check ingredients) and blackberries, for serving

1. Place the avocado, blackberries, honey, juice, vanilla, and salt in a food processor or high-powered blender and process until smooth.

2. Transfer to four small jars or containers and serve each with a scoop of coconut yogurt and fresh berries. If not serving immediately, cover and keep in the refrigerator for up to 3 days.

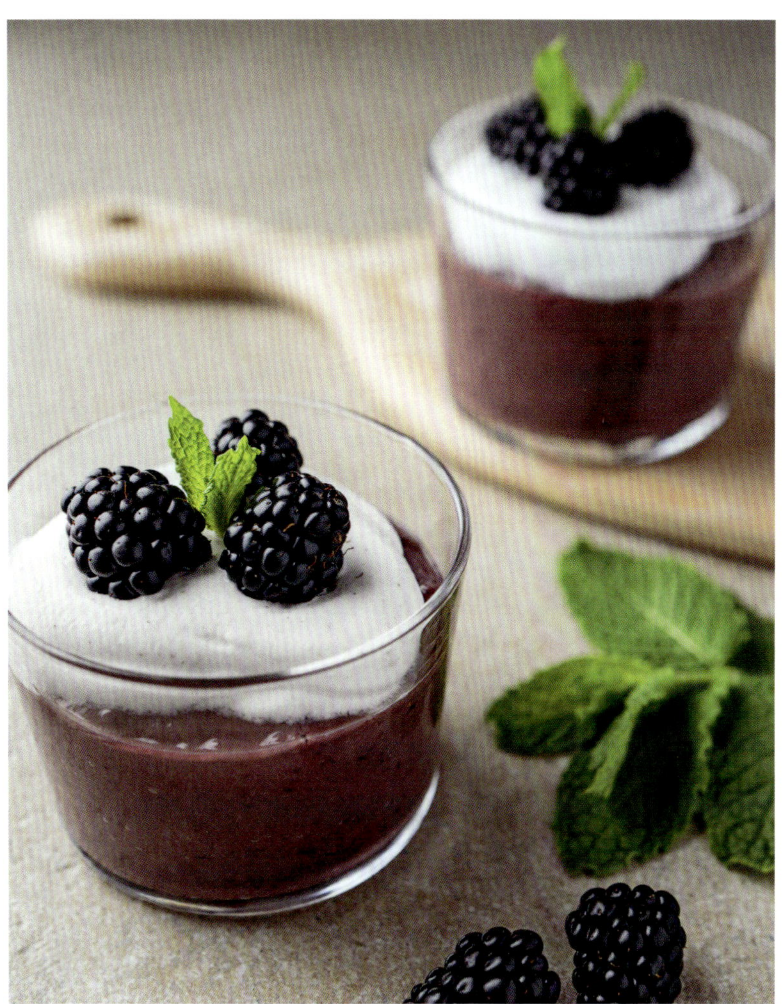

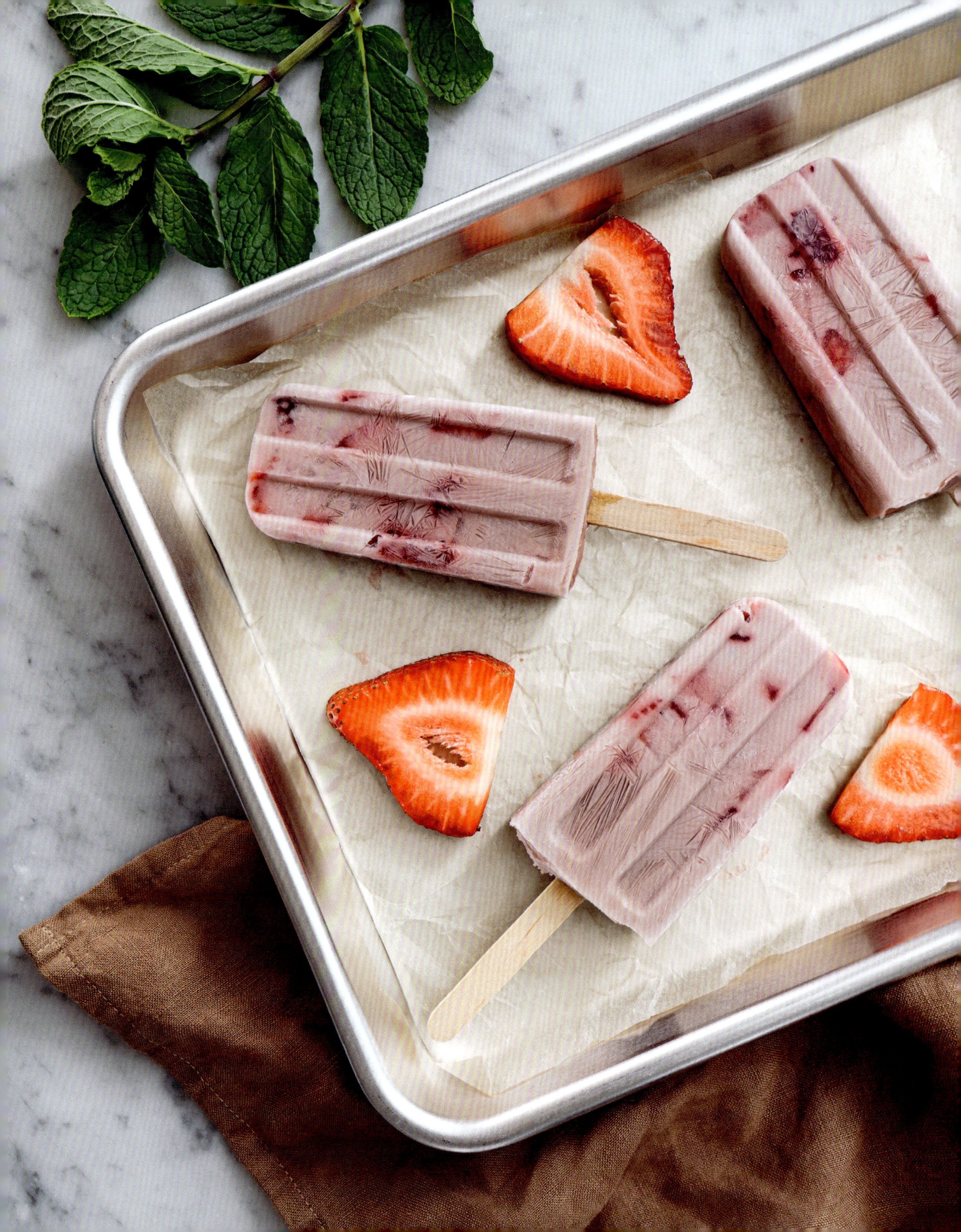

15 MINUTES, PLUS 6 HOURS TO FREEZE

MAKES 10 ICE POPS

Maple Strawberry Probiotic Pops

12 ounces plain unsweetened coconut yogurt (check ingredients)

¾ cup pomegranate or cranberry juice

⅓ cup maple syrup

1 teaspoon vanilla extract

Pinch sea salt

1½ cups diced strawberries

1. Place the yogurt, juice, maple syrup, vanilla, and salt in a medium bowl and whisk to combine. Set aside.

2. Spoon the strawberries into the bottom of your ice pop molds in equal portions, then pour the yogurt mixture about halfway into each mold. Use a stick to gently stir the bottom of each mold, incorporating the strawberries and yogurt mixture. Top off each mold with the yogurt mixture and add sticks.

3. Freeze for at least 6 hours before enjoying. They keep for up to 1 month in an airtight container in the freezer.

CHAPTER 12

Core AIP 4-Week Meal Plan and Shopping Lists

In this chapter you'll find four complete weeks of done-for-you meal plans and corresponding shopping lists to help you get started right away. Some notes:

- **Servings:** Each week of the meal plans serve one person for generous servings of breakfasts, lunches, and dinners. If you find the quantities are too large, freeze any extra servings for later. (If you need a meal plan that serves two people, visit THEAUTOIMMUNEPROTOCOL.COM/PRINTABLES for a downloadable meal plan that serves two.)
- **Schedule:** Cooking from scratch is mostly required on nights and weekends; many meals simply need to be reheated or assembled quickly. Scratch-cooked meals are noted in color and bold type with the corresponding page number for the recipe. Meals to be eaten as leftovers are shown in regular font.
- **Prep day:** The day before the meal plan starts and every subsequent Sunday is designated as prep day—most weeks you'll do some extra batch-cooking on these days. Take note of which meals are to be prepped ahead on prep day.
- **Bone broth:** You can either purchase or make broth for cooking recipes called for in the plans (see page 119 for my recipe). Bones are on the shopping lists, but you can eliminate them if you purchase or have a stash of broth already.
- **Storage:** You will need to freeze and thaw portions of meals for use later in the meal plan; it is always handy to freeze in single-serving portions, but I've noted where you can freeze three or four servings together if you want. I've given you two days' thawing time for single portions of meals that will need only a quick reheat when the time comes to enjoy them. You can reduce this if you use a microwave to quickly thaw your meals.

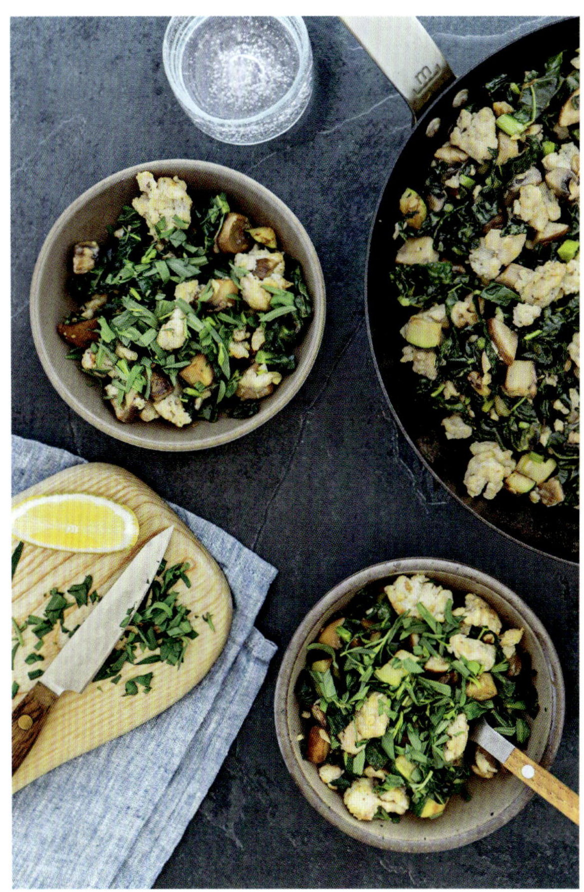

- **Shopping for fresh items:** You will need to shop before cooking dinner on Sundays and Wednesdays—if you want to shop on different days, adjust accordingly. Always cross-reference your shopping list with what you have left over from the previous shopping session to make sure you don't buy anything you may still have in stock (especially things like lemons or fresh herbs).
- **Shopping for pantry items:** Before each shopping session, compare the provided shopping list with items you have in your pantry and add as needed.

CORE AIP MEAL PLAN: Week 1

	BREAKFAST	LUNCH	DINNER	NOTES
SUNDAY PREP	**LEMONGRASS GINGER BREAKFAST SOUP,** page 143 **MAPLE LIME STEAK AND RADICCHIO SALAD,** page 157 **HEALING BONE BROTH,** page 119 (optional)			*Freeze 4 portions of Lemongrass Ginger Breakfast Soup (3 together and 1 individually)* *Portion 2 cups of broth to keep in the refrigerator for use next week; freeze the rest*
MONDAY	Lemongrass Ginger Breakfast Soup	Maple Lime Steak and Radicchio Salad	**NOURISHING CORE CHILI,** page 150	*Freeze 2 portions of Nourishing Core Chili (together or individually)*
TUESDAY	Lemongrass Ginger Breakfast Soup	Maple Lime Steak and Radicchio Salad	Nourishing Core Chili	
WEDNESDAY	Lemongrass Ginger Breakfast Soup	Maple Lime Steak and Radicchio Salad	Nourishing Core Chili	
THURSDAY	Lemongrass Ginger Breakfast Soup	Maple Lime Steak and Radicchio Salad	**PORK TENDERLOIN WITH CABBAGE,** page 172	
FRIDAY	**LEMON TARRAGON TURKEY SKILLET,** page 137	Pork Tenderloin with Cabbage	**CURRIED BEEF VEGETABLE PIE,** page 171	*Freeze 4 portions of Curried Beef Vegetable Pie (together or individually)*
SATURDAY	Lemon Tarragon Turkey Skillet	Pork Tenderloin with Cabbage	Curried Beef Vegetable Pie	
SUNDAY	Lemon Tarragon Turkey Skillet	Pork Tenderloin with Cabbage	Curried Beef Vegetable Pie	
SUNDAY PREP	**NUTRIVORE BREAKFAST BATCH COOK,** page 144 **BACON CHICKEN RANCH SALAD,** page 153			*These meals can be batch-cooked anytime on Sunday for the following week*

CORE AIP MEAL PLAN: Week 2

	BREAKFAST	LUNCH	DINNER	NOTES
MONDAY	Nutrivore Breakfast	Bacon Chicken Ranch Salad	Curried Beef Vegetable Pie	
TUESDAY	Nutrivore Breakfast	Bacon Chicken Ranch Salad	**RUSTIC CHICKEN AND KALE STEW,** page 149	*Freeze 3 portions of Rustic Chicken Stew (together or individually)*
WEDNESDAY	Nutrivore Breakfast	Bacon Chicken Ranch Salad	Rustic Chicken and Kale Stew	*Pull out 2 portions of Nourishing Core Chili to thaw for Friday*
THURSDAY	Nutrivore Breakfast	Bacon Chicken Ranch Salad	Rustic Chicken and Kale Stew	
FRIDAY	Nutrivore Breakfast	Nourishing Core Chili	**CHICKEN NOODLE PESTO BOWL,** page 169	
SATURDAY	Nutrivore Breakfast	Nourishing Core Chili	Chicken Noodle Pesto Bowl	
SUNDAY	**PORK BREAKFAST SKILLET,** page 139	Chicken Noodle Pesto Bowl	**HERB ROASTED SALMON WITH ASPARAGUS,** page 180	*Pull out 4 portions of Curried Beef Vegetable Pie to thaw for Tuesday*

CORE AIP MEAL PLAN: Week 3

	BREAKFAST	LUNCH	DINNER	NOTES
MONDAY	Pork Breakfast Skillet	Chicken Noodle Pesto Bowl	Herb Roasted Salmon with Asparagus	*Pull out 3 portions of Lemongrass Ginger Breakfast Soup to thaw for Wednesday*
TUESDAY	Pork Breakfast Skillet	Herb Roasted Salmon with Asparagus	Curried Beef Vegetable Pie	
WEDNESDAY	Lemongrass Ginger Breakfast Soup	Herb Roasted Salmon with Asparagus	Curried Beef Vegetable Pie	
THURSDAY	Lemongrass Ginger Breakfast Soup	Curried Beef Vegetable Pie	**HEARTY PORK AND CABBAGE STEW,** page 158	*Freeze 3 portions of Hearty Pork and Cabbage Stew (together or individually)* *Pull out 3 portions of Rustic Chicken and Kale Stew to thaw for Saturday*
FRIDAY	Lemongrass Ginger Breakfast Soup	Curried Beef Vegetable Pie	Hearty Pork and Cabbage Stew	
SATURDAY	**SALMON AND APPLE BREAKFAST BOWL,** page 135	Hearty Pork and Cabbage Stew	Rustic Chicken and Kale Stew	
SUNDAY	Salmon and Apple Breakfast Bowl	Rustic Chicken and Kale Stew	**ONE-PAN ROASTED CHICKEN WITH BROCCOLINI AND LEMON,** page 175	*Pull out 3 portions of Hearty Cabbage Stew to thaw for Tuesday*
SUNDAY PREP	**NUTRIVORE BREAKFAST BATCH COOK,** page 144			*This meal can be batch-cooked anytime on Sunday for the following week*

CORE AIP MEAL PLAN: Week 4

	BREAKFAST	LUNCH	DINNER	NOTES
MONDAY	Nutrivore Breakfast	Rustic Chicken and Kale Stew	One-Pan Roasted Chicken with Broccolini and Lemon	
TUESDAY	Nutrivore Breakfast	One-Pan Roasted Chicken with Broccolini and Lemoni	Hearty Pork and Cabbage Stew	
WEDNESDAY	Nutrivore Breakfast	One-Pan Roasted Chicken with Broccolini and Lemoni	Hearty Pork and Cabbage Stew	
THURSDAY	Nutrivore Breakfast	Hearty Pork and Cabbage Stew	**BACON CHICKEN RANCH SALAD,** page 153	
FRIDAY	Nutrivore Breakfast	**ZESTY ORANGE GINGER BEEF AND BROCCOLI BOWL,** page 179	**CAULI-SHRIMP STIR-FRY,** page 167	*Pull out 1 portion of Lemongrass Ginger Breakfast Soup to thaw for Sunday*
SATURDAY	Nutrivore Breakfast	Zesty Orange Ginger Beef and Broccoli Bowl	Cauli-Shrimp Stir-Fry	
SUNDAY	Lemongrass Ginger Breakfast Soup	Zesty Orange Ginger Beef and Broccoli Bowl	Cauli-Shrimp Stir-Fry	

CORE AIP SHOPPING LIST: Week 1

PANTRY ITEMS

OILS/VINEGARS
- ☐ Apple cider vinegar
- ☐ Avocado oil
- ☐ Olive oil

SPICES
- ☐ Baking soda
- ☐ Bay leaves
- ☐ Cinnamon (ground)
- ☐ Garlic powder
- ☐ Ginger powder
- ☐ Onion powder
- ☐ Sea salt
- ☐ Tamarind paste
- ☐ Turmeric powder

OTHER
- ☐ Fish sauce
- ☐ Honey
- ☐ Maple syrup
- ☐ Unsweetened, dried tart cherries or raisins (check ingredients)

BROTH
- ☐ 2 cups bone broth, homemade (page 119) or store-bought

SUNDAY

MEAT
- ☐ 3 pounds bone-in, skin-on chicken thighs
- ☐ 1½ pounds 1-inch-thick flank steak
- ☐ 1 pound ground beef
- ☐ 1 pound ground pork
- ☐ 4 slices thick-cut uncured bacon (check ingredients)

PRODUCE
- ☐ 2 yellow onions
- ☐ 2 large sweet potatoes
- ☐ 3 large carrots
- ☐ 1 beet
- ☐ 1 bunch celery
- ☐ 2 large zucchinis
- ☐ 5 ounces spinach
- ☐ 5 ounces arugula
- ☐ 1 head radicchio
- ☐ 2 bunches green onions
- ☐ 12 ounces button mushrooms
- ☐ 1 lemon
- ☐ 1 lime
- ☐ 2 avocados

HERBS AND SPICES
- ☐ 1 head garlic
- ☐ 4 inches fresh ginger
- ☐ 3 lemongrass stalks
- ☐ Fresh oregano (¼ cup)
- ☐ Fresh rosemary

OTHER
- ☐ 1 (14-ounce) can pumpkin puree

WEDNESDAY

MEAT
- ☐ 1½ pounds pork tenderloin
- ☐ 2 pounds ground beef
- ☐ 1 pound ground turkey

PRODUCE
- ☐ 1 yellow onion
- ☐ 4 shallots
- ☐ 2 pounds light-fleshed sweet potatoes
- ☐ 1 small sweet potato
- ☐ 2 pounds parsnips
- ☐ 1 large carrot
- ☐ 1½ pounds red cabbage (½ a whole cabbage)
- ☐ 1 large or 2 small zucchinis
- ☐ 1 bunch Tuscan kale
- ☐ 1 pound mushrooms
- ☐ 1 lemon
- ☐ 1 green apple

HERBS AND SPICES
- ☐ 1 head garlic
- ☐ 1 bunch cilantro
- ☐ Fresh tarragon (¼ cup)
- ☐ Fresh thyme

CORE AIP SHOPPING LIST: Week 2

PANTRY ITEMS

OILS/VINEGARS

- ☐ Apple cider vinegar
- ☐ Avocado oil
- ☐ Olive oil

SPICES

- ☐ Bay leaves
- ☐ Cinnamon (ground)
- ☐ Garlic powder
- ☐ Ginger powder
- ☐ Onion powder
- ☐ Sea salt

OTHER

- ☐ Coconut aminos

BROTH

- ☐ ½ cup bone broth, homemade (page 119) or store-bought

SUNDAY

MEAT

- ☐ 3 pounds bone-in, skin-on chicken thighs
- ☐ 1½ pounds chicken breasts
- ☐ 1 pound ground beef
- ☐ 1 pound ground pork
- ☐ 4 slices thick-cut uncured bacon (check ingredients)

PRODUCE

- ☐ 1 yellow onion
- ☐ 1 red onion
- ☐ 3 pounds sweet potatoes
- ☐ 3 carrots
- ☐ 1 small beet
- ☐ 3 bunches kale
- ☐ 1 large head romaine lettuce
- ☐ 1 bunch radishes
- ☐ 2 lemons
- ☐ 5 avocados

HERBS

- ☐ 1 head garlic
- ☐ Fresh dill
- ☐ Fresh oregano
- ☐ Fresh parsley
- ☐ Fresh thyme

OTHER

- ☐ 12 ounces sauerkraut or other fermented vegetables, homemade (page 120) or store-bought (check ingredients)
- ☐ 4 ounces plain unsweetened coconut yogurt (check ingredients)
- ☐ 4 ounces olives (check ingredients)

WEDNESDAY

MEAT

- ☐ 1½ pounds boneless, skinless chicken thighs
- ☐ 1 pound ground pork

PRODUCE

- ☐ 1 yellow onion
- ☐ 3 shallots
- ☐ 1 sweet potato
- ☐ 2 carrots
- ☐ 2 zucchinis
- ☐ 8 ounces mushrooms
- ☐ 2 limes

HERBS

- ☐ 1 bunch cilantro
- ☐ Fresh marjoram (or sub oregano)

CORE AIP SHOPPING LIST: Week 3

PANTRY ITEMS

OILS/VINEGARS
- ☐ Olive oil

SPICES
- ☐ Bay leaves
- ☐ Sea salt

BROTH
- ☐ 3 cups bone broth, homemade (page 119) or store-bought

SUNDAY

MEAT
- ☐ 1½ pounds salmon fillet, skin-on

PRODUCE
- ☐ 1 large head cauliflower
- ☐ 1 bunch thin asparagus spears
- ☐ 1 bunch green onions
- ☐ 1 lemon

HERBS
- ☐ 1 head garlic
- ☐ 1 bunch cilantro
- ☐ Fresh parsley
- ☐ Fresh mint

WEDNESDAY

MEAT
- ☐ 2 pounds ground pork
- ☐ 2 (6-ounce) cans boneless, skinless salmon

PRODUCE
- ☐ 1 yellow onion
- ☐ 2 large carrots
- ☐ 2 large parsnips
- ☐ ½ green cabbage
- ☐ 1 bunch celery
- ☐ 1 bunch green onions
- ☐ 1 lemon
- ☐ 1 avocado
- ☐ 1 green apple

HERBS
- ☐ Fresh dill

OTHER
- ☐ 8 ounces sauerkraut, homemade (page 120) or store-bought (check ingredients)
- ☐ 4 ounces plain unsweetened coconut yogurt (check ingredients)

CORE AIP SHOPPING LIST: Week 4

PANTRY ITEMS

OILS/VINEGARS

- ☐ Apple cider vinegar
- ☐ Avocado oil
- ☐ Olive oil

SPICES

- ☐ Cinnamon (ground)
- ☐ Garlic powder
- ☐ Ginger powder
- ☐ Onion powder
- ☐ Sea salt

OTHER

- ☐ Coconut aminos

BROTH

- ☐ ½ cup bone broth, homemade (page 119) or store-bought

SUNDAY

MEAT

- ☐ 3 pounds bone-in, skin-on chicken thighs
- ☐ 1 pound ground beef
- ☐ 1 pound ground pork

PRODUCE

- ☐ 1 red onion
- ☐ 3 pounds sweet potatoes
- ☐ 1 pound carrots
- ☐ 2 bunches kale
- ☐ 1 pound Broccolini
- ☐ 1 lemon
- ☐ 3 avocados

HERBS

- ☐ Fresh oregano
- ☐ Fresh thyme

OTHER

- ☐ 12 ounces sauerkraut or fermented vegetables, homemade (page 120) or store-bought (check ingredients)

WEDNESDAY

MEAT

- ☐ 1½ pounds chicken breast
- ☐ 1 pound medium shrimp, peeled, deveined and without tails
- ☐ 4 slices thick-cut uncured bacon (check ingredients)

PRODUCE

- ☐ 1 red onion
- ☐ 1 white onion
- ☐ 1 large head romaine lettuce
- ☐ 14 ounces frozen riced cauliflower
- ☐ 6 ounces shiitake mushrooms (or sub button mushrooms)
- ☐ 1 bunch radishes
- ☐ 1 bunch green onions
- ☐ 1 lemon
- ☐ 2 avocados

HERBS

- ☐ 1 head garlic
- ☐ 1 inch fresh ginger
- ☐ Fresh dill
- ☐ Fresh parsley
- ☐ Fresh cilantro (for garnish)

OTHER

- ☐ 4 ounces plain unsweetened coconut yogurt (check ingredients)

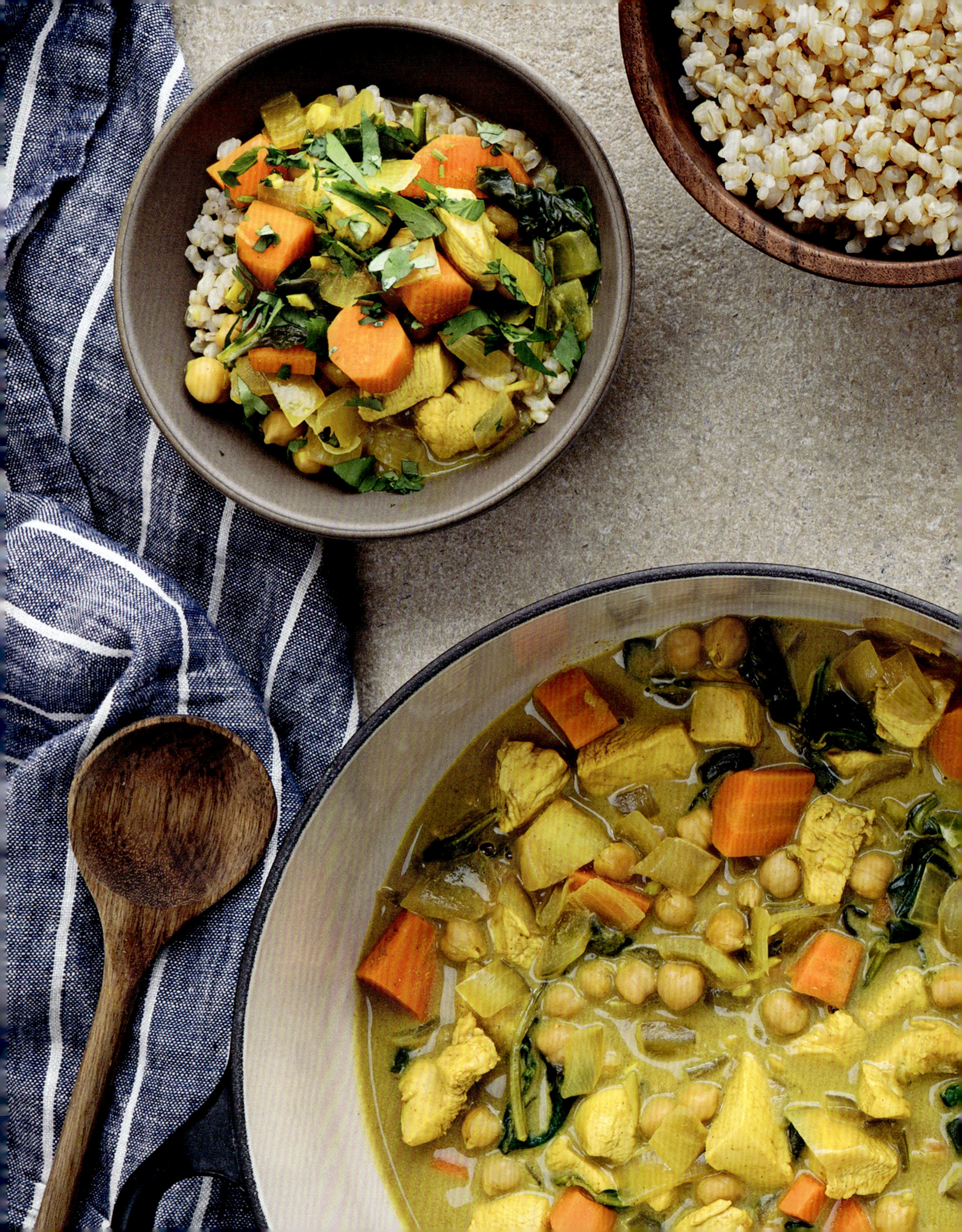

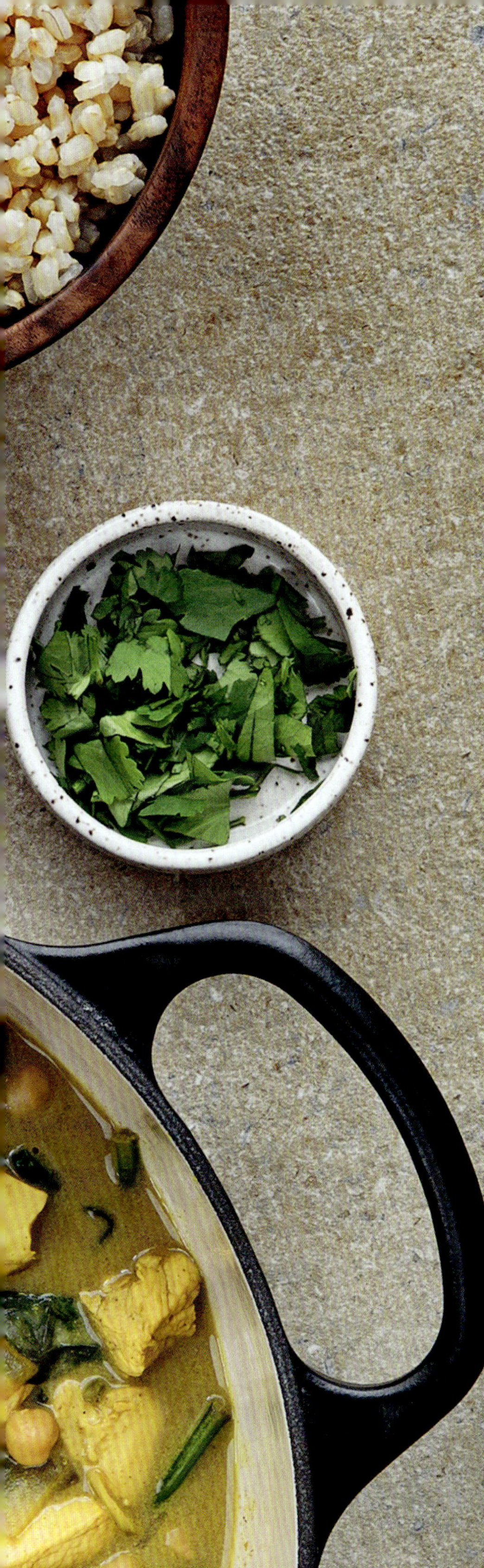

PART III

Modified AIP Recipe Collection

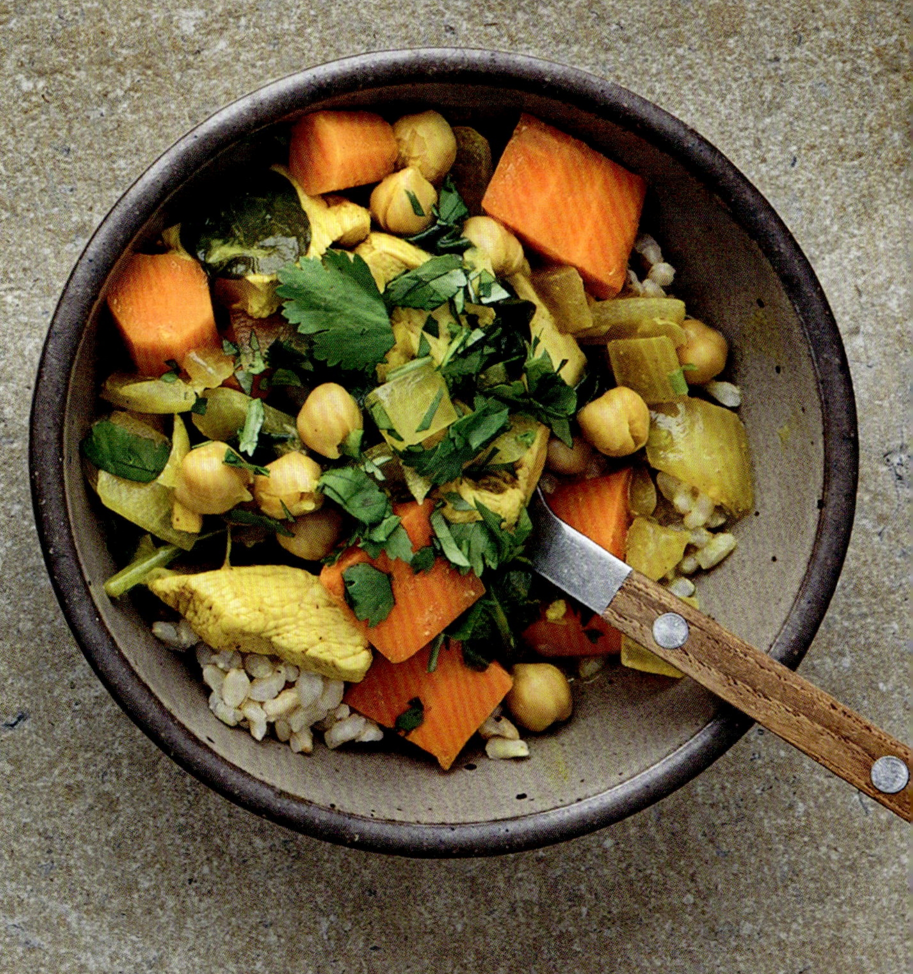

Welcome to the Modified AIP recipe collection, where I've gathered all my favorite recipes that incorporate the additional foods included in this version of the elimination diet—ghee, rice, pseudo-grains, legumes, and seeds. Just as with the Core AIP collection, these recipes were crafted with a focus on foods that promote healing while offering lots of variety as you maintain your Modified AIP elimination phase.

The inclusion of a few more ingredients allows you to conveniently start your day with a nourishing *Cherry-Cacao Shake* (page 222) or a comforting *Chicken and Black Bean Breakfast Bowl* (page 221), and for dinner, enjoy something heartier, like *Savory Beef and Bean Chili* (page 235) or the aromatic *Thai-Inspired Sunflower Shrimp* (page 251). Whether you're craving a rich dessert, like *Spiced Pear Upside-Down Cake* (page 270), or looking for a satisfying, quick meal, like *Verdant Lentil Vegetable Soup* (page 242), this collection offers the tools to maintain your health while embracing new flavors and textures along your Modified AIP journey.

A reminder: If you are on Core AIP, even though these recipes aren't included during your elimination phase, they come in handy when it is time for you to start reintroductions and expand your diet.

CHAPTER 13

Modified Basics

30 MINUTES

MAKES
1½ CUPS

Homemade Ghee (Clarified Butter)

1 pound unsalted butter, cut into 1-inch pieces

Cheesecloth, for straining

1. Place the butter in a heavy-bottomed saucepan over medium-low heat. Melt the butter completely.

2. Once the butter has melted, allow it to come to a gentle simmer. It will start to bubble as the water content evaporates. Turn the heat to low to maintain a gentle simmer and cook for 10 to 15 minutes.

3. After the butter has simmered for enough time, the milk solids will begin to separate. The butter will turn golden and the milk solids will start sinking to the bottom while a foamy layer forms on top. When you reach this stage, stir often to prevent burning.

4. Once the milk solids turn light brown, the liquid is clear and golden, and it has a nutty aroma, your ghee is finished cooking. Remove from the heat and carefully pour the ghee through a cheesecloth into a container. Discard the solids.

5. Let the ghee cool completely before sealing the jar. Use ghee for sautéing, roasting, and stir-frying. Store at room temperature for up to 3 months or refrigerate for up to 1 year.

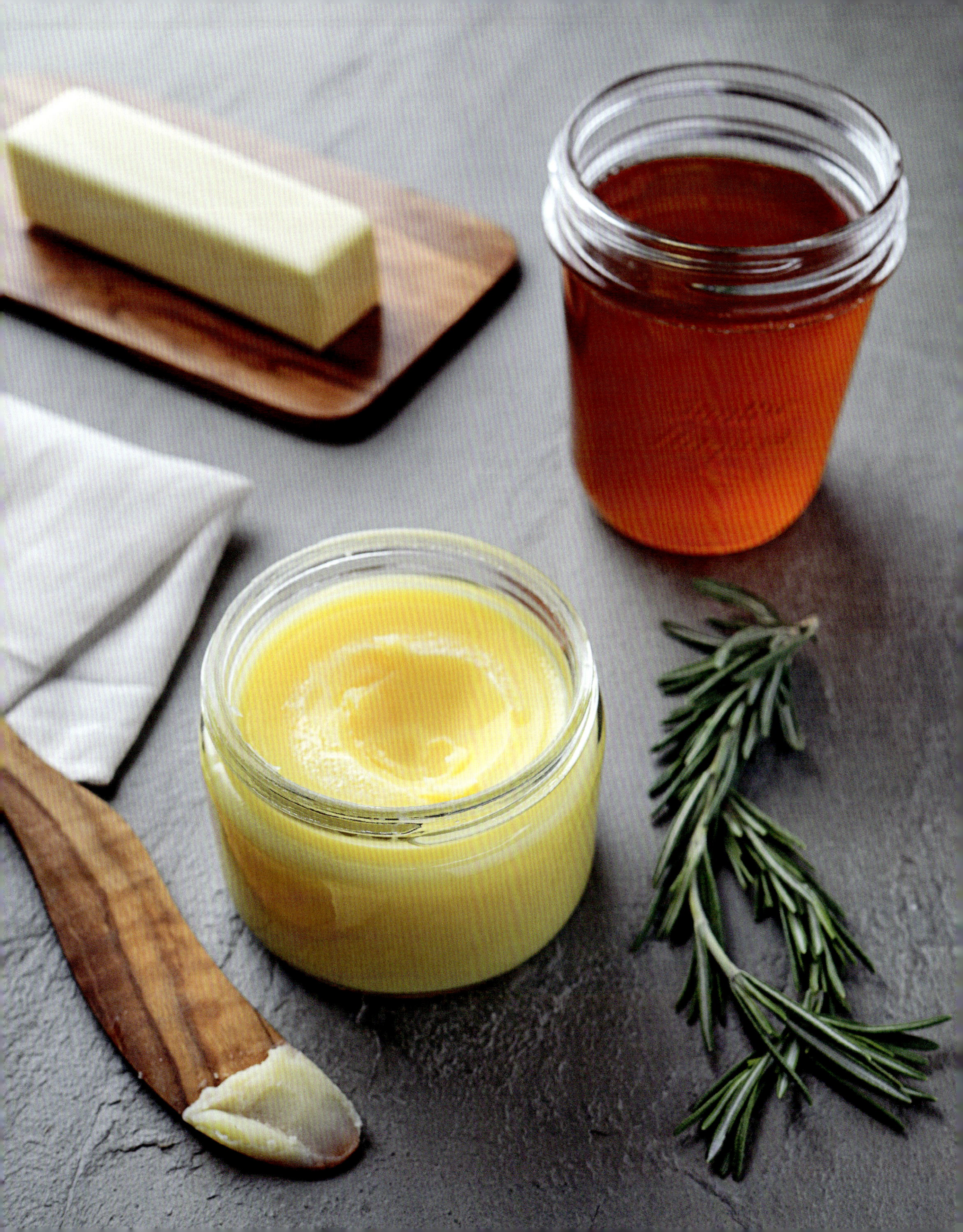

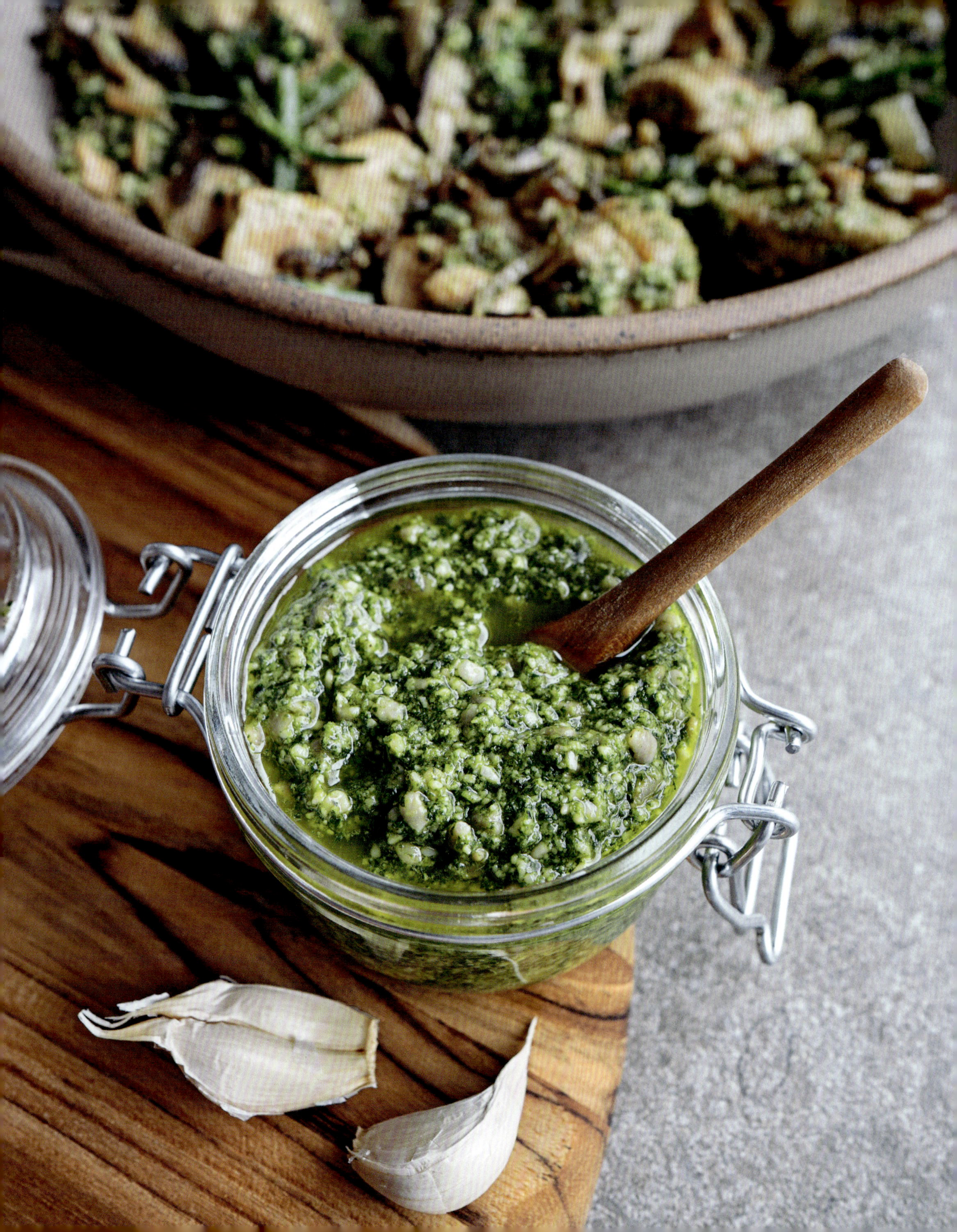

5 MINUTES
MAKES 2 CUPS

Sunflower Seed Pesto

4 ounces fresh basil (about 4 cups)

1 ounce fresh mint (about 1 cup)

2 garlic cloves

1 cup olive oil

3 tablespoons lemon juice (about 1 lemon)

1 teaspoon sea salt

1 cup sunflower seeds, divided

1. Place the basil, mint, garlic, oil, lemon juice, salt, and ½ cup of the sunflower seeds in a blender or food processor and blend on high speed for 15 seconds, stopping to scrape the sides if needed. Once the herbs are fully processed, add the remaining sunflower seeds and pulse to combine until a slightly chunky texture remains.

2. Use the pesto as a flavorful topping for grilled or sautéed meats or roasted vegetables, or with noodles compliant with the elimination phase. If not using immediately, transfer to a storage container and keep in the refrigerator for up to 5 days.

Hummus

15 MINUTES

MAKES
6 SERVINGS

2 (14-ounce) cans chickpeas, drained and rinsed

½ cup tahini (sesame butter)

½ cup olive oil

4 garlic cloves

⅓ cup lemon juice (about 3 lemons)

1½ teaspoons sea salt

Fresh parsley and additional olive oil, for garnish

1. Place the chickpeas, tahini, oil, garlic, lemon juice, and salt in a food processor and process on high speed for about 1 minute, stopping to scrape the sides of the bowl if needed. Continue to process until a smooth paste forms; if it's too thick, add water 1 tablespoon at a time until desired consistency is reached.

2. If not using immediately, transfer to a storage container and keep in the refrigerator for up to 1 week. Serve garnished with parsley and a drizzle of oil.

Super Seed Crackers

1 HOUR
45 MINUTES

MAKES
6 SERVINGS

¾ cup sunflower seeds

⅓ cup flax seeds

⅓ cup sesame seeds

¼ cup pumpkin seeds

2 tablespoons chia seeds

1 cup boiling water

¼ cup tapioca flour (or substitute arrowroot starch)

1 tablespoon ground flax seeds

¾ teaspoon sea salt

¼ cup olive or avocado oil

1. Preheat the oven to 300°F. Line a large baking sheet with parchment paper and set aside.

2. In a medium bowl, combine the sunflower, flax, sesame, pumpkin, and chia seeds. Add the boiling water, stir, and allow to sit for 10 minutes.

3. Meanwhile, in a small bowl, combine the tapioca flour, ground flax, and salt and stir to combine. When the seeds are finished soaking, add the flour mixture and oil and stir to combine until a thick mixture forms. Spread out on the baking sheet, using a spatula to work as evenly as possible throughout the entire surface, avoiding gaps or holes. Once the spread is even, use the spatula to gently push down the seeds and create a flat surface. The more even your spread, the more even your crackers will turn out.

4. Bake for 75 to 90 minutes, rotating the pan once or twice. The crackers will start to brown and firm up when they are finished. Allow to cool in the pan for 10 minutes, then carefully transfer to a cutting board using the parchment paper and cut into rectangles. Allow to cool completely. They keep in a sealed container at room temperature for up to 2 weeks.

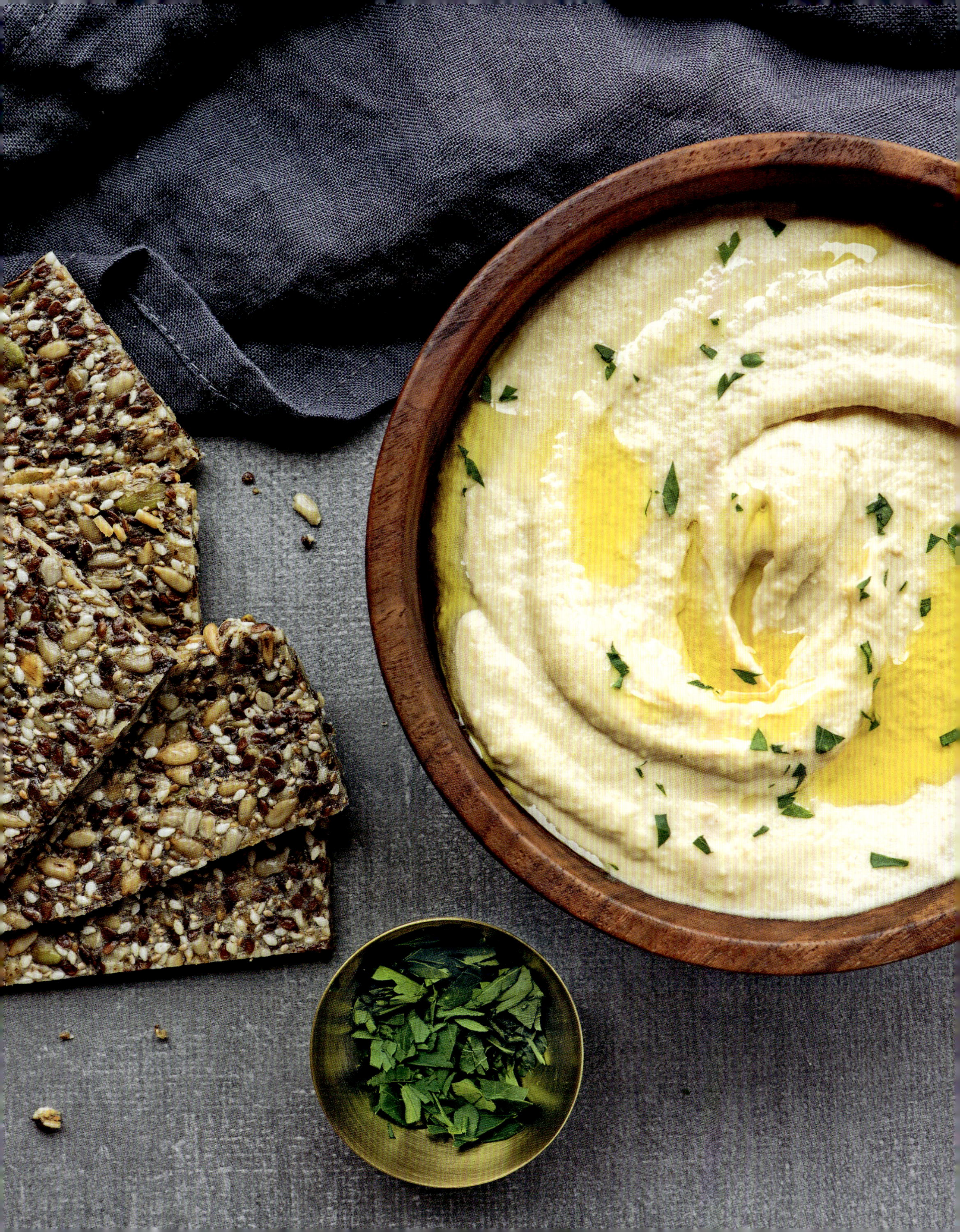

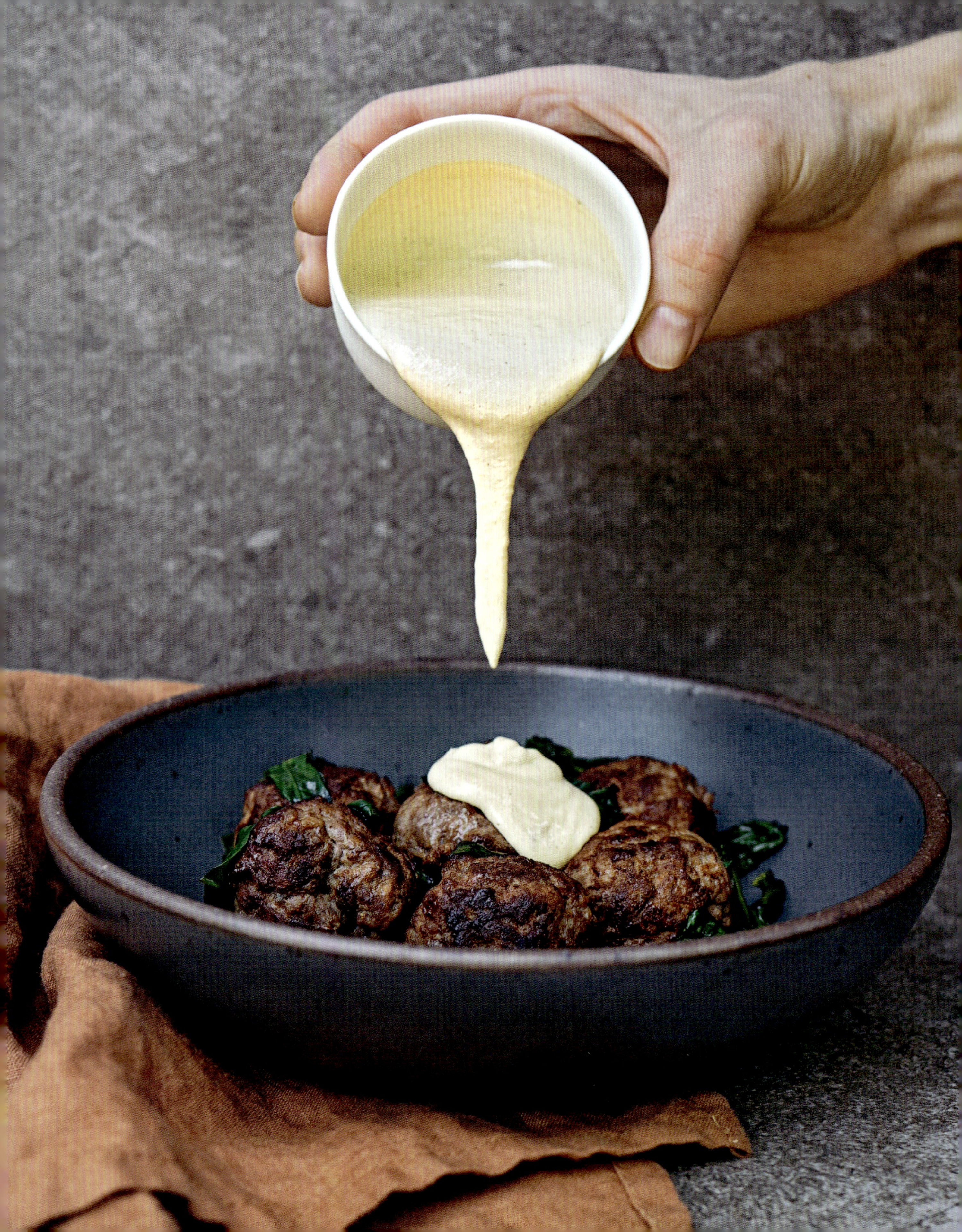

15 MINUTES
MAKES 1 CUP

Tahini Ginger Sauce

½ cup tahini (sesame butter)

⅓ cup lemon juice
(from about 3 lemons)

¼ cup water, plus more if needed

1 garlic clove

1 teaspoon minced ginger
(from a 1-inch piece of root)

1 tablespoon honey

½ teaspoon sea salt

1. Place all the ingredients in a blender and blend until smooth. Add additional water 1 tablespoon at a time until desired consistency is reached.

2. Use the sauce to drizzle over meats, vegetables, salad, or noodles compliant with the elimination phase. If not using immediately, transfer to a storage container and keep in the refrigerator for up to 1 week.

CHAPTER 14

Modified Breakfasts

Buckwheat Breakfast Porridge

15 MINUTES (AFTER OVERNIGHT SOAKING)

MAKES 4 SERVINGS

1 cup buckwheat groats, soaked overnight*

1 (14-ounce) can coconut milk (check ingredients)

¼ teaspoon sea salt

¼ cup hulled hemp seeds

¼ cup ground flax seeds

1 serving plain pea, hemp, or rice protein powder

3 tablespoons coconut or maple sugar

½ teaspoon ground cinnamon

Fresh fruit, coconut yogurt (check ingredients), seeds, and/or coconut flakes, for serving

**The night before, place the buckwheat in a container with 2 cups of water and store in the refrigerator. When it is time to make the recipe, drain and rinse the buckwheat well.*

1. Place the soaked, drained, and rinsed buckwheat in a large saucepan along with the coconut milk and salt and bring to a boil over high heat. Turn down the heat to maintain a simmer and cook, covered, for 10 minutes.

2. Stir in the hemp seeds, ground flax, protein powder, coconut sugar, and cinnamon. If the mixture is too thick for your liking, you can add some more water until the desired consistency is reached.

3. Serve with any desired toppings, such as fresh fruit, coconut yogurt, seeds or seed butters, or coconut flakes. The porridge keeps in the refrigerator for up to 5 days.

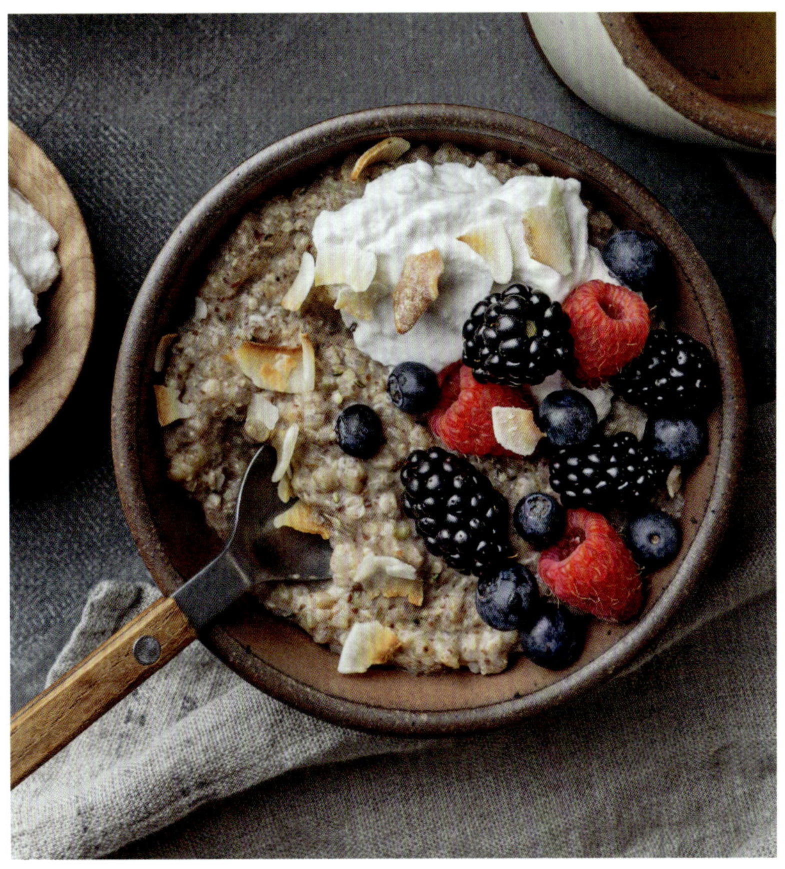

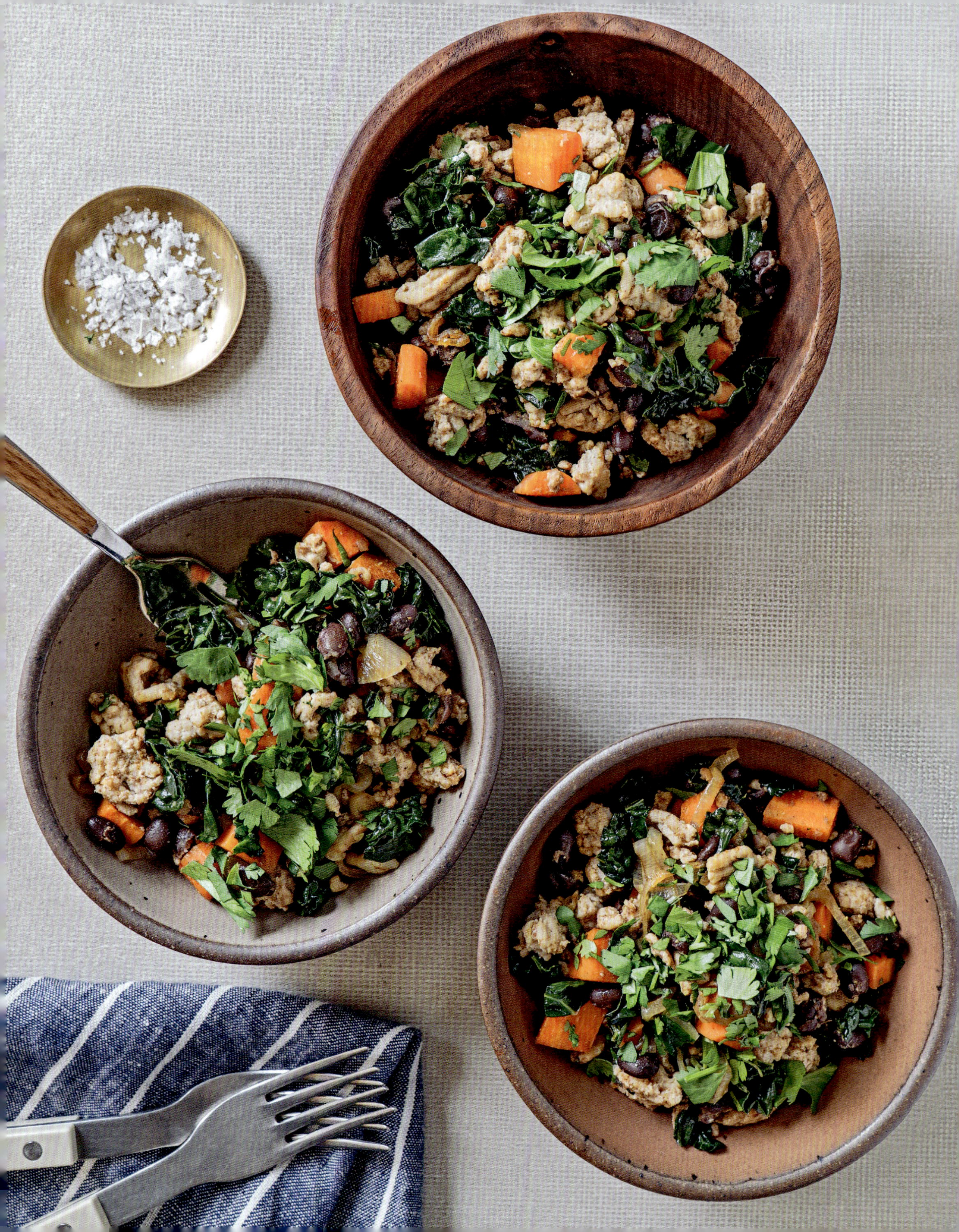

30 MINUTES

MAKES
3 SERVINGS

Chicken and Black Bean Breakfast Bowl

3 tablespoons avocado oil, divided

2 shallots, thinly sliced

2 carrots, chopped (about 2 cups)

1 bunch kale, stemmed and sliced into thin ribbons

1 teaspoon sea salt, divided

1 pound ground chicken

1 (14-ounce) can black beans, drained and rinsed

1 teaspoon ground cumin

½ teaspoon ground coriander

¼ teaspoon ground cinnamon

¼ teaspoon ground black pepper

1 tablespoon apple cider vinegar

Fresh cilantro, for garnish (optional)

1. Heat 1 tablespoon of the oil in a large skillet over medium heat. When the pan is hot, add the shallots and cook, stirring, for 3 minutes, or until beginning to brown. Add the carrots and cook for another 3 minutes, stirring occasionally. Add the kale and ½ teaspoon of the salt and cook for 3 more minutes, or until the kale is wilted and the carrots are cooked. Transfer to a bowl and set aside.

2. In the same skillet, heat the remaining 2 tablespoons oil over medium heat. Add the chicken, quickly stirring and breaking it up into pieces. Cook for 3 to 5 minutes, until the chicken is fully cooked throughout. Add the black beans, the remaining ½ teaspoon salt, the cumin, coriander, cinnamon, and pepper to the mixture. Stir to combine thoroughly and cook for another 2 minutes.

3. Add the vinegar, return the vegetables to the skillet, and stir to combine. When warmed and incorporated, turn off the heat. Serve topped with cilantro, if using. It keeps for up to 5 days in the refrigerator.

5 MINUTES
MAKES 2 CUPS

Super Berry Protein Smoothie

1¼ cups cranberry or pomegranate juice

1 medium banana

¾ cup frozen blueberries

1 serving plain pea, hemp, or rice protein powder

1 tablespoon ground flax seeds

Place all the ingredients in a blender and blend until smooth. Serve immediately.

5 MINUTES
MAKES 2 CUPS

Cherry-Cacao Shake

½ cup plain unsweetened coconut yogurt (check ingredients)

¾ cup water

1 medium banana

1 serving plain pea, hemp, or rice protein powder

1 tablespoon cacao powder

¾ cup frozen sweet cherries

Place all the ingredients in a blender and blend until smooth. Serve immediately.

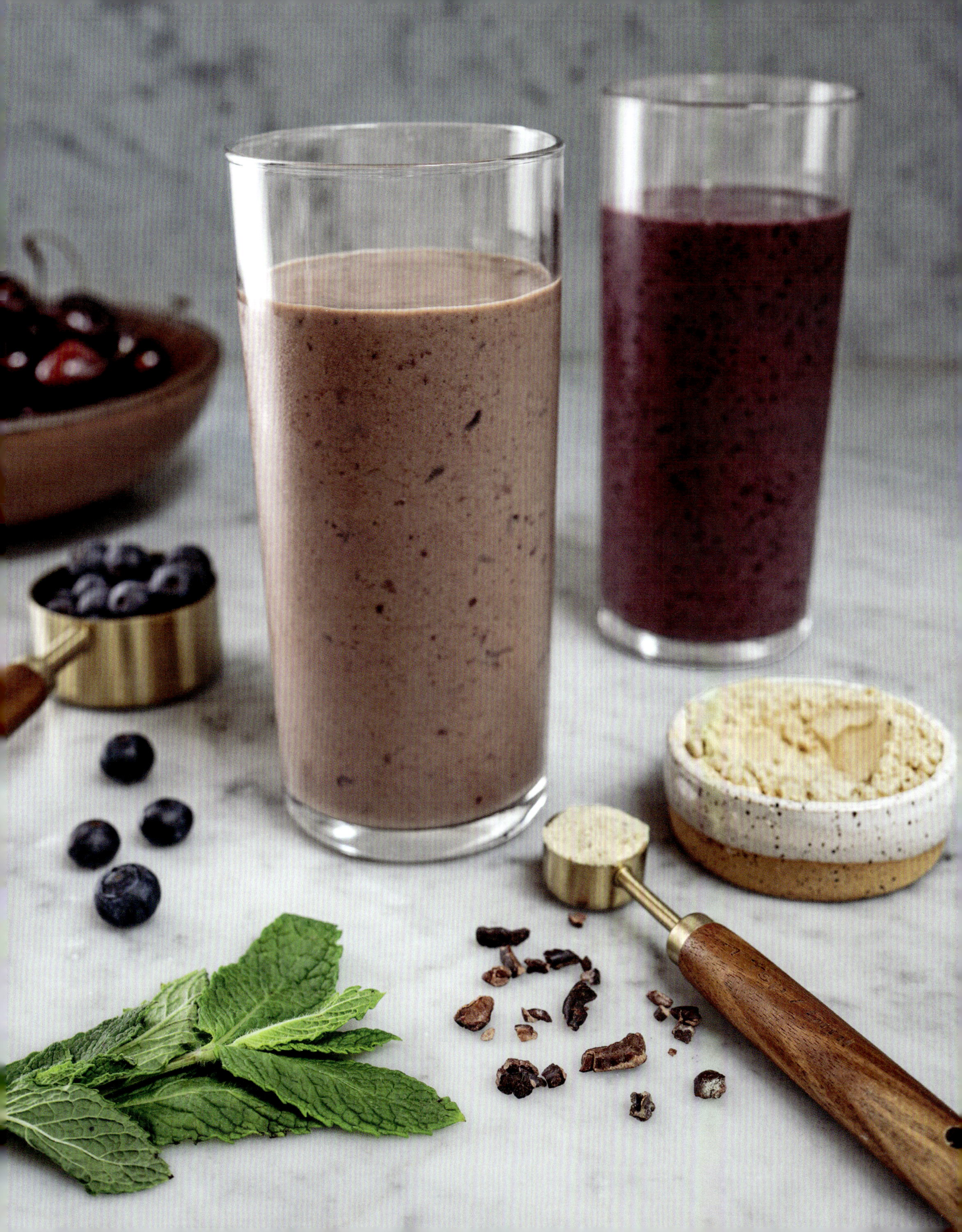

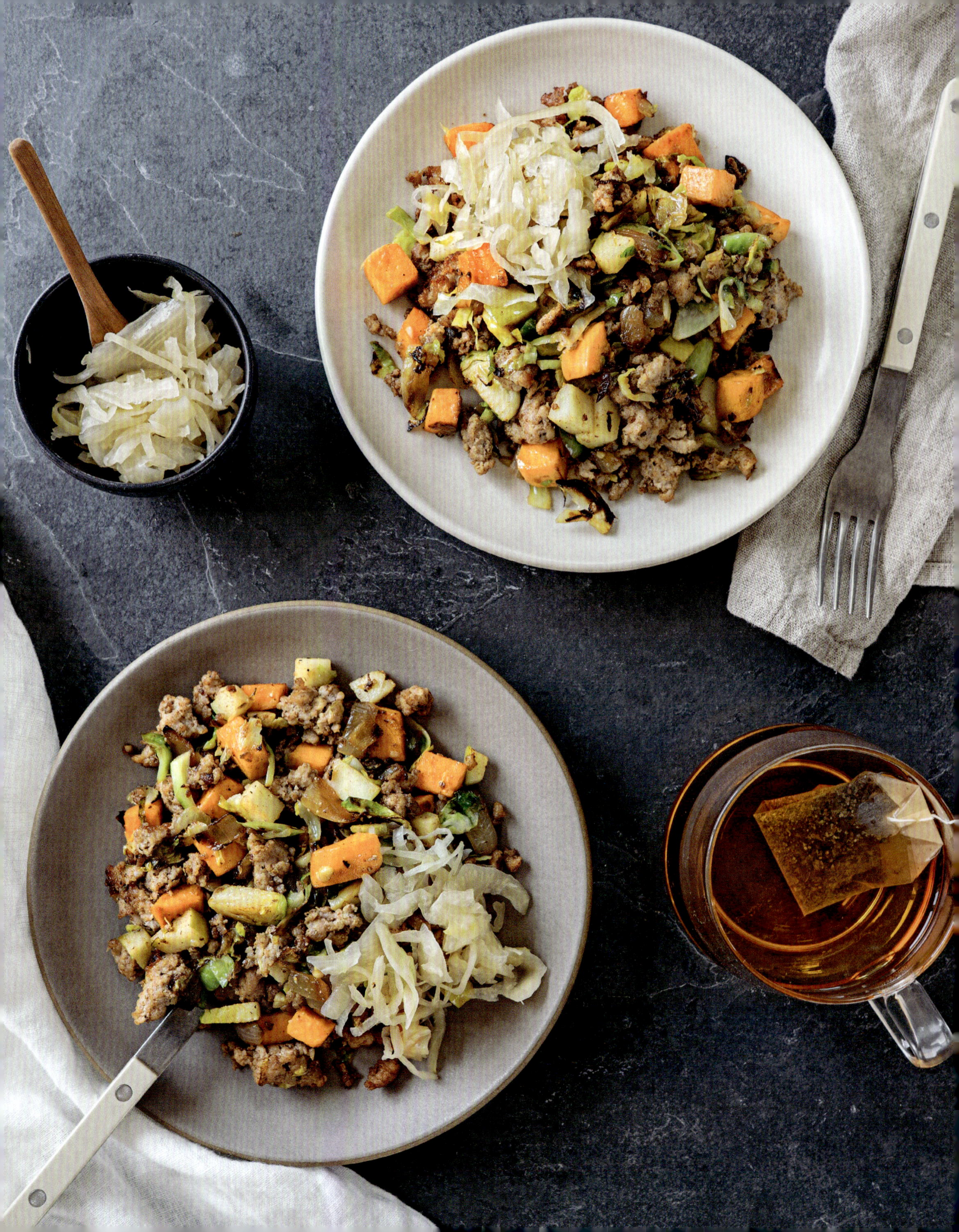

45 MINUTES

MAKES
3 SERVINGS

Spiced Pork Skillet Breakfast

2 tablespoons avocado oil (or substitute olive oil)

½ onion, chopped

1 sweet potato, peeled and diced (about 2 cups)

6 ounces brussels sprouts, ends removed, halved, and thinly sliced (about 2 cups)

3 garlic cloves, minced

1¼ teaspoons sea salt, divided

1 pound ground pork

¾ teaspoon ground ginger

½ teaspoon ground cumin

½ teaspoon ground cinnamon

¼ teaspoon ground black pepper

⅛ teaspoon ground coriander

⅛ teaspoon ground cardamom

½ green apple, cored and diced

1 tablespoon maple syrup

¾ cup sauerkraut, homemade (page 120) or store-bought (check ingredients)

1. Heat the oil in a large skillet over medium heat. When the pan is hot, add the onion and cook, stirring, for 3 minutes, or until beginning to brown. Add the sweet potato and cook, stirring occasionally, for 7 minutes, or until softened but still firm. Add the brussels sprouts, garlic, and ¼ teaspoon of the salt and cook for another 3 to 5 minutes, until all the vegetables are tender. Transfer to a bowl and set aside.

2. Add the pork to the same skillet over medium heat, using a spoon to break the meat into pieces. Cook for 5 to 7 minutes, until the meat is cooked throughout, while continuing to stir and break it into smaller pieces. Meanwhile, combine the ginger, cumin, cinnamon, pepper, coriander, and cardamom in a small bowl and set aside.

3. When the meat has finished cooking, add the remaining 1 teaspoon of salt, apple, spice mixture, and maple syrup, stir to combine, and cook for another 1 to 2 minutes. Add the vegetable mixture back to the pan and give it a good stir. Turn off the heat and serve warm topped with a large scoop of sauerkraut. It keeps in the refrigerator for up to 5 days.

1 HOUR

MAKES
6 SERVINGS

Rise and Shine Cardamom Granola

1¼ cups buckwheat groats

¼ cup hulled hemp seeds

½ cup pumpkin seeds

½ cup unsweetened large-flake coconut

2 tablespoons ground flax seeds

2 tablespoons maple sugar (or substitute coconut or date sugar)

¼ teaspoon sea salt

⅛ teaspoon ground cardamom

¼ cup avocado oil

⅓ cup sunflower seed butter

¼ cup maple syrup

1 teaspoon vanilla extract

⅓ cup raisins or dried cranberries (check ingredients)

1. Preheat the oven to 300°F. Line a large baking sheet with parchment paper; set aside.

2. Place the buckwheat groats and the hemp together in a fine-mesh strainer and rinse thoroughly with cold water. Set aside to drain.

3. In a large bowl, combine the pumpkin seeds, coconut, flax, maple sugar, salt, and cardamom.

4. In a small saucepan, combine the oil, sunflower seed butter, maple syrup, and vanilla. Place over low heat and stir until warm enough to combine thoroughly, about 5 minutes.

5. Add the rinsed and drained buckwheat and hemp to the bowl with the pumpkin seed mixture (it is fine if they still have some residual moisture). Give a good stir, then add the oil and seed butter mixture and stir again to combine fully. Stir in the dried fruit.

6. Transfer the mixture to the prepared baking sheet, spreading it out evenly so there are some pieces with space in between for even browning. Bake for 40 to 45 minutes, until toasted on top and mostly firm to the touch. Allow to cool for 20 minutes, then transfer into a storage container; do not cover until completely cooled. It keeps for up to 4 weeks stored in an airtight container at room temperature.

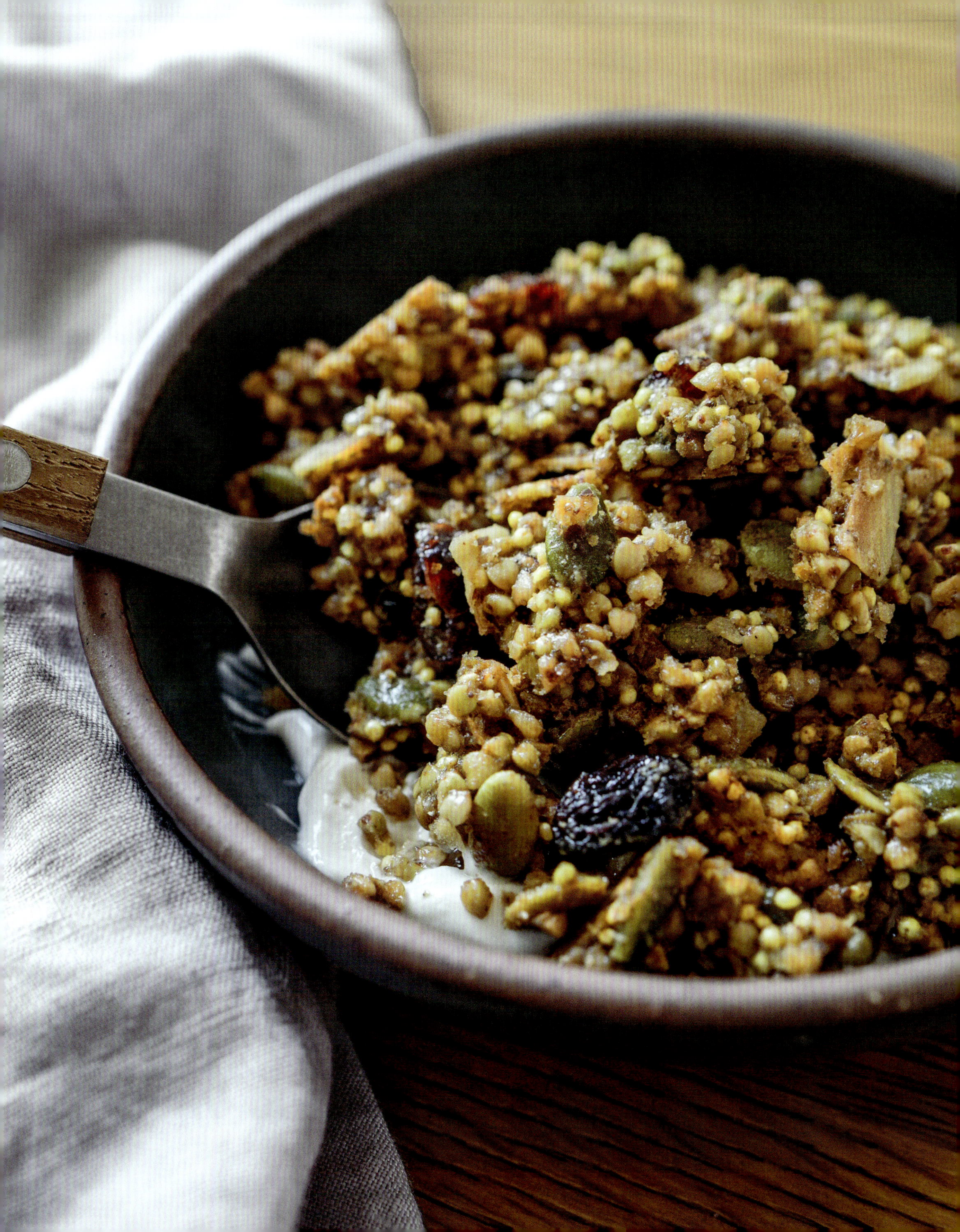

CHAPTER 15

Modified Soups, Stews, and Salads

30 MINUTES

MAKES
4 SERVINGS

Thai Lime Chicken Lettuce Cups

2 tablespoons avocado oil

1½ pounds ground chicken

2 shallots, thinly sliced

½ teaspoon minced fresh ginger

2 tablespoons coconut aminos

1 tablespoon fish sauce

1 bunch cilantro greens or Thai basil leaves, chopped (about 2 cups)

2 ounces mint, chopped (about 2 cups)

1 lemongrass stalk, end and outer leaves removed, bottom 1 inch minced

2 tablespoons lime juice (about 1 juicy lime)

2 tablespoons toasted rice powder*

1 head romaine, lettuce leaves washed and separated

***TO MAKE YOUR OWN TOASTED RICE POWDER:** *Place ¼ to ½ cup uncooked jasmine rice in a small skillet over medium heat and toast, stirring, until golden brown, about 10 minutes. Allow to cool completely, then grind in a spice grinder to a grainy powder.*

1. Put the oil and ground chicken in a cold skillet and use a spoon to break it up into pieces. Turn the heat to medium and cook, continuing to stir and break it up into smaller pieces, until the meat is fully cooked, about 10 minutes. Add the shallots, ginger, coconut aminos, and fish sauce and cook, stirring, for 2 more minutes. Turn off the heat and set aside to cool for 10 minutes while you make the salad.

2. Place the cilantro or basil, mint, lemongrass, and lime juice in a medium bowl and stir to combine.

3. When the meat mixture has cooled, transfer to the bowl with the salad and stir to combine thoroughly. Add the toasted rice powder and stir to coat evenly. Serve with fresh lettuce leaves. It keeps in the refrigerator for 5 days.

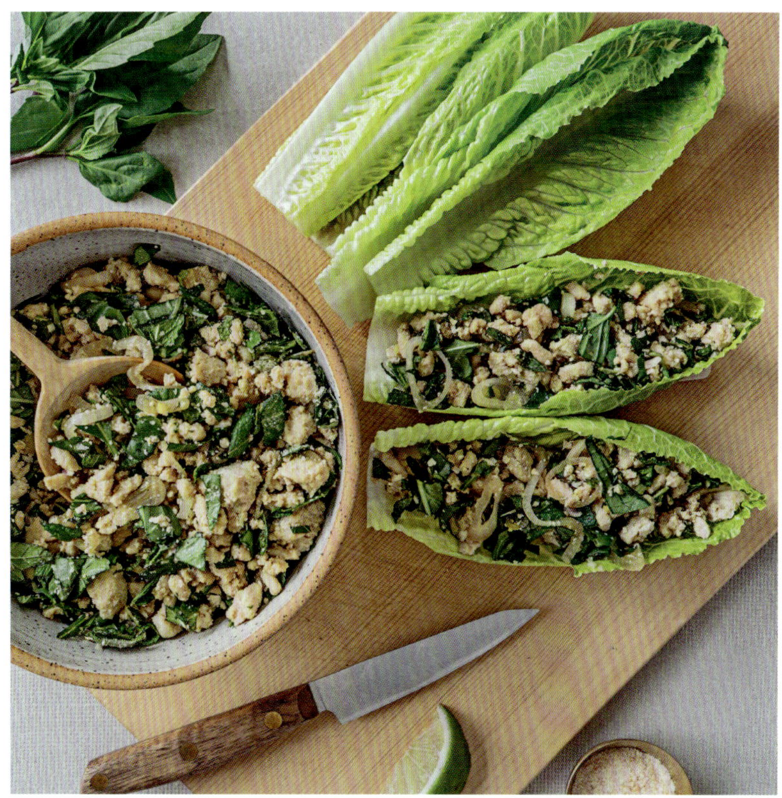

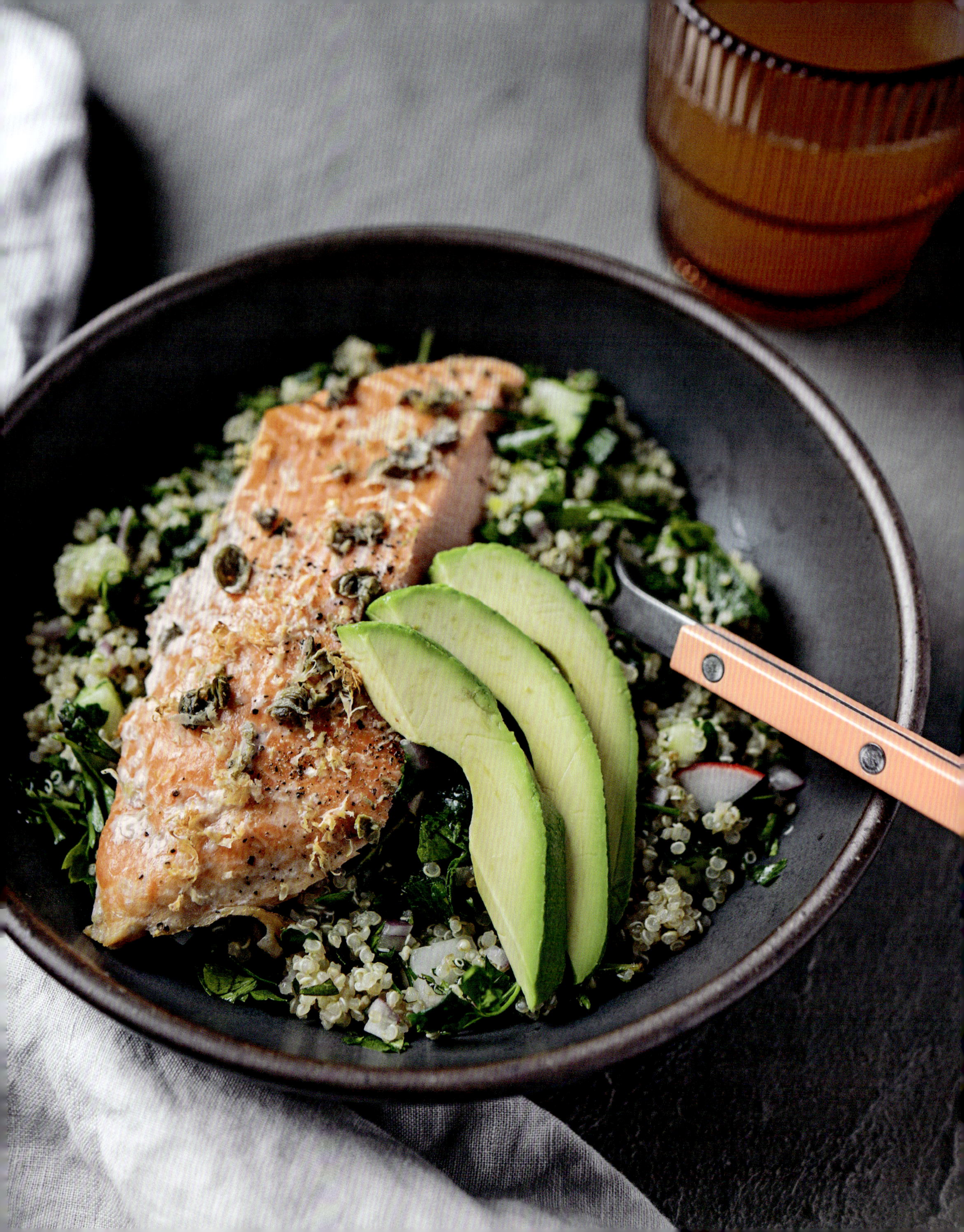

45 MINUTES

MAKES
4 SERVINGS

Herbed Quinoa Bowl with Roasted Salmon

1½ cups quinoa, rinsed and drained

2½ cups water

2 bunches parsley, stems removed and minced

½ cup mint leaves, minced

½ red onion, minced

1 cucumber, diced

3 radishes, diced

1 lemon

½ cup olive oil

¼ teaspoon sea salt, divided, plus more if needed

1½-pound salmon fillet, skin on

1 tablespoon capers, finely chopped (check ingredients; can substitute olives)

Freshly ground black pepper

2 avocados

1. Preheat the oven to 400°F.

2. Place the quinoa and water in a medium pot and bring to a boil over high heat. Turn down the heat to maintain a simmer and cook, covered, for 10 to 15 minutes, or until the liquid is absorbed. Transfer to a bowl and set aside to cool while you prepare the rest of the salad.

3. In a medium bowl, combine the parsley, mint, onion, cucumber, and radishes and stir to combine. Before adding the dressing ingredients, zest some of the lemon to add to the fish later. Then add the oil, lemon juice, and the salt to the salad and toss to coat. Set aside while the quinoa cools and you cook the salmon.

4. Place the salmon fillet skin-side down on the parchment-lined baking sheet. Sprinkle with the capers, lemon zest, some pepper, and additional salt to taste (if you are using salt-cured capers, you might not need to add salt). Cook for 10 to 12 minutes, until the salmon is just cooked through and flakes when probed with a fork. Remove from the oven and cool.

5. When cooled, add the quinoa to the salad mixture and stir to combine. Serve a portion of the dressed salad with some salmon and half an avocado, sliced. It keeps for up to 3 days in the refrigerator.

PREP NOTE: *For greater flexibility, batch-cook the quinoa salad and enjoy with a serving of seafood canned in oil, like sardines, mackerel, or oysters.*

1 HOUR

MAKES
4 SERVINGS

Aromatic Vietnamese Noodle Bowl

1 tablespoon avocado oil

1 onion, chopped, divided

3 (2-inch) pieces fresh ginger

3 cinnamon sticks

5 whole star anise

3 whole cardamom pods

5 whole cloves

1 teaspoon whole coriander or fennel seeds (optional)

3 quarts bone broth, homemade (page 119) or store-bought

2 teaspoons fish sauce

2 teaspoons coconut sugar (or substitute date sugar)

2 teaspoons smoked sea salt, plus more if needed

2 carrots, chopped (about 2 cups)

1 pound broccoli florets, chopped

4 ounces mushrooms, thinly sliced

1 pound pho-style rice noodles

1 pound thinly sliced lean beef

8 ounces mung bean sprouts

1 bunch Thai basil, stems removed

2 limes, quartered

1. Heat the oil in a large stockpot over medium heat. When the pan is hot, add half of the onion and cook, stirring, for 3 minutes. Add the ginger pieces, cinnamon, star anise, cardamom, cloves, and coriander seeds (if using) and cook until fragrant, about 1 minute. Add the broth, increase the heat to high, and bring to a boil, then turn down the heat to maintain a simmer. Cook, covered, for 30 minutes. Carefully strain the broth into a second pot, being careful not to mistakenly send it down the drain. Discard the onion and spice solids and return the pot with the broth to the stovetop.

2. Add the fish sauce, coconut sugar, salt, carrots, broccoli, mushrooms, and remaining onion to the broth and cook for 5 minutes, or until the vegetables are tender. Meanwhile, prepare the rice noodles according to package instructions. When the vegetables are finished cooking, taste the broth and add salt if necessary; set aside.

3. Portion each bowl with rice noodles and a serving of sliced beef, then pour the hot broth with the vegetables on top; this will cook the meat. Serve with sprouts, basil leaves, and lime wedges on the side to be added to each bowl. The broth and vegetables keep for up to 5 days in the refrigerator; they also freeze well.

PREP NOTE: *If batch-cooking this meal ahead, cook the broth and vegetables for storage. Before serving a portion, prepare the noodles fresh, reheat the broth and vegetables, and pour them over a serving of beef, then garnish with fresh toppings.*

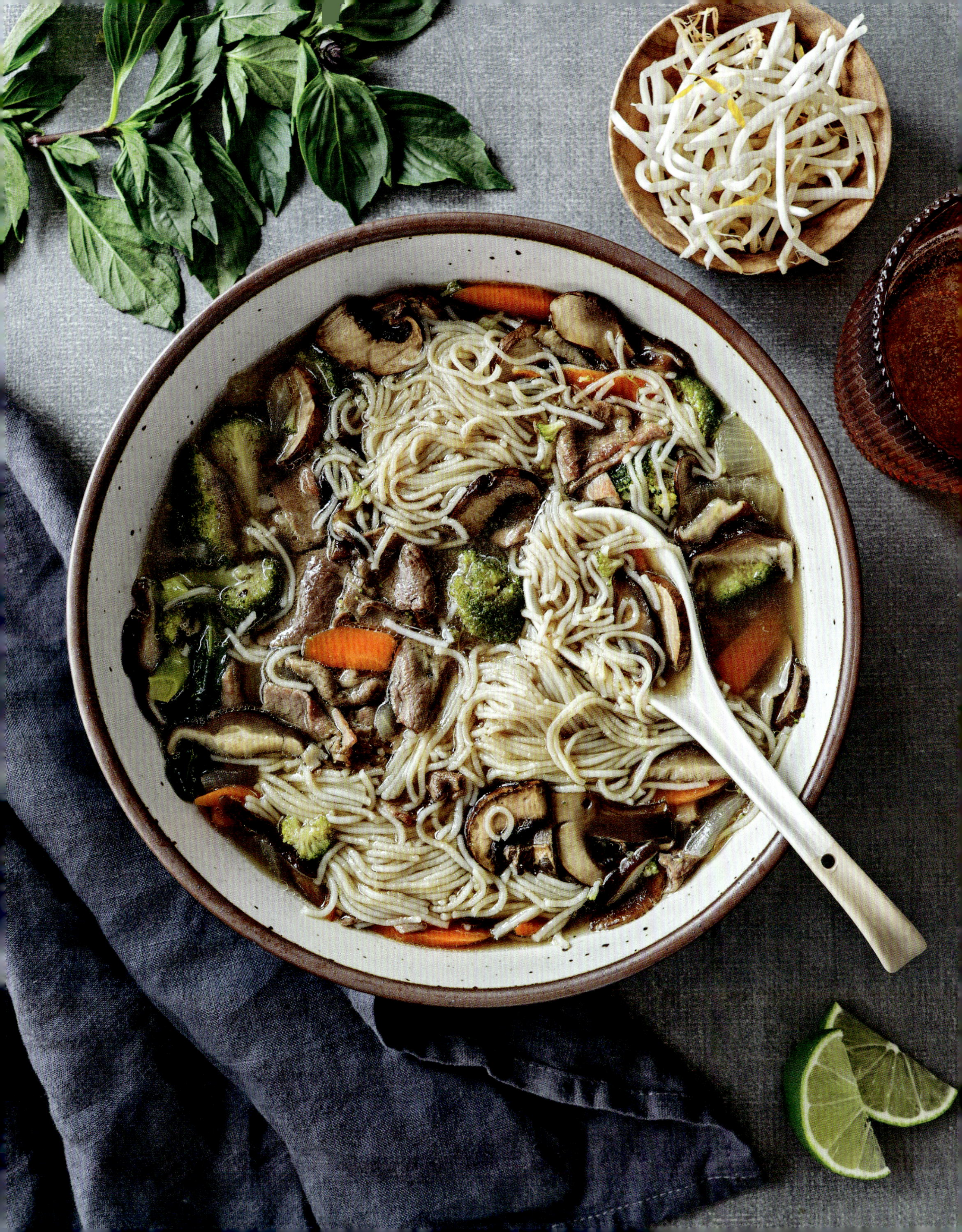

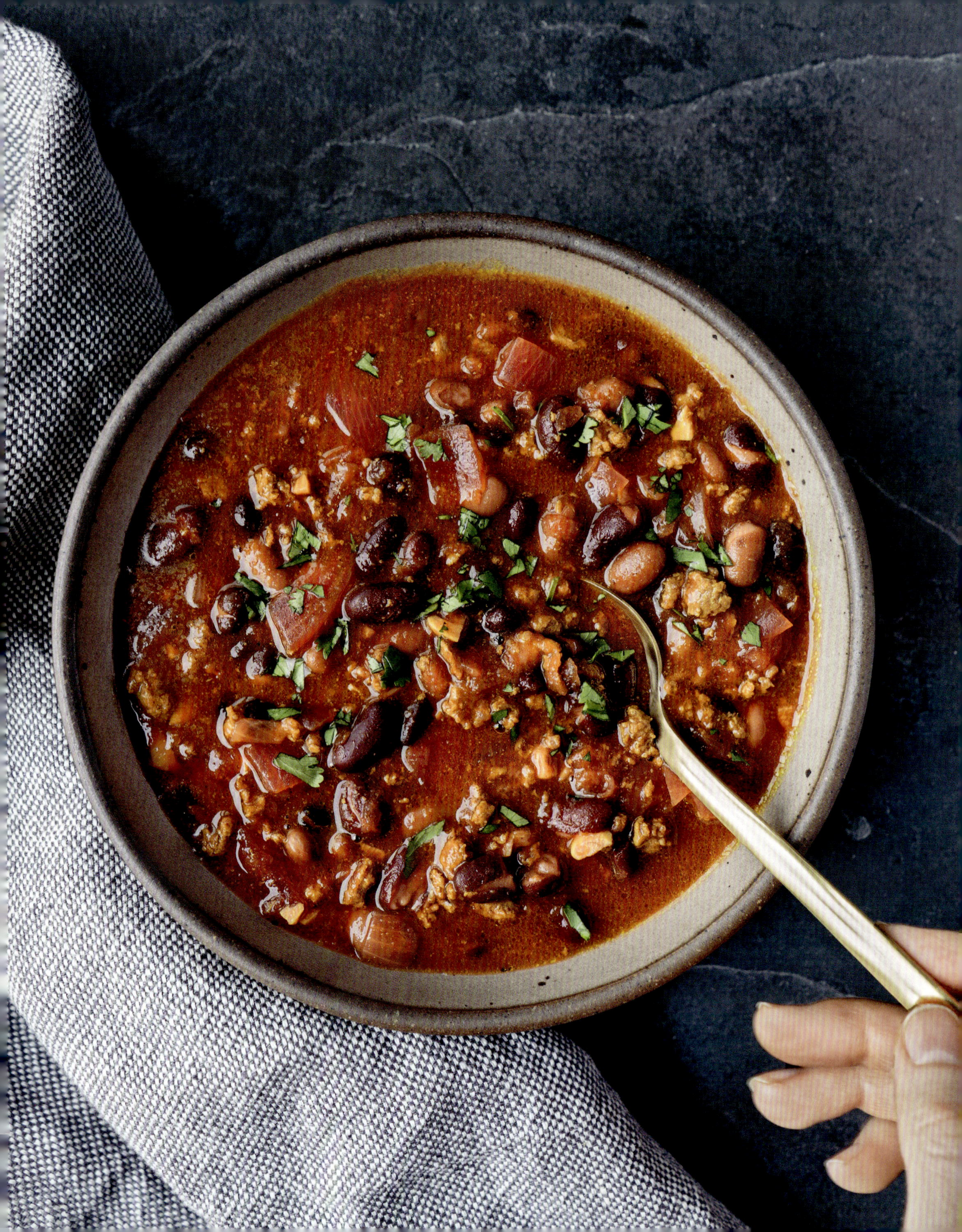

50 MINUTES

MAKES 8 SERVINGS

Savory Beef and Bean Chili

2 pounds ground beef

1 large yellow onion, chopped

1 head garlic, peeled and minced

2 cups bone broth, homemade (page 119) or store-bought

1 quart water

1 large beet, peeled and shredded or diced

1 (14-ounce) can pumpkin puree

2 ½ teaspoons smoked sea salt

2 teaspoons ground cumin

2 teaspoons onion powder

2 teaspoons garlic powder

½ teaspoon ground coriander

¼ teaspoon ground turmeric

⅛ teaspoon ground cinnamon

3 (14-ounce) cans beans (a mix of black, pinto, and/or kidney), drained and rinsed

3 tablespoons apple cider vinegar

1 tablespoon fish sauce

Black pepper

Fresh cilantro, for garnish (optional)

1. Place the ground beef in a large, heavy-bottomed pot over medium heat. Cook for about 10 minutes, using a spoon to break the beef into pieces and stir as it cooks. When the beef is lightly browned and cooked throughout, transfer to a bowl using a slotted spoon and set aside, reserving the pan juices for cooking.

2. Increase the heat to medium-high and add the onion. Cook, stirring, for about 5 minutes, until beginning to brown. Add the garlic and cook for another 30 seconds, or until fragrant. Add the broth, water, beet, pumpkin, smoked salt, cumin, onion powder, garlic powder, coriander, turmeric, and cinnamon to the pot with the cooked beef. Bring to a simmer, then lower the heat to maintain a simmer and cook for 10 minutes.

3. Add the beans, vinegar, and fish sauce, season with pepper, and stir to combine. Serve garnished with cilantro, if using. It keeps for up to 1 week in the refrigerator; it also freezes well.

Cozy White Bean Stew

1 HOUR
30 MINUTES, PLUS
8 HOURS FOR
SOAKING

MAKES
6 SERVINGS

1 pound dry Great Northern beans

1½ tablespoons plus 1 teaspoon sea salt, divided

3 quarts water, divided

¼ cup olive oil or ghee (see page 210)

1 large yellow onion, diced

1 head garlic, peeled and minced

6 celery ribs, thinly sliced (about 3 cups)

2 large parsnips, diced (about 4 cups)

1 carrot, diced (about 1 cup)

4 cups bone broth, homemade (page 119) or store-bought

2 teaspoons ground cumin

½ teaspoon ground coriander

⅛ teaspoon ground black pepper

2 cups oyster mushrooms, diced (or substitute button mushrooms)

3 tablespoons lemon juice (about 1 lemon)

1 bunch cilantro, bottom stems removed, chopped

TIME-SAVING TIP: *You can make this recipe using canned beans by cooking the vegetables as above and adding 4, 14-ounce cans of rinsed beans about 30 minutes into simmering.*

1. About 8 to 12 hours before beginning to cook, soak the beans in 2 quarts of the water and 1½ tablespoons of the salt. I like to do this the night before if I will be cooking the recipe for lunch, or in the morning of if I will be cooking it for dinner. When you're ready to begin, drain and rinse the beans well with cool water and set aside.

2. Heat the oil in a large, heavy-bottomed soup pot over medium heat. When the pan is hot, add the onion and cook, stirring, for about 3 minutes, until just starting to brown. Add the garlic and cook for another minute, or until fragrant. Add the celery, parsnips, and carrot and cook, stirring, for 3 minutes to give the vegetables a little color.

3. Add the broth, remaining 1 quart water, the cumin, coriander, pepper, and soaked beans to the pot. Bring to a boil, cover, then turn down the heat to maintain a simmer. Cook, stirring occasionally, for 50 minutes, or until the beans are tender.

4. Add the mushrooms and cook for another 10 minutes. Test the beans to ensure they are cooked throughout; if not, continue cooking until they are tender. Add the lemon juice and cilantro and stir to combine. It keeps in the refrigerator for up to 1 week; it also freezes well.

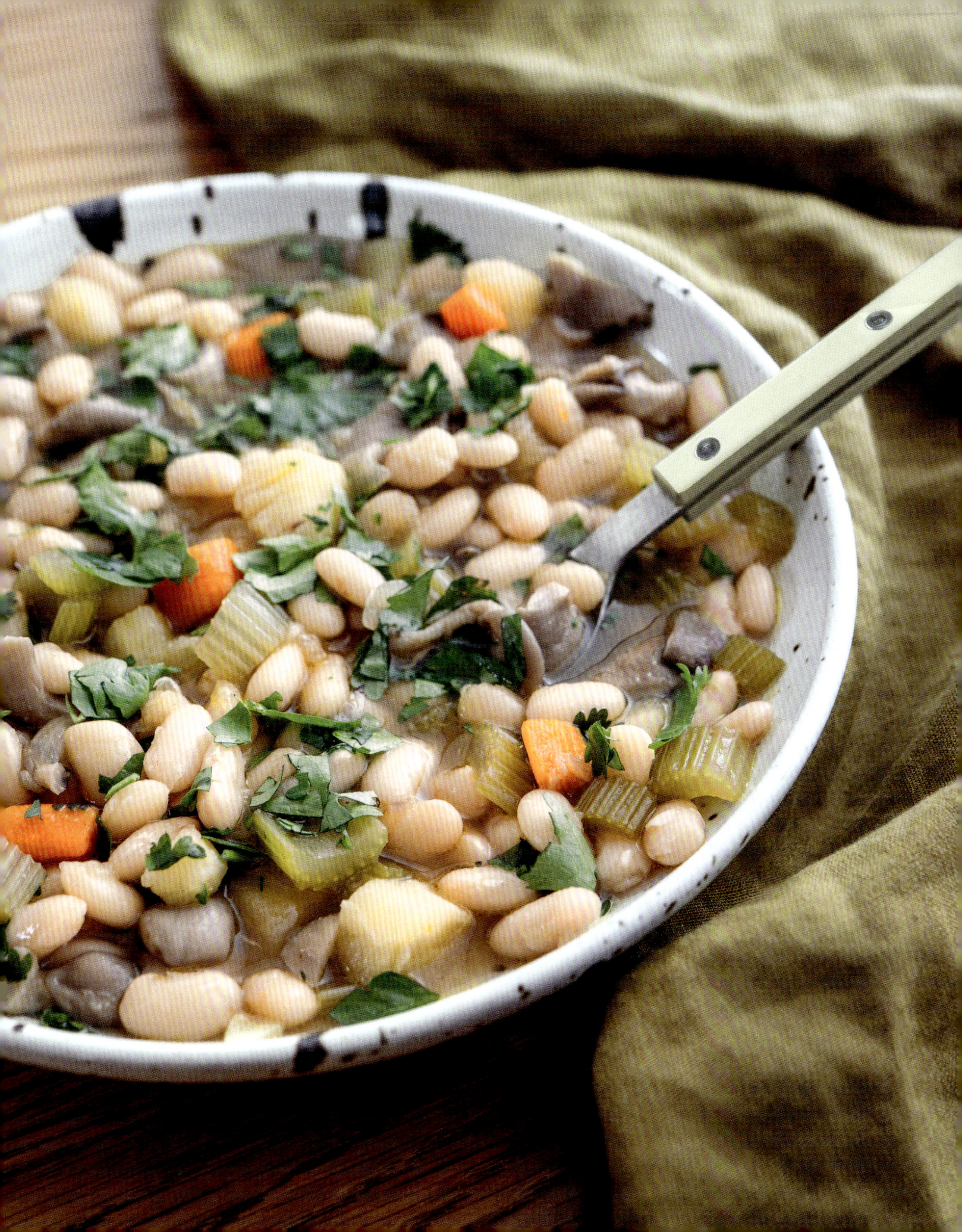

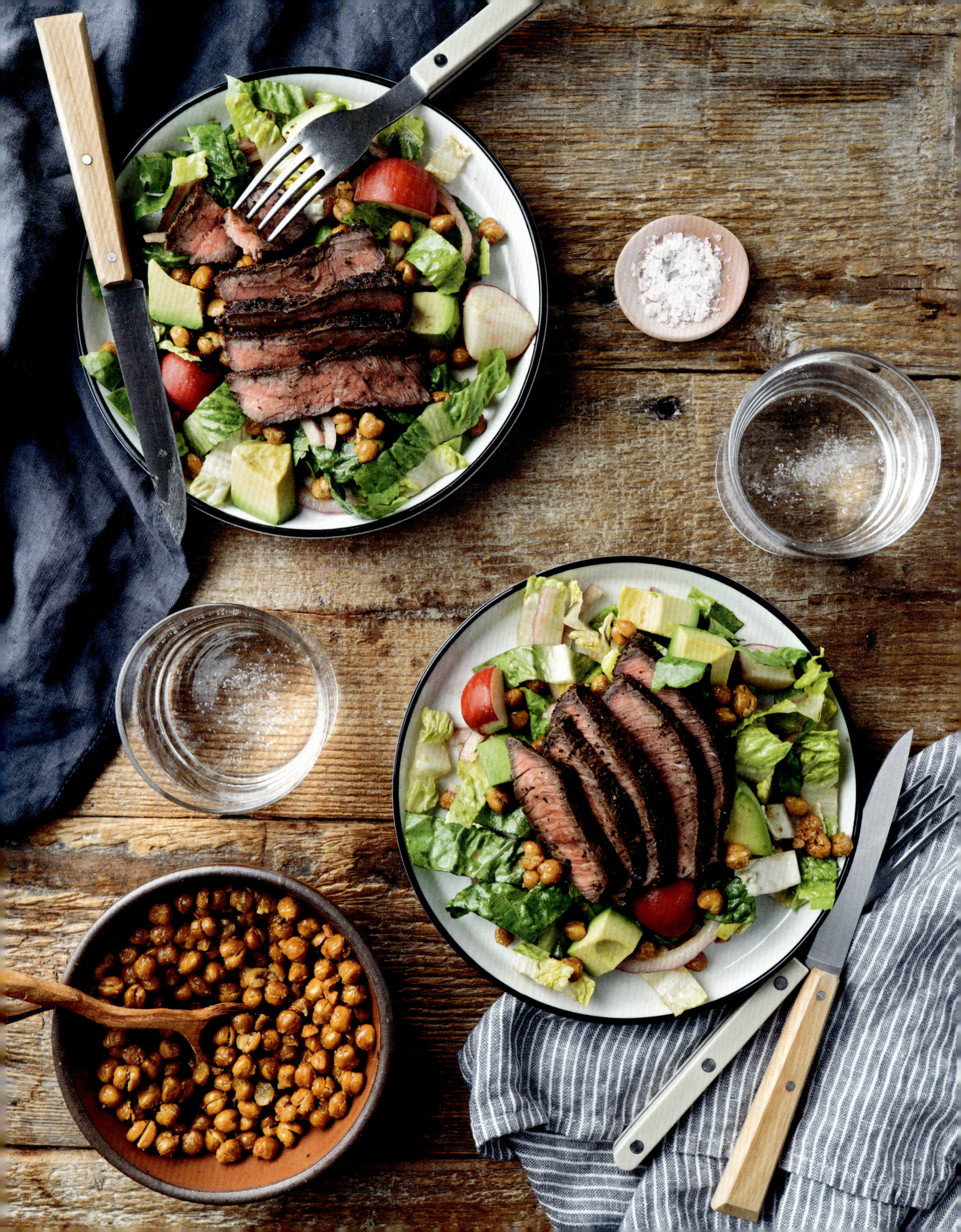

1 HOUR

MAKES
4 SERVINGS

Coffee-Rubbed Steak Salad with Balsamic Dressing

CHICKPEA CROUTONS

1 (14-ounce) can chickpeas, drained and rinsed

1 tablespoon olive oil

½ teaspoon garlic powder

¼ teaspoon sea salt

COFFEE RUB AND STEAK

1 tablespoon ground coffee

1 teaspoon coconut or maple sugar

1 teaspoon sea salt

1 teaspoon ground black pepper

1½ pounds 1-inch-thick beef sirloin steaks

1 tablespoon avocado oil

STEAK SALAD

2 large heads romaine lettuce, chopped

½ red onion, thinly sliced

1 bunch radishes, quartered

2 avocados, flesh cubed

¼ cup olive oil

2 tablespoons balsamic vinegar (or substitute red wine vinegar)

¼ teaspoon sea salt

1. Preheat the oven to 400°F.

2. Place the chickpeas in a dry towel and gently squeeze to remove excess water; remove the skins and arrange the chickpeas on a baking sheet. Roast for 20 minutes.

3. Meanwhile, place the coffee rub ingredients in a small bowl and stir to combine. Rub the steak with the spice mixture and allow to sit at room temperature while the beans bake.

4. When the chickpeas have roasted for 20 minutes, transfer them to a medium bowl with the oil, garlic powder, and salt, toss to combine, then arrange them back on the same baking sheet. Roast for an additional 10 minutes, or until crispy and browned. Remove from the oven and set aside.

5. Next, make the salad: Combine the lettuce, onion, radishes, and avocado in a large bowl and toss with the olive oil, vinegar, and salt. Set aside while you cook the steak.

6. Heat the avocado oil in a large skillet over medium-high heat. When the pan is hot, add the steak and cook for 4 to 5 minutes untouched, until a nice brown crust has developed on the first side. Flip and cook for another 4 to 5 minutes, until the internal temperature reaches 125°F (for medium-rare), longer if your steak is more than 1 inch thick. Transfer to a cutting board, cover with a piece of foil, and rest for 5 minutes.

7. Serve each portion of salad topped with chickpea croutons and slices of steak.

PREP NOTE: *If batch-cooking this ahead, store the greens, dressing, and cooked steak separately for storage; cube the avocado and toss each portion fresh for serving. It keeps for up to 3 days in the refrigerator.*

Rustic Beans and Greens with Bacon

1 HOUR
30 MINUTES, PLUS
8 HOURS FOR
SOAKING

MAKES
6 SERVINGS

1 pound dry black beans

2 quarts plus 3 cups water, divided

1½ tablespoons plus 1 teaspoon sea salt, divided

6 slices thick-cut uncured bacon (check ingredients)

1 onion, chopped

4 garlic cloves, minced

3 cups bone broth, homemade (page 119) or store-bought

1 bay leaf

1 teaspoon ground cumin

2 tablespoons rice vinegar

1 bunch collard greens, stemmed and cut into thin ribbons

2 avocados, pitted and sliced

TIME-SAVING TIP: *You can make this recipe using canned beans by skipping the 45-minute cooking time in step 3 and adding 4, 14-ounce cans of rinsed black beans to the final step, when you add the collard greens.*

1. About 8 to 12 hours before beginning to cook, soak the beans in 2 quarts of the water and 1½ tablespoons of the salt. I like to do this the night before if I will be cooking the recipe for lunch, or the morning of if I will be cooking it for dinner. When ready to begin, drain and rinse the beans well with cool water and set aside.

2. Place the bacon in a cold, heavy-bottomed pot. I like to cut the slices in half so they more easily cover the bottom surface of the pan. Turn the heat to medium-low and cook, turning occasionally, until browned and slightly crisp, about 10 minutes. Transfer to a paper towel–lined plate to cool, leaving the rendered fat in the pan.

3. Add the onion, turn up the heat to medium, and cook for 5 minutes, or until starting to brown. Add the garlic and cook for 1 minute, or until fragrant. Add the broth, remaining 3 cups water, the soaked beans, chopped bacon, bay leaf, cumin, and remaining 1 teaspoon salt to the pot. Bring to a simmer and cook, covered, for 45 minutes, or until the beans are just tender.

4. Add the vinegar and collard greens and cook for 15 minutes, or until the beans are fully tender. Remove the bay leaf. Slice the avocados just before serving and top each bowl with the fresh slices. It keeps in the refrigerator for up to 1 week; it also freezes well.

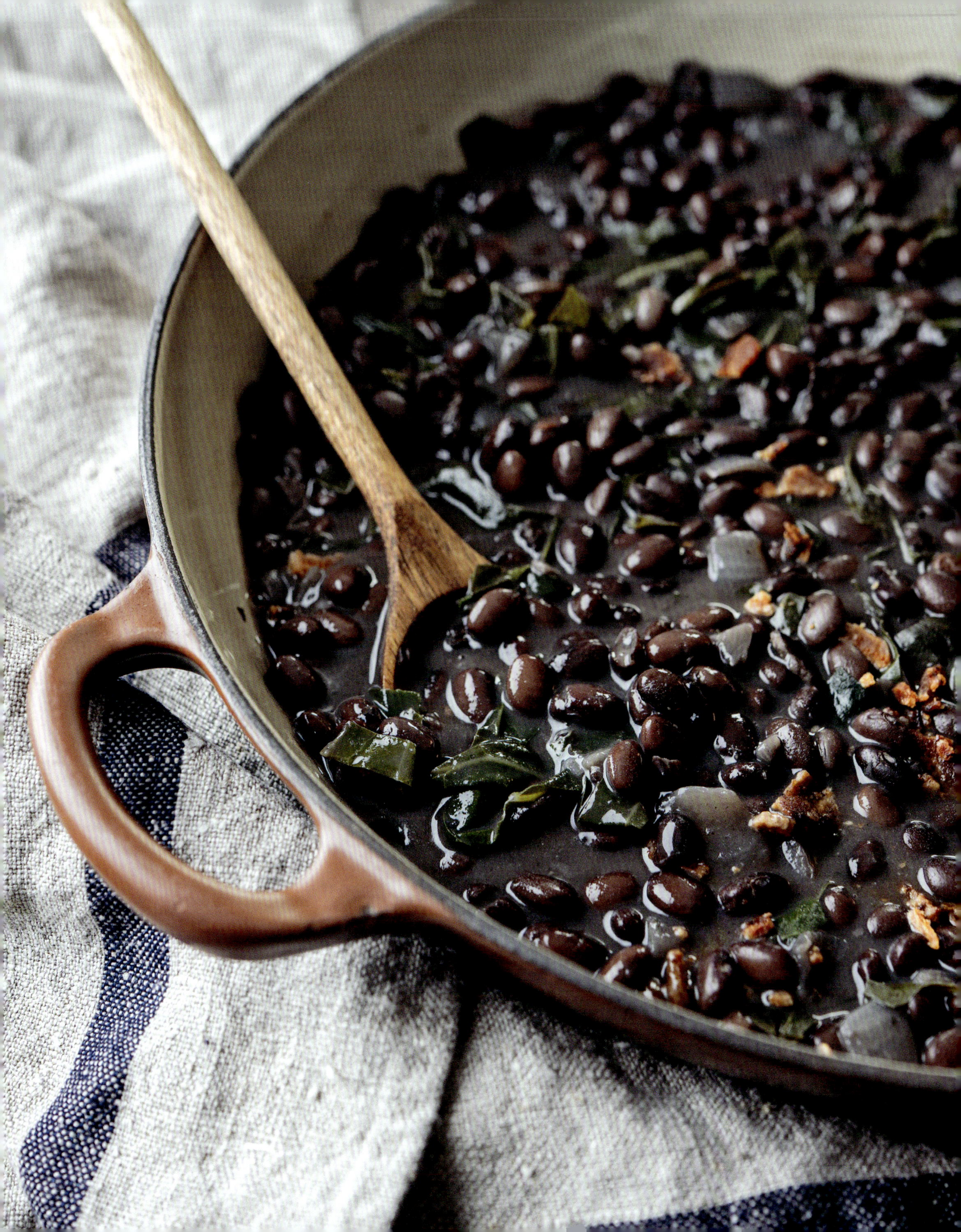

1 HOUR

MAKES
6 SERVINGS

Verdant Lentil Vegetable Soup

¼ cup olive oil or ghee (see page 210)

1 onion, diced

3 celery ribs, diced (about 1 cup)

2 carrots, diced (about 2 cups)

4 garlic cloves, minced

3 cups bone broth, homemade (page 119) or store-bought

4 ½ cups water, divided

3 cups dry green lentils

1 teaspoon ground cumin

½ teaspoon ground coriander

12 ounces mushrooms, diced

1 teaspoon salt

Black pepper

3 tablespoons lemon juice (about 1 lemon)

5 ounces baby spinach

1 bunch cilantro, bottom stems removed, chopped

1. Heat the oil in a large, heavy-bottomed soup pot over medium heat. When the pan is hot, add the onion and cook, stirring, for 3 minutes, or until just starting to brown. Add the celery and carrots and cook for another 5 minutes. Add the garlic and cook for another minute, or until fragrant.

2. Add the broth, 4 cups of the water, the lentils, cumin, and coriander to the pot and bring to a simmer. Cook, covered, for 15 minutes. Add the mushrooms, salt, and pepper to taste and cook for another 3 minutes, or until the lentils and vegetables are tender.

3. While the lentils are cooking, combine the lemon juice, spinach, and remaining ½ cup water in a blender and blend until smooth.

4. When the lentils are finished cooking, stir the spinach mixture and the cilantro into the soup and serve. It keeps in the refrigerator for up to 1 week; it also freezes well for up to 3 months.

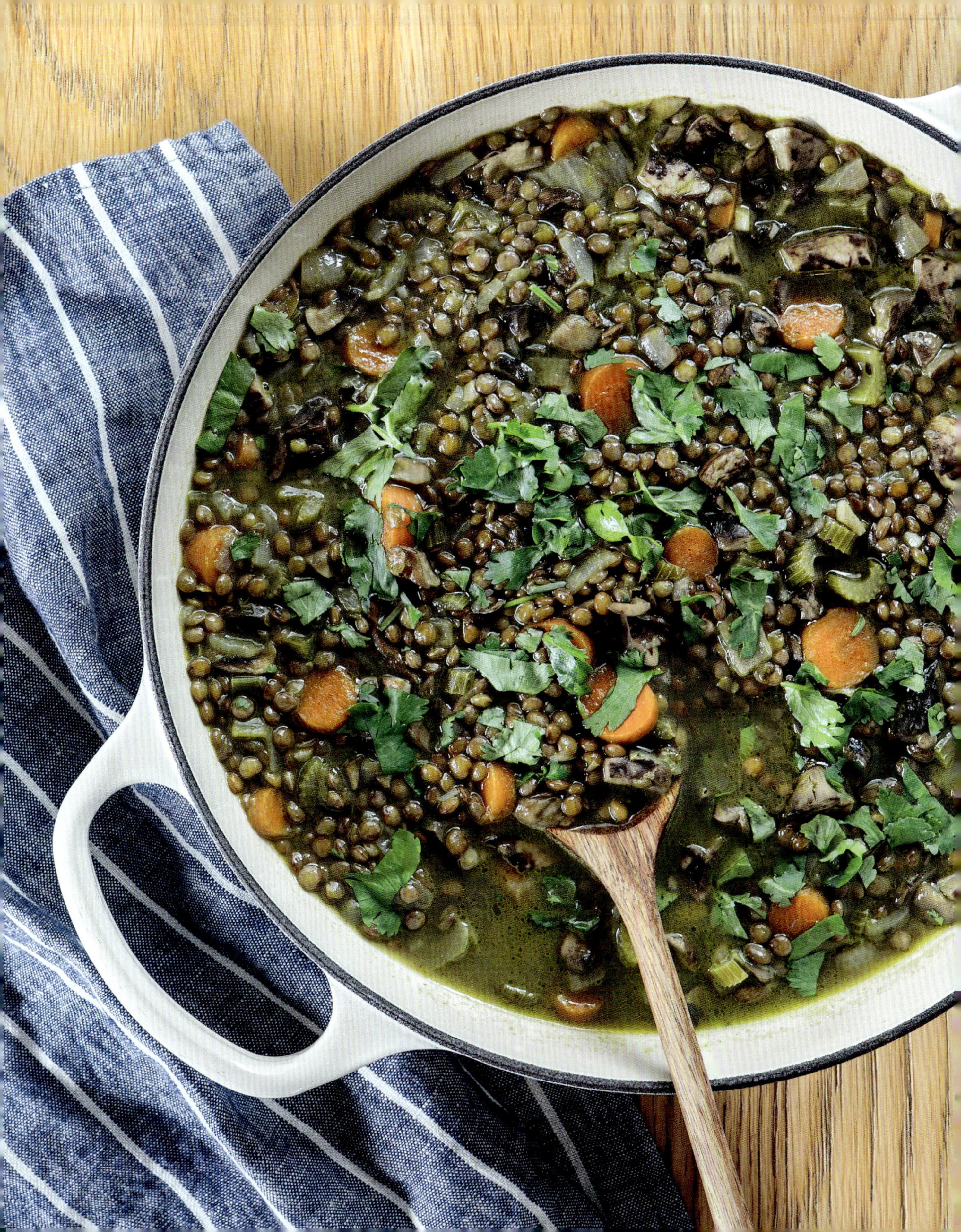

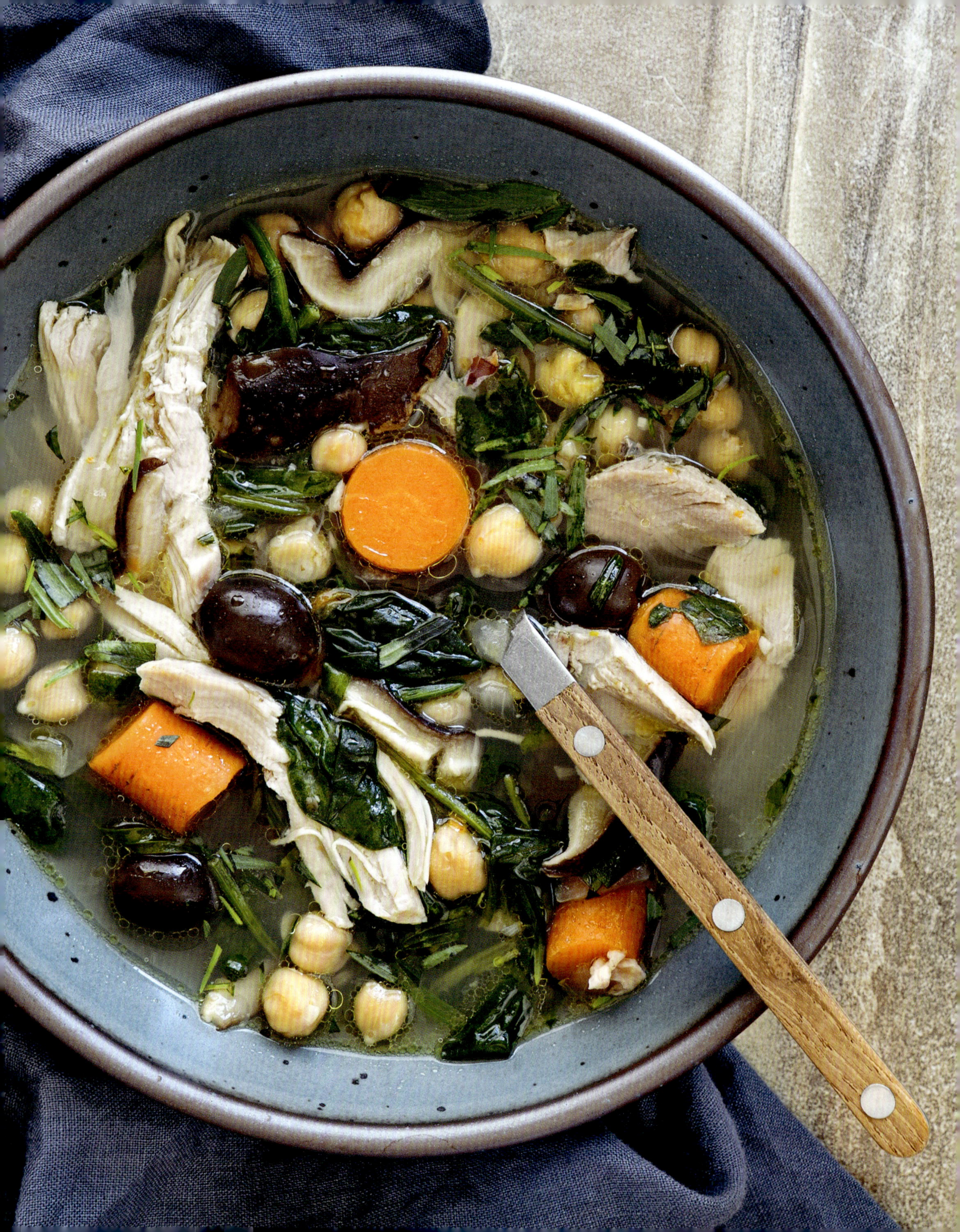

1 HOUR
45 MINUTES

MAKES
8 SERVINGS

Tarragon Chicken Soup with Chickpeas

¼ cup olive oil or ghee (see page 210)

1 onion, chopped

8 ounces mushrooms, chopped

4 garlic cloves, minced

2 quarts water

2 pounds bone-in, skin-on chicken thighs

2 carrots, chopped (about 2 cups)

½ cup pitted black olives (check ingredients)

1 tablespoon sea salt (reduce if using salt-cured olives)

1 bay leaf

2 (14-ounce) cans chickpeas, drained and rinsed

5 ounces spinach

¼ cup fresh tarragon leaves, finely chopped

1½ tablespoons lemon juice (about ½ lemon)

1. Heat the oil in a large, heavy-bottomed soup pot over medium heat. When the pan is hot, add the onion and mushrooms and cook, stirring, for 5 minutes, or until starting to brown. Add the garlic and cook until fragrant, about 1 minute.

2. Add the water, chicken, carrots, olives, salt, and bay leaf to the pot. Bring to a gentle boil, then cover tightly and lower the heat to maintain a bare simmer. Cook until the meat is tender and falling off the bone, 45 minutes to 1 hour—a low simmer ensures your chicken will come out perfectly tender.

3. Use tongs to remove the chicken from the pot and set aside to cool. Remove the bay leaf and discard. Add the chickpeas, spinach, tarragon, and lemon juice to the soup. Let the soup rest to develop flavor while the chicken cools.

4. When the chicken has cooled enough to handle, use your hands to remove the meat off the bone and add it back to the soup, discarding the skin and saving the bones for future batches of bone broth (see page 119). Reheat, if necessary, before serving. It keeps for up to 1 week in the refrigerator; it also freezes well.

CHAPTER 16

Modified Main Meals

45 MINUTES

MAKES 6 SERVINGS

Chicken and Chickpea Curry

2 cups brown rice

5 ½ cups water, divided

2 tablespoons coconut oil or ghee (see page 210)

1 yellow onion, diced

4 garlic cloves, minced

1 (1-inch) piece ginger, minced

1 lemongrass stalk, end and outer leaves removed, bottom 2 inches minced

3 carrots, chopped (about 3 cups)

1 ½ teaspoons tamarind paste

¾ teaspoon sea salt

1 ½ teaspoons ground turmeric

¾ teaspoon ground cumin

¼ teaspoon ground coriander

¼ teaspoon ground cinnamon

1 (14-ounce) can coconut milk (check ingredients)

2 pounds chicken breast, cut into 1½-inch pieces

1 (14-ounce) can chickpeas, drained and rinsed

5 ounces baby spinach (or substitute 8 ounces frozen green peas)

2 tablespoons lime juice (about 1 juicy lime)

Fresh cilantro, for garnish

1. Place the rice in a fine-mesh strainer and rinse under cold water for a minute, then drain. Place the rice in a medium saucepan with 4 cups of the water. Bring to a boil over high heat, then turn down the heat to maintain a simmer and cook, covered, for 30 minutes, or until all the water is absorbed.

2. Heat the oil in a lidded, heavy-bottomed pot over medium heat. When the pan is hot and the fat is melted, add the onion and cook, stirring, for 3 minutes, or until just starting to brown. Add the garlic, ginger, and lemongrass and cook, stirring, for 1 minute, or until fragrant. Add the remaining 1½ cups water, the carrots, tamarind paste, salt, turmeric, cumin, coriander, and cinnamon. Bring to a simmer and cook for 5 minutes.

3. Stir in the coconut milk and bring back to a simmer. Add the chicken, lower the heat to maintain a simmer, and cook, covered, for 10 to 12 minutes, until the chicken is cooked throughout. Add the chickpeas, spinach, and lime juice and stir to combine and wilt the spinach (or thaw the peas, if using). Turn off the heat. Serve a portion of chicken curry over rice and garnish with cilantro. It keeps for up to 5 days in the refrigerator.

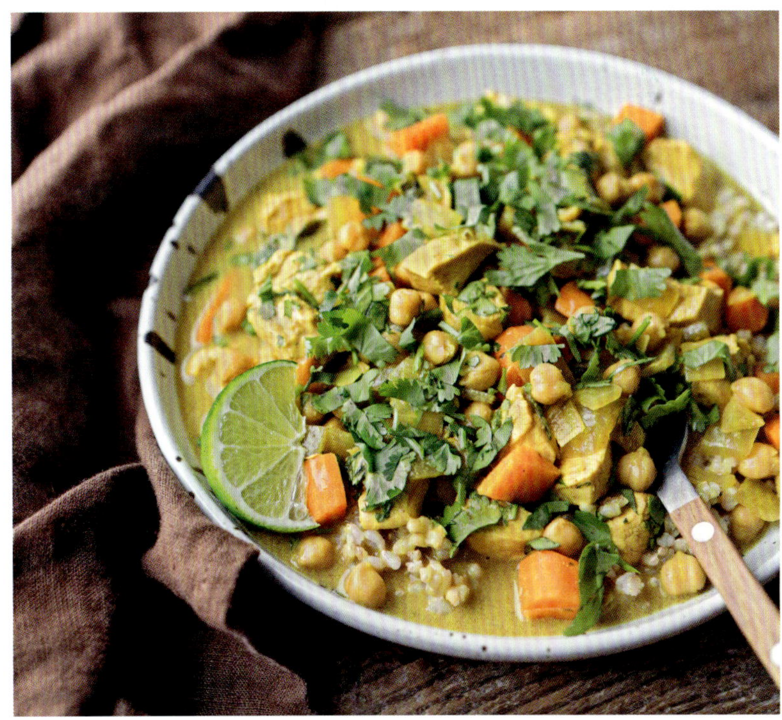

45 MINUTES

MAKES
4 SERVINGS

Soba Noodle Bowl with Chicken and Shiitake Mushrooms

1 pound 100% buckwheat soba noodles

3 tablespoons avocado oil, divided

2 tablespoons coconut aminos

2 tablespoons rice vinegar

2 teaspoons fish sauce

2 tablespoons lime juice (about 1 juicy lime)

1 (2-inch) piece ginger, minced

3 garlic cloves, minced

1 bunch cilantro, bottom stems removed, chopped

2 large shallots, thinly sliced

1 bunch Broccolini, roughly chopped

8 ounces shiitake mushrooms, thinly sliced (substitute button mushrooms)

1½ pounds chicken breast, cut into 1½-inch pieces

½ teaspoon sea salt

Green onions and radishes, thinly sliced, and sesame seeds, for garnish

1. Bring a pot of water to boil, add the soba noodles, and cook according to the package instructions. Meanwhile, combine 1 tablespoon of the oil, the coconut aminos, vinegar, fish sauce, lime juice, ginger, garlic, and cilantro in a blender and blend until combined. When the noodles are finished cooking, drain and immediately rinse with cold water. Allow to continue draining for a few minutes, then transfer to a bowl and toss well with the sauce to prevent sticking. Set aside.

2. Heat 1 tablespoon of the oil in a large skillet over medium-high heat. When hot, add the shallots and cook, stirring, for 2 minutes. Add the Broccolini and mushrooms and cook, stirring, for 5 minutes, or until browned and tender. Turn off the heat, transfer to a medium bowl, and set aside.

3. Sprinkle the chicken with the salt. In the same skillet, heat the remaining 1 tablespoon oil over medium heat. When hot, add the chicken and cook, stirring, until cooked through, 7 to 8 minutes.

4. Serve each bowl of noodles with a scoop of vegetables and a portion of chicken and garnish with green onions, radishes, and sesame seeds. It keeps for up to 3 days in the refrigerator.

PREP NOTE: *If you are batch-cooking this recipe, store the noodles mixed with the sauce and the chicken and vegetables separately.*

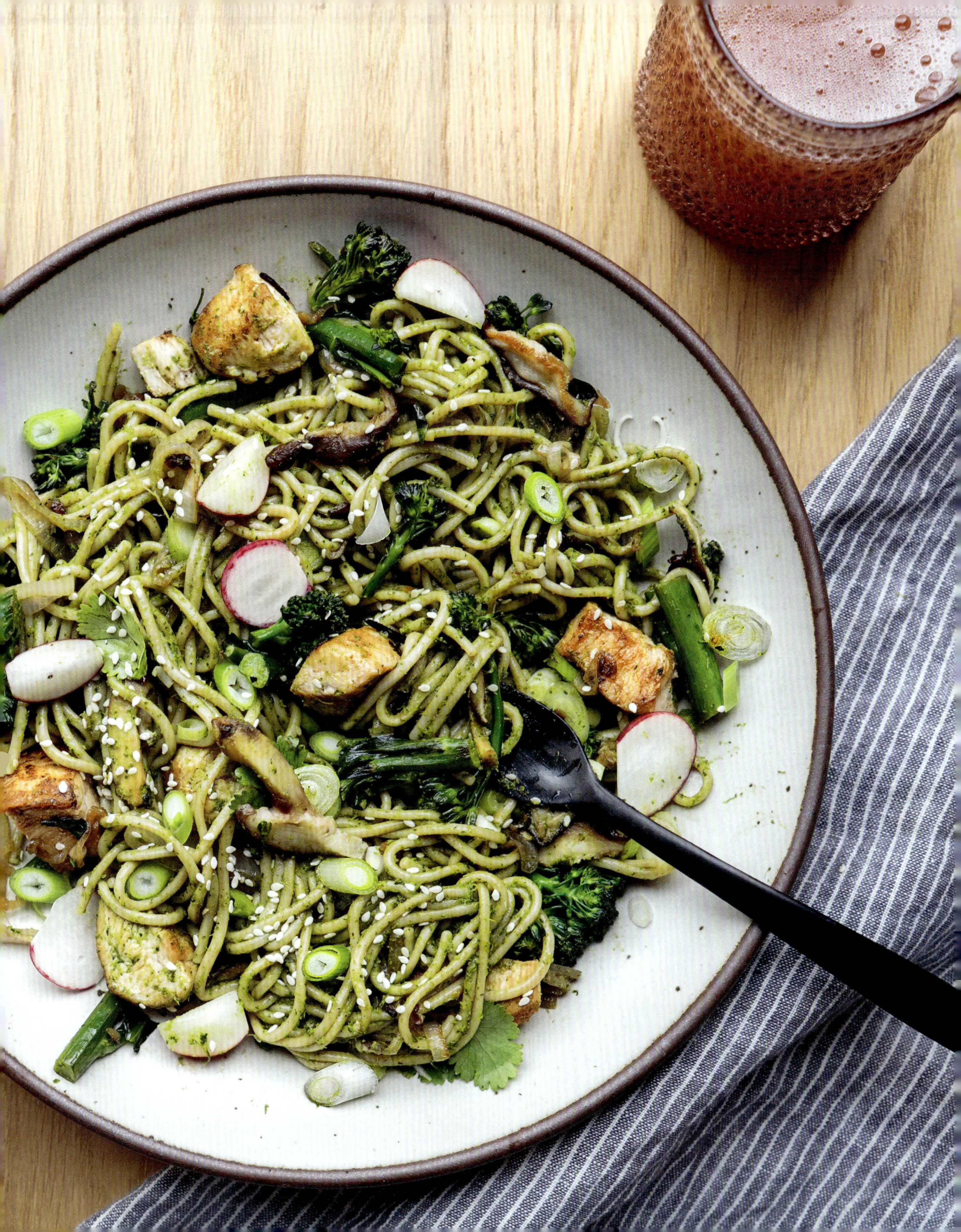

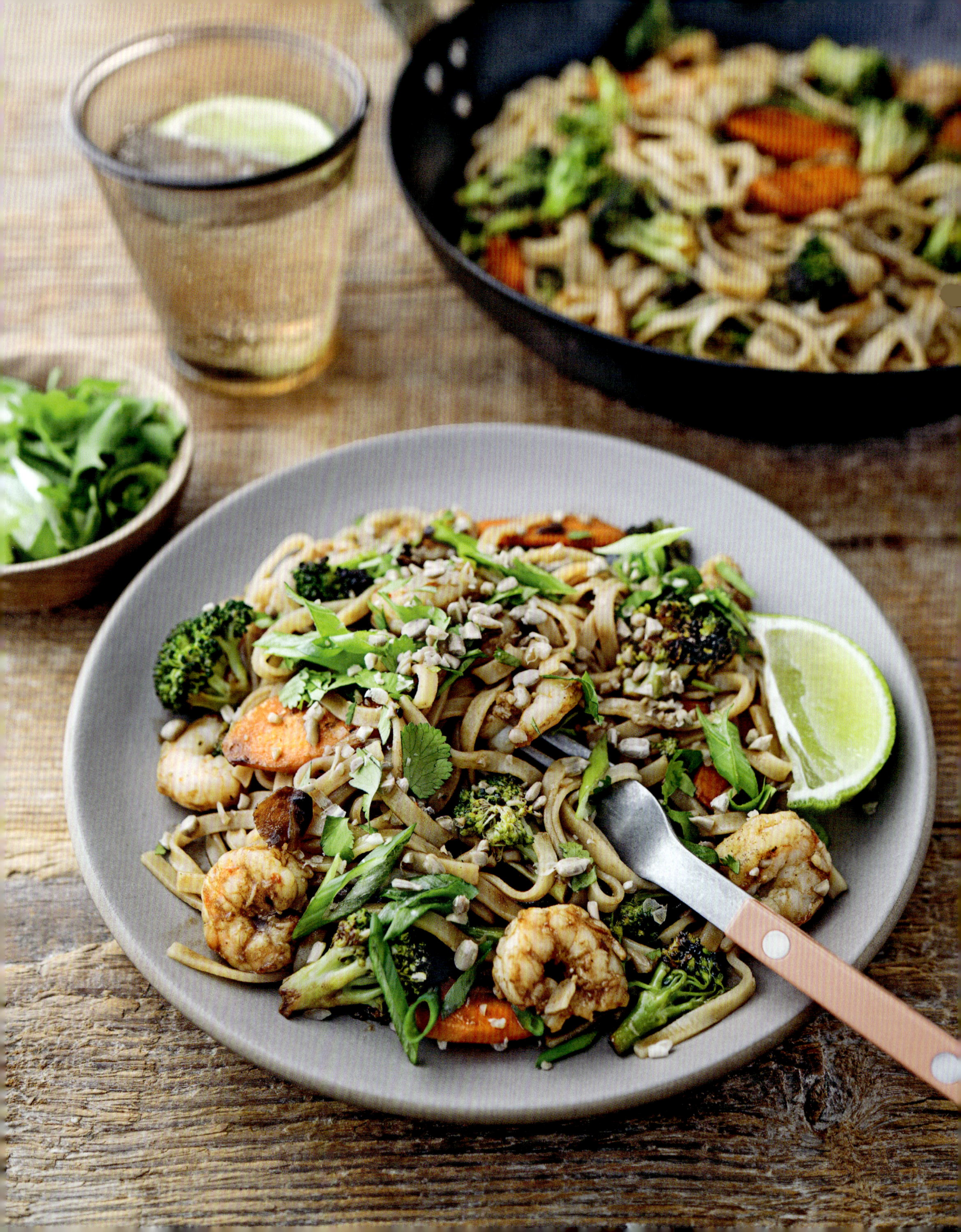

45 MINUTES
MAKES
4 SERVINGS

Thai-Inspired Sunflower Shrimp

8 ounces rice pad Thai noodles

2 tablespoons tamarind paste

1½ tablespoons fish sauce

1½ tablespoons coconut sugar

1½ tablespoons coconut aminos

2 tablespoons avocado oil

½ yellow onion, diced

1 pound broccoli florets, chopped

2 large carrots, cut diagonally into thin slices (about 3 cups)

4 garlic cloves, minced

1 pound medium shrimp, peeled, deveined, and without tails

¼ cup sunflower seeds, minced

1 bunch cilantro, bottom stems removed, chopped

1 bunch green onions, white and green parts, thinly sliced on the diagonal

1 lime, quartered

1. Bring a pot of water to boil, add the rice noodles, and cook according to the package instructions. While the noodles are cooking, make the sauce by whisking the tamarind paste, fish sauce, coconut sugar, and coconut aminos in a large bowl to combine. When the noodles are finished cooking, drain, rinse with cold water, and add to the bowl with the sauce, mixing to combine. Set aside while you cook the vegetables and shrimp.

2. Heat the oil in a large skillet over medium-high heat. When the pan is hot, add the onion and cook, stirring, for 5 minutes, or until starting to brown. Add the broccoli and carrots and cook, stirring occasionally, for about 10 minutes, until browned and just tender. Add the garlic and shrimp and cook, stirring, for about 1 minute, until shrimp are fully cooked. Turn off the heat and add the vegetable mixture to the noodles; mix to coat in the sauce.

3. Serve each plate of noodles and vegetables topped with minced sunflower seeds, cilantro, green onions, and a lime wedge. It keeps for up to 3 days in the refrigerator.

1 HOUR

MAKES
4 SERVINGS

Fall Veggies and Beef with Quinoa and Tahini Sauce

1 pound butternut squash, peeled and cubed

1 red onion, cut into large pieces

1 pound brussels sprouts, ends removed and quartered

2 tablespoons avocado oil

1½ teaspoons sea salt, divided

1 pound ground beef

½ teaspoon ground cumin

½ teaspoon onion powder

⅛ teaspoon garlic powder

⅛ teaspoon ground black pepper

Pinch ground coriander

1½ cups quinoa, rinsed and drained

3 cups water

4 ounces plain unsweetened coconut yogurt (check ingredients)

¼ cup tahini (sesame butter)

1. Preheat the oven to 425°F.

2. In a large bowl, combine the squash, onion, brussels sprouts, oil, and ½ teaspoon of the salt; toss to combine. Arrange evenly on a large baking tray and set aside.

3. In the same bowl, combine the beef, ½ teaspoon of the remaining salt, the cumin, onion powder, garlic powder, pepper, and coriander. Work the seasonings into the meat using your hands, then arrange 2-inch pieces of the beef mixture on top of the vegetables to cook together. Place in the oven and cook for 15 minutes, or until the vegetables are fork-tender and the beef is fully cooked.

4. In the meantime, cook the quinoa. Place the quinoa in a medium saucepan with the water. Bring to a boil, then turn down the heat to maintain a simmer and cook, covered, for 10 to 15 minutes, until all the liquid is absorbed.

5. To make the sauce, whisk together the yogurt, tahini, and remaining ½ teaspoon salt in a small bowl. Serve each bowl of quinoa topped with beef and vegetables and a scoop of sauce. It keeps in the refrigerator for up to 5 days.

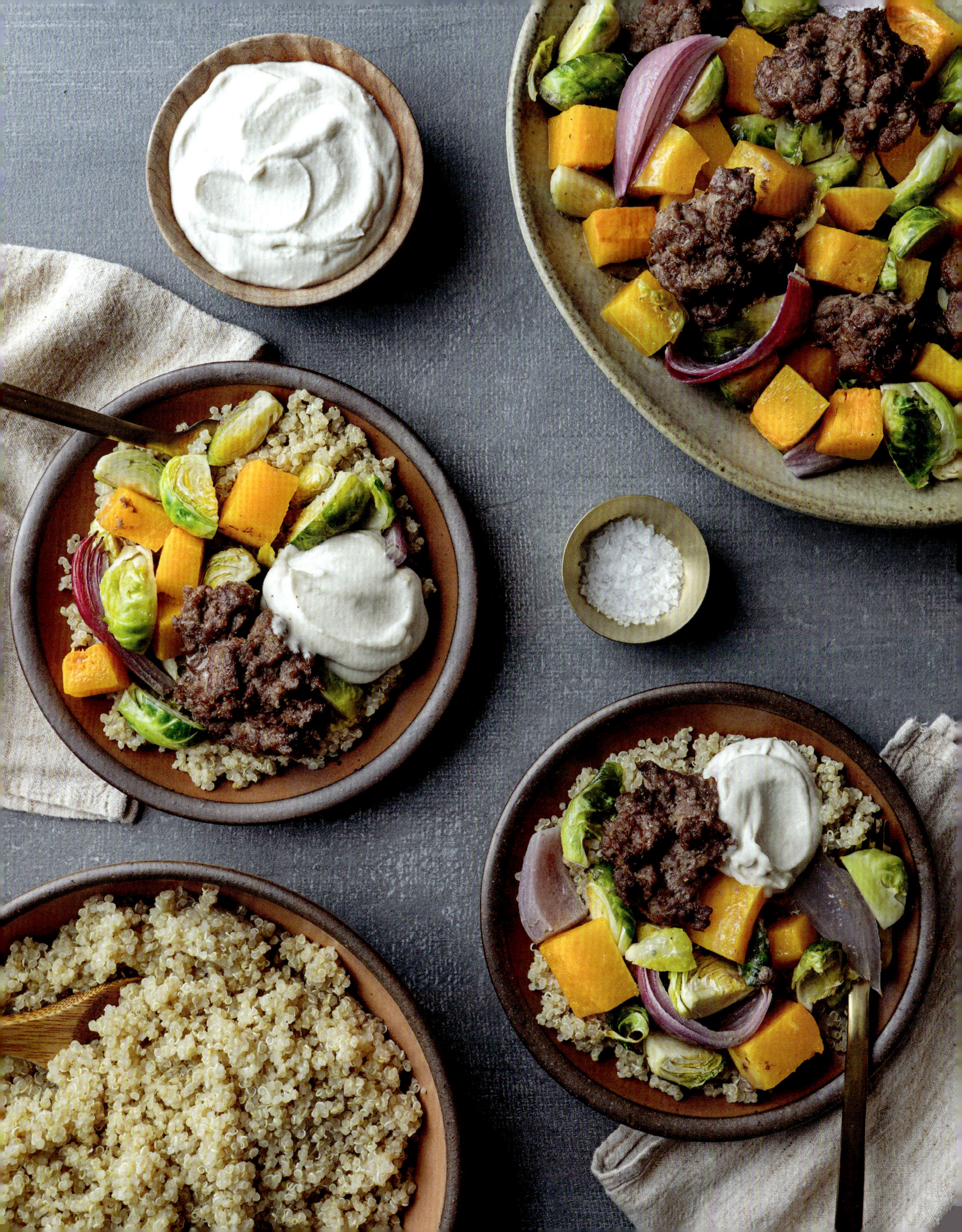

1 HOUR

MAKES
6 SERVINGS

Coconut-Tahini Turkey Meatballs

1½ cups brown rice

3 cups water

2 tablespoons coconut flour

1 teaspoon sea salt

1 teaspoon garlic powder

1 teaspoon onion powder

1 teaspoon ground cumin

½ teaspoon ground black pepper

2 pounds ground turkey (or substitute ground chicken)

2 tablespoons coconut oil (or substitute avocado oil), divided

1 onion, halved and thinly sliced

4 garlic cloves, minced

1 (1-inch) piece ginger, minced

1 cup coconut cream

2 tablespoons tahini (sesame butter)

2 tablespoons coconut aminos

1 tablespoon lime juice (about ½ juicy lime)

1 teaspoon fish sauce

1 bunch Swiss chard, stems removed and cut into ribbons

Fresh cilantro and green onions, for garnish

1. Place the rice in a fine-mesh strainer and rinse under cold water for a minute, then drain. Place the rice in a medium saucepan with the water and bring to a boil over high heat, then turn down the heat to maintain a simmer. Cook, covered, for 30 minutes, or until all the water is absorbed. Remove from the heat and keep covered to steam as you finish the meal.

2. While the rice is cooking, make the meatballs. In a medium bowl, combine the coconut flour, the salt, the garlic powder, onion powder, cumin, and pepper and stir to combine. Add the turkey, mix thoroughly, and form into 1½-inch meatballs.

3. Heat 1 tablespoon of the oil in a lidded, heavy-bottomed pot over medium heat. When the fat has melted and the pan is hot, add the meatballs and brown for 5 minutes, turning each one occasionally to ensure each side is browned. Transfer to a bowl and set aside.

4. Add the remaining 1 tablespoon oil to the pot you used to cook the meatballs, still on medium heat. Add the onion and cook, stirring, for 5 minutes, or until beginning to brown. Add the garlic and ginger and cook, stirring, until fragrant, about 1 minute. Add the coconut cream, tahini, coconut aminos, lime juice, and fish sauce, then add the meatballs back to the pot. Bring to a simmer, cover, and cook for 10 minutes, stirring occasionally.

5. Add the chard to the pot and cook for another 2 minutes, or until the meatballs reach 165°F. Serve the meatballs on a bed of rice generously garnished with cilantro and green onions. It keeps for up to 5 days in the refrigerator.

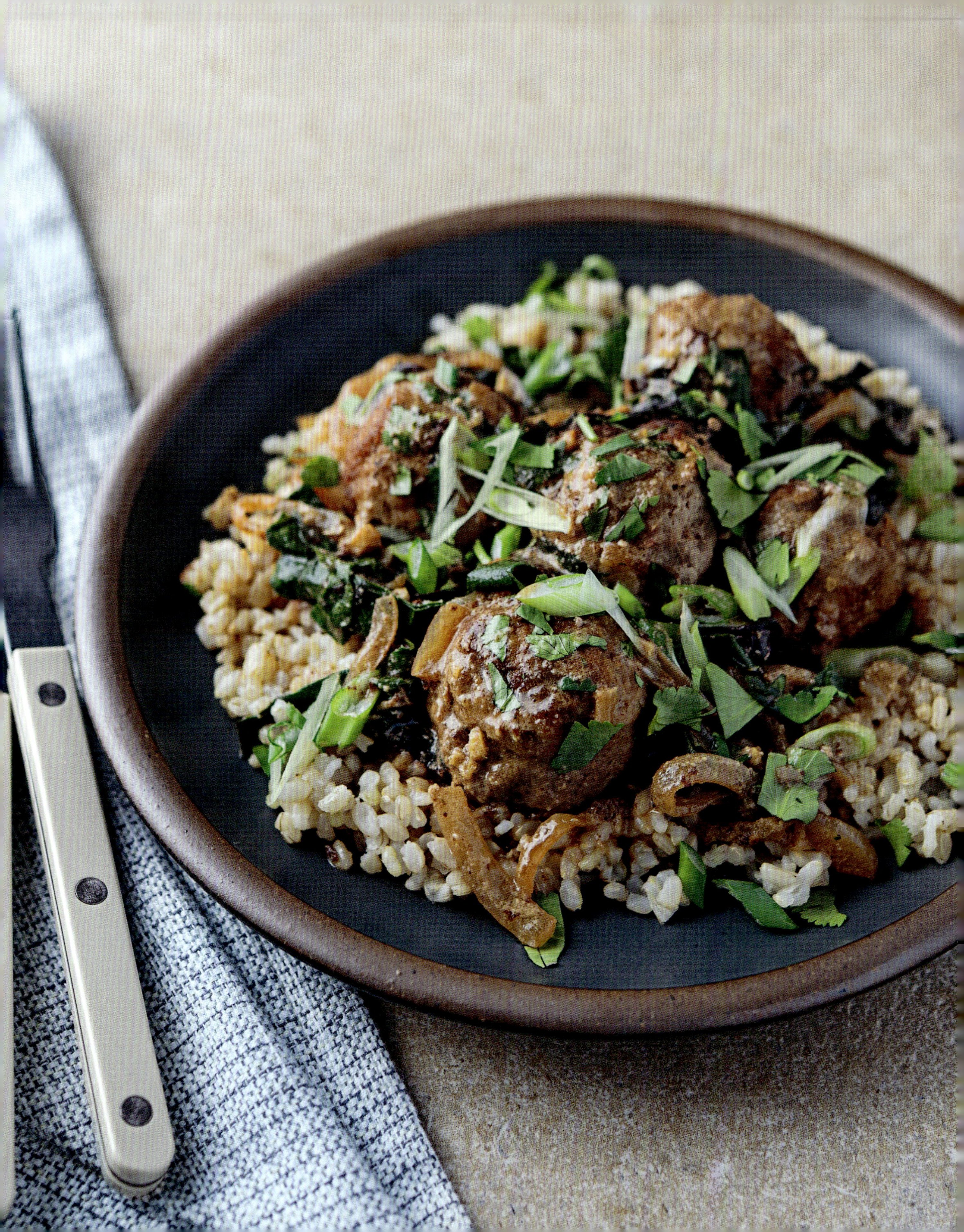

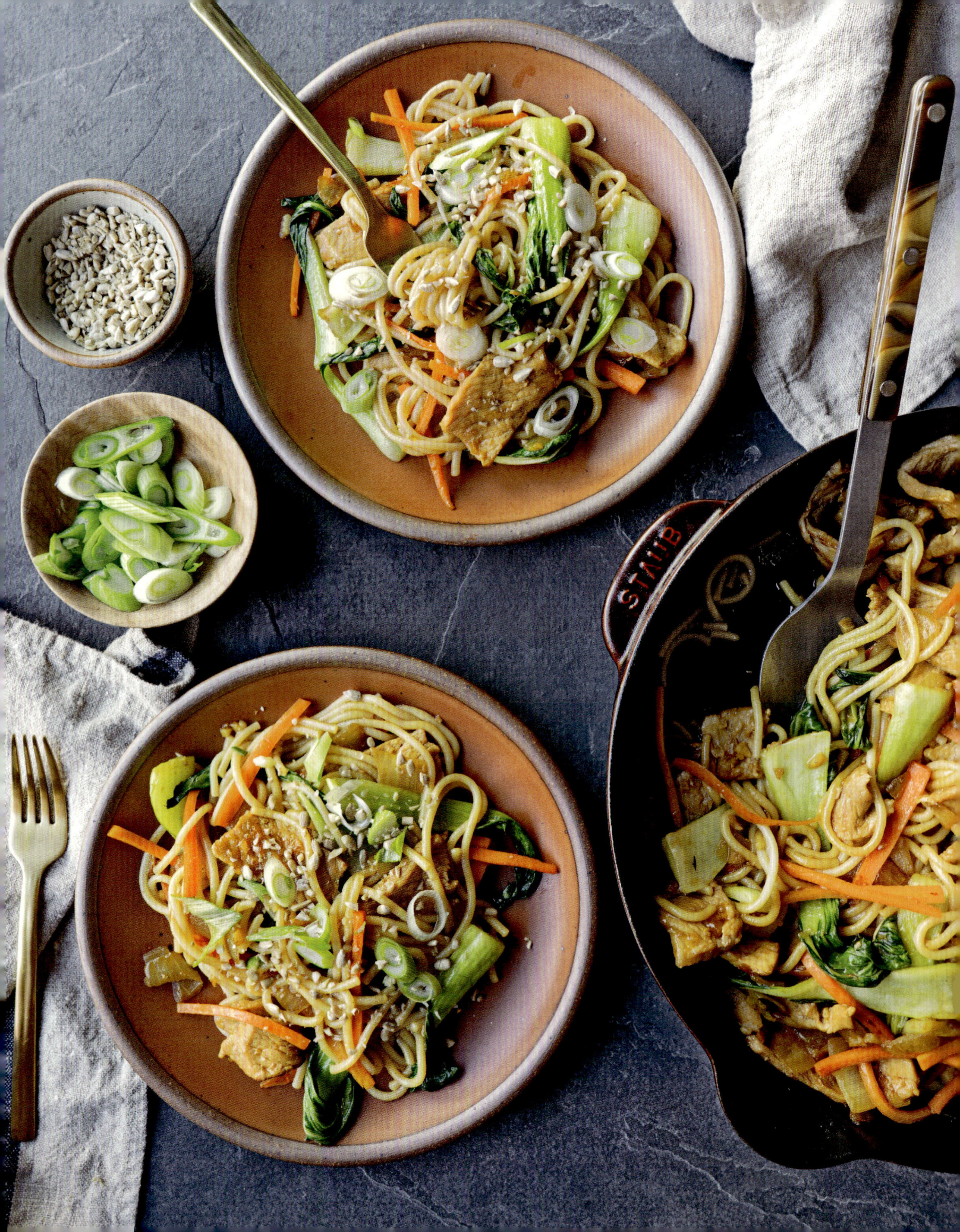
STAUB

45 MINUTES

MAKES
3 SERVINGS

Pork Udon Stir-Fry

8 ounces brown rice udon noodles

2 tablespoons avocado oil, divided

1 onion, chopped

1 carrot, cut into matchsticks

2 baby bok choy, ends removed and leaves halved lengthwise

1½ pounds pork loin chops or tenderloin, cut into strips for stir-fry

¼ teaspoon sea salt

1 (1-inch) piece ginger, minced

4 garlic cloves, minced

½ cup coconut aminos

1 tablespoon arrowroot powder

1 tablespoon rice vinegar

1 bunch green onions, white and green parts, thinly sliced on the diagonal

2 tablespoons sunflower seeds, minced

Sesame seeds, for garnish

1. Bring a pot of water to boil, add the udon noodles, and cook according to the package instructions. Drain and rinse with cold water, then set aside.

2. Heat 1 tablespoon of the oil in a large skillet over medium heat. When the pan is hot, add the onion and cook, stirring, for 3 minutes, or until beginning to brown. Add the carrot and cook for 2 minutes. Add the bok choy and cook for 2 to 3 more minutes, until the greens are wilted and just cooked. Transfer to a bowl and set aside.

3. In the same skillet, heat the remaining 1 tablespoon oil over medium-high heat. When the pan is hot, add the pork and sprinkle with the salt. Cook for 2 to 3 minutes, stirring minimally to allow the pork pieces to brown a bit. Add the ginger and garlic and cook, stirring, for 30 seconds, or until fragrant. Add the coconut aminos to the pan, turn down the heat to medium, and cook the pork and sauce for 3 to 4 minutes, until the sauce has reduced by about half and the pork is cooked throughout.

4. Add the arrowroot powder and vinegar and stir to combine thoroughly as the sauce thickens. Add the noodles and vegetables to the pan and heat, stirring, until fully warm. Serve each portion garnished with green onions, sunflower seeds, and sesame seeds. It keeps in the refrigerator for up to 3 days.

45 MINUTES

MAKES
4 SERVINGS

Tropical Chicken and Rice Bowl

1½ cups long-grain white rice

3 cups water

1 teaspoon sea salt, divided

1½ pounds skinless chicken breast, cut into 1-inch pieces

4 tablespoons avocado oil, divided

1 onion, diced

3 carrots, diced (about 3 cups)

1 cup diced pineapple

1 cup frozen green peas

4 garlic cloves, minced

2 tablespoons coconut aminos

1 teaspoon fish sauce

½ bunch cilantro, bottom stems removed, chopped

2 tablespoons lime juice (about 1 juicy lime)

1. Place the rice in a fine-mesh strainer and rinse under cold water for a minute, then drain. Place the rice and water in a large soup pot or Dutch oven over medium heat and bring to a boil. Turn down the heat to maintain a simmer and cook, covered, for 15 minutes.

2. While the rice is cooking, sprinkle ½ teaspoon of the salt over the chicken and set aside while you make the vegetables. Heat 2 tablespoons of the oil in a large skillet over medium-high heat. When the pan is hot, add the onion and carrots and cook, stirring occasionally, for 5 minutes, or until beginning to brown. Add the pineapple, peas, and garlic and cook for an additional 2 minutes. Turn off the heat and set aside until the rice is finished.

3. When the rice is finished cooking, add the vegetable mixture to the pot with the rice, mix, and cover. Set aside while you cook the chicken. Heat the remaining 2 tablespoons oil in the skillet you cooked the vegetables in over medium heat. When the pan is hot, add the chicken and cook, stirring occasionally, for 5 to 7 minutes, until the chicken is browned and cooked throughout.

4. Add the chicken to the rice and vegetable mixture along with the coconut aminos, fish sauce, cilantro, and lime juice and stir to combine. It keeps for up to 5 days in the refrigerator.

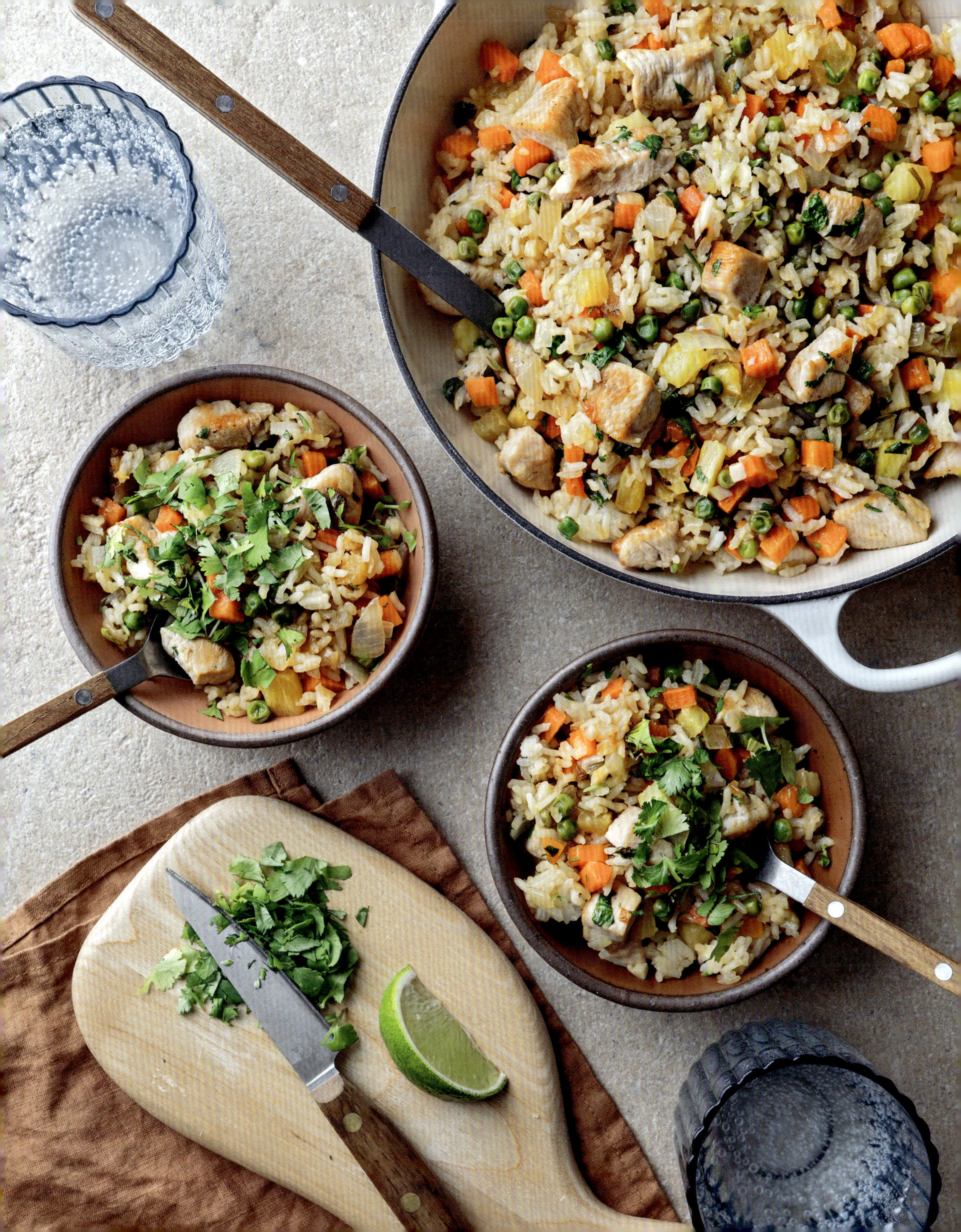

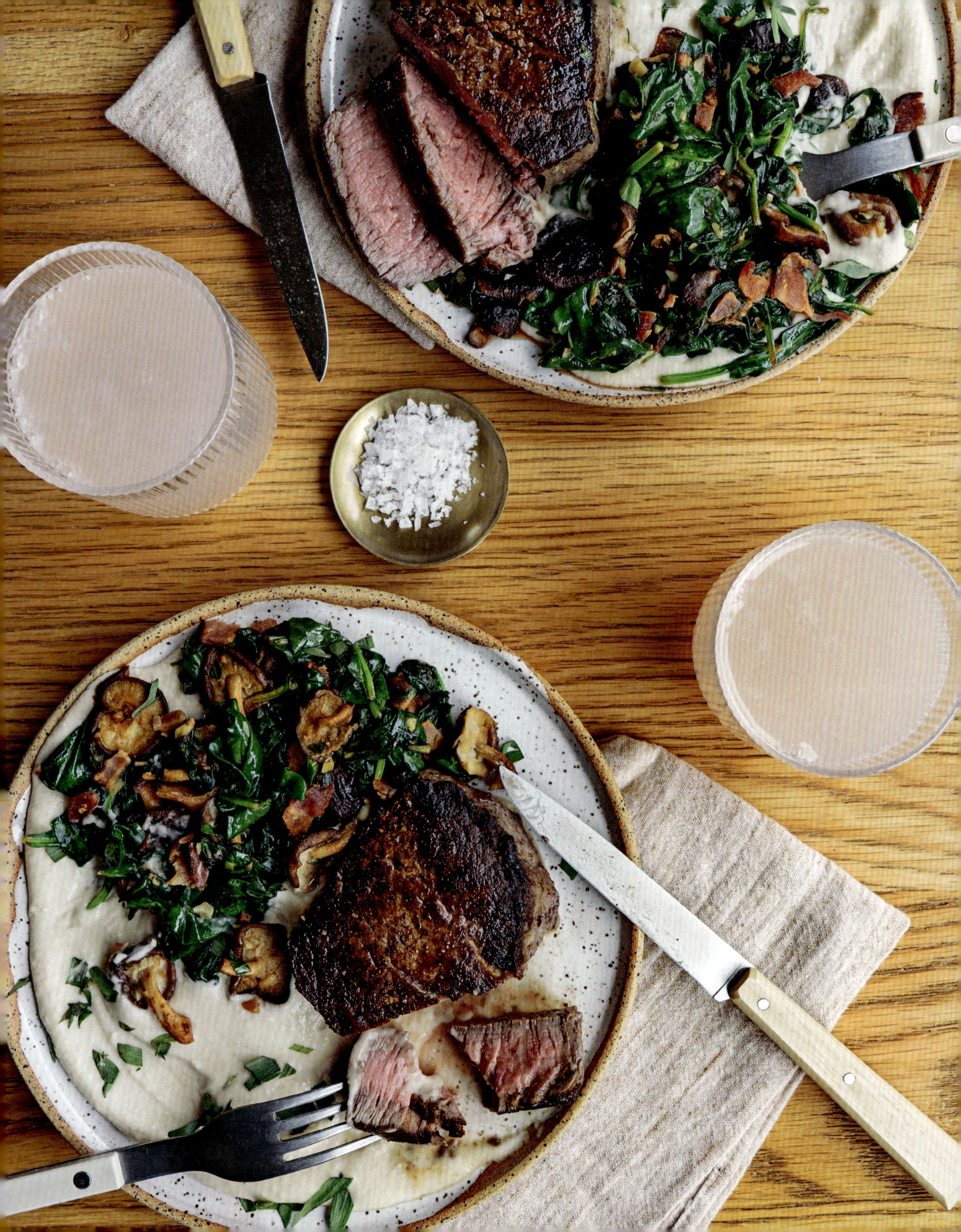

40 MINUTES

MAKES
2 SERVINGS

Steakhouse Dinner with Tarragon and Bacon

2 beef tenderloin steaks, 2½ inches thick (about 12 ounces)

1½ teaspoons sea salt, divided

½ teaspoon ground black pepper

1 (14-ounce) can navy beans, drained and rinsed

¼ cup olive oil

1½ tablespoons lemon juice (about ½ lemon)

2 tablespoons water, plus more if needed

1 garlic clove

4 slices thick-cut uncured bacon (check ingredients)

4 ounces shiitake mushrooms (or substitute button mushrooms), cut into 2-inch pieces

4 garlic cloves, minced

5 ounces baby spinach leaves

1½ tablespoons lemon juice (about ½ lemon)

¼ cup fresh tarragon leaves, chopped and divided

1. Preheat the oven to 425°F. Rub the steaks all over with 1 teaspoon of the salt and the pepper and set aside.

2. To make the bean puree, combine the beans, oil, lemon juice, water, garlic, and ¼ teaspoon of the remaining salt in a blender or food processor and blend until smooth. If the consistency is too thick, add water 1 tablespoon at a time until desired consistency is reached. Transfer to a small saucepan and set aside.

3. Next, cook the bacon slices in a large skillet, flipping as needed, until the slices are crisp, about 10 minutes. Transfer to a paper towel–lined plate to cool and carefully transfer about 1 tablespoon of fat to a separate ovenproof skillet to use with the steaks, reserving the rest of the fat in the original skillet (you'll use this in a few minutes to cook the vegetables).

4. Before beginning to cook the steaks, check that your oven is at temperature. Turn the heat under the ovenproof skillet with 1 tablespoon of the fat to medium-high. When hot, add the steaks and allow to cook, untouched, for 4 to 5 minutes, until a nice crust has formed on one side. Flip the steaks and place directly in the oven; cook for another 5 to 7 minutes, until the internal temperature is 125°F (for medium-rare; cook to 135°F for a medium steak). Immediately transfer to a cutting board, cover with foil, and rest for at least 5 minutes.

5. While the steak is cooking, heat the bean puree and chop the bacon so they are ready to serve. While the steak is resting, make the vegetables. Turn the heat under the pan you cooked the bacon in to medium. When hot, add the mushrooms and cook for 3 minutes. Add the garlic and cook, stirring, until fragrant, about 30 seconds. Add the spinach and cook until wilted, 1 to 2 minutes, then add the lemon juice, chopped bacon, the remaining ¼ teaspoon salt, and half of the tarragon; stir to combine.

6. Serve a portion of bean puree topped with vegetables and steak. Garnish with the remaining tarragon.

CHAPTER 17

Modified Sweet Treats

1 HOUR
MAKES 8 BARS

Hemp and Buckwheat Bliss Bars

¼ cup tahini (sesame butter)

¼ cup maple syrup

¼ cup avocado oil

2 tablespoons ground flax seeds

2 tablespoons tapioca or arrowroot starch

1 cup hulled hemp seeds

1 cup buckwheat groats

½ cup pumpkin seeds

2 tablespoons maple, coconut, or date sugar

½ teaspoon sea salt

½ teaspoon ground cinnamon

½ teaspoon ground ginger

¼ cup dark chocolate chips (check ingredients)

1. Preheat the oven to 325°F. Line an 8-inch square baking dish with parchment paper and set aside.

2. Combine the tahini, maple syrup, and oil in a small saucepan over low heat. Heat, stirring, until warm and the ingredients are combined. Stir in the flax seeds and tapioca or arrowroot starch; set aside.

3. In a large bowl, combine the hemp seeds, buckwheat, pumpkin seeds, maple sugar, salt, cinnamon, and ginger and stir to combine. Add the tahini mixture and mix thoroughly. Stir in the chocolate chips. Transfer the mixture to the prepared baking dish, using a spatula to gently tamp down and work evenly into each corner. Bake for 45 minutes, or until beginning to turn golden brown.

4. Allow to cool fully in the pan, then cut into 8 bars. It keeps for up to 2 weeks in an airtight container at room temperature.

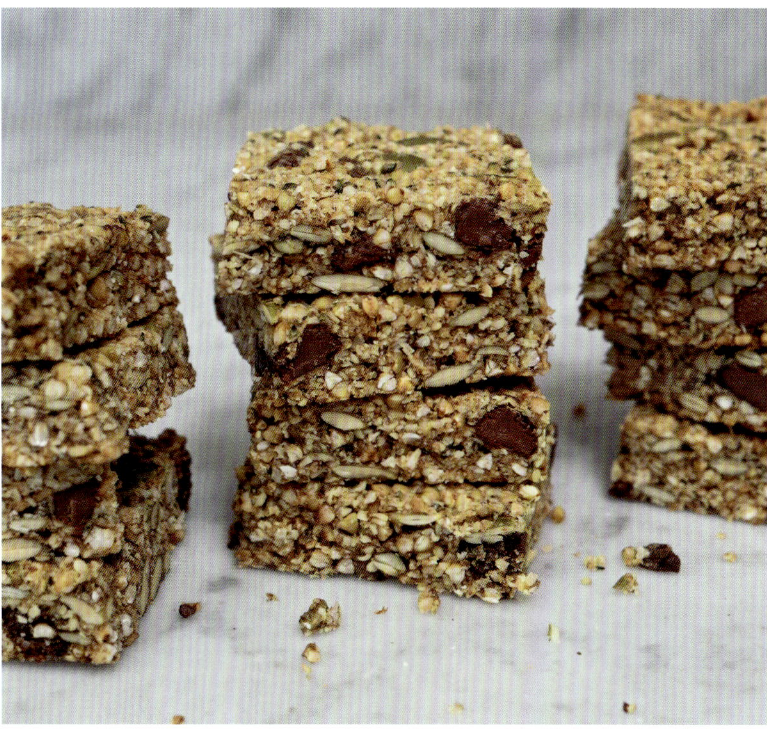

35 MINUTES
MAKES 2 DOZEN COOKIES

Vanilla Tahini Cookies

1 cup (160 grams) sweet white rice flour

½ cup (60 grams) tapioca flour

½ teaspoon baking soda

½ teaspoon sea salt

½ cup tahini (sesame butter)

½ cup maple syrup

1 tablespoon vanilla extract

¼ cup sesame seeds

1. Preheat the oven to 350°F. Line a baking sheet with parchment paper.

2. In a medium bowl, combine the rice flour, tapioca flour, baking soda, and salt. Set aside.

3. In a large bowl, combine the tahini, maple syrup, and vanilla and mix until smooth. Add the dry ingredients and stir until a slightly crumbly dough forms. You may need to use your hands to work the final bits together. Form into a large ball and set aside.

4. Spread the sesame seeds on a small plate. Using your hands, roll about 1 tablespoon of the mixture into a ball and gently flatten with the bottom of a glass. Press one side to coat with sesame seeds, then arrange on the baking sheet. Bake for 15 to 18 minutes, until cracked on top and slightly browned beneath.

5. Allow the cookies to cool for at least 10 minutes before serving. They keep for up to 1 week in an airtight container at room temperature.

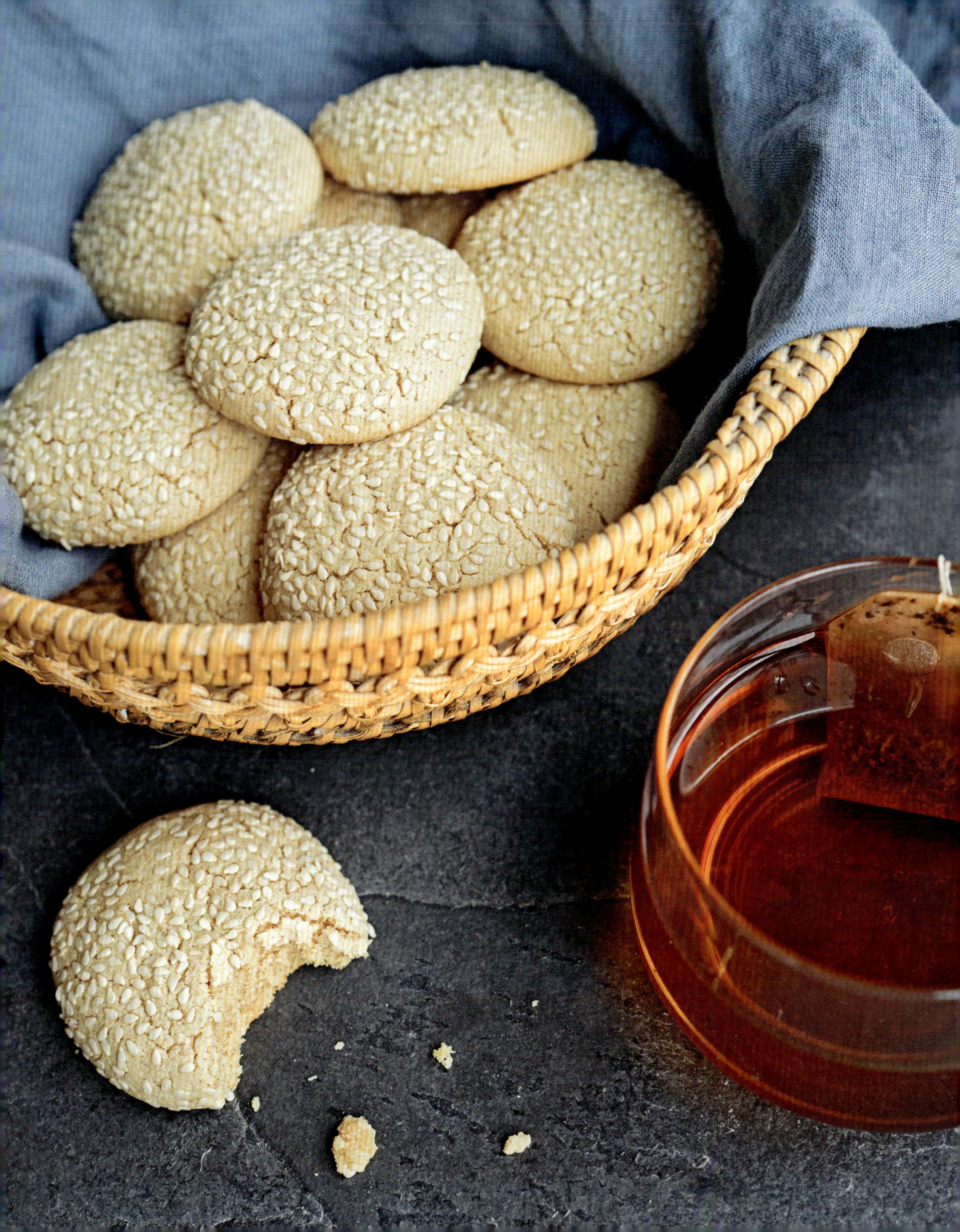

45 MINUTES

MAKES
12 BROWNIES

Fudgy Maple Cacao Brownies

3 tablespoons ground flax seeds

¾ cup water

½ cup avocado oil

3 tablespoons tahini (sesame butter)

⅓ cup maple syrup

2 teaspoons vanilla extract

1 cup (160 grams) sweet white rice flour

¾ cup maple sugar (or substitute coconut sugar)

⅓ cup (40 grams) tapioca flour

⅓ cup cacao powder

½ teaspoon baking soda

½ teaspoon sea salt

⅓ cup dark chocolate chips (check ingredients)

1. Preheat the oven to 350°F. Line an 8-inch square baking pan with parchment paper; set aside.

2. In a small bowl, add the flax seeds and water and whisk to combine. Set aside for 5 minutes so the flax can absorb some of the water. In a medium bowl, combine the oil, tahini, maple syrup, and vanilla and use an electric mixer on low speed or a whisk to combine. Set aside.

3. In a large bowl, combine the rice flour, sugar, tapioca flour, cacao powder, baking soda, and salt. Add both the oil and flax mixtures to the bowl and mix well until a thin batter forms.

4. Pour into the prepared baking dish and sprinkle the chocolate chips evenly across the surface, letting them sink into the mixture. For a chewy texture, bake for 25 minutes, or until a top crust has formed and a knife is mostly clean (but not completely dry) when inserted. For a cake-like texture, bake for 30 minutes, or until a knife inserted comes out clean. Allow to cool completely before enjoying. It keeps for up to 5 days in an airtight container at room temperature.

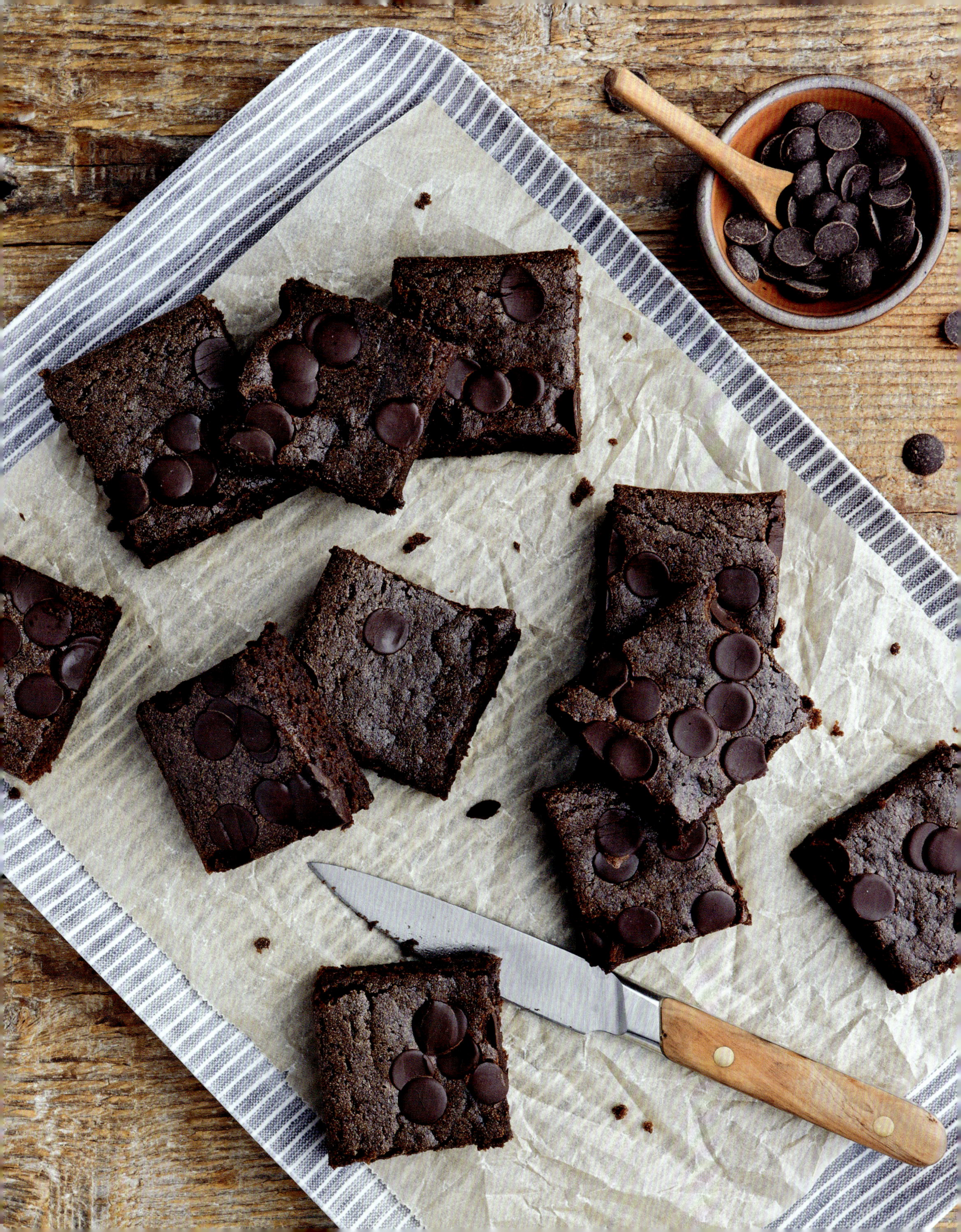

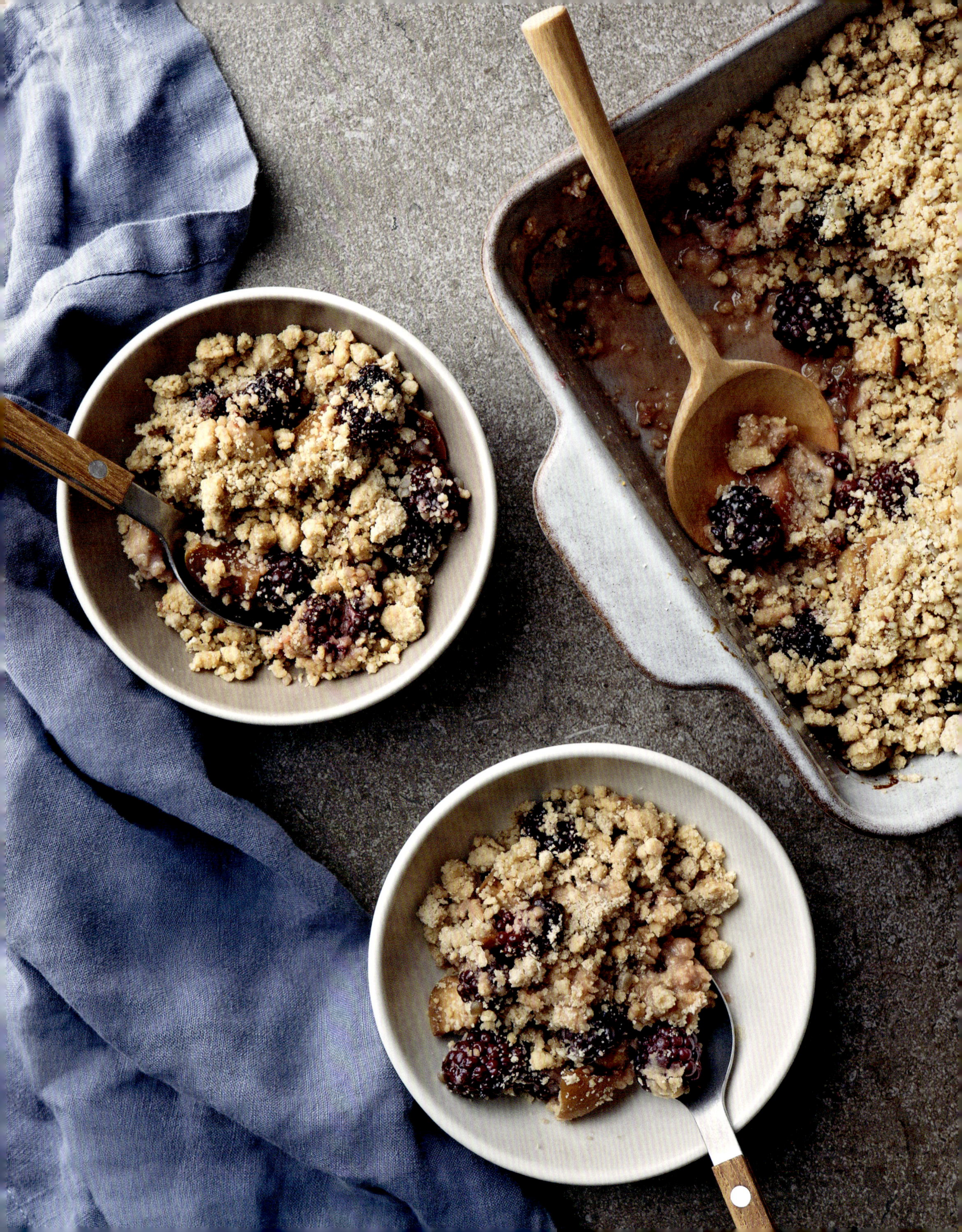

1 HOUR
30 MINUTES

MAKES
6 SERVINGS

Stone Fruit and Seed Crumble

FILLING

5 firm nectarines or peaches, pitted and cut into pieces

3 cups blackberries (fresh or frozen)

2 to 3 tablespoons maple sugar (or substitute coconut or date sugar)

TOPPING

1 cup (150 grams) cassava flour

⅓ cup maple sugar (or substitute coconut or date sugar)

¼ cup (28 grams) arrowroot flour

1 teaspoon ground ginger

¼ teaspoon ground cardamom

¼ teaspoon sea salt

½ cup vegetable shortening or ghee (see page 210)

2 to 3 tablespoons water

1 teaspoon vanilla extract

2 tablespoons sunflower seeds, minced

NOTE: *If you need to serve a crowd, double this recipe and bake it in a 9 by 13-inch baking dish.*

1. Preheat the oven to 350°F.

2. In a large bowl, combine the nectarines, berries, and 2 tablespoons of the maple sugar and stir to combine thoroughly (if your fruit is more tart than usual, use 3 tablespoons). Transfer to an 8-inch square baking pan, using a spatula to gently level it. Set aside.

3. To make the topping, combine the cassava flour, maple sugar, arrowroot, ginger, cardamom, and salt in a medium bowl. Add the shortening, 2 tablespoons water, and the vanilla and work with your hands to combine until small, pea-size granules form. If your mixture is on the dry side, add the remaining 1 tablespoon water. Keep working until the mixture forms a dry dough that can be broken apart into smaller pieces. When the consistency is right, add the sunflower seeds.

4. Use your hands to distribute the topping evenly over the fruit mixture, without disrupting the granules too much. Bake for 45 to 50 minutes, until the topping is just browned. Cool to room temperature before serving. It keeps for up to 5 days in the refrigerator.

3 HOURS, WITH TIME TO SET

MAKES 6 SERVINGS

Spiced Pear Upside-Down Cake

TOPPING

⅓ cup avocado oil

⅓ cup maple syrup

⅓ cup maple sugar

1 teaspoon ground cinnamon

½ teaspoon ground ginger

⅛ teaspoon ground allspice

⅛ teaspoon ground cardamom

Pinch ground cloves

¼ teaspoon sea salt

2 firm pears, cored and cut into thin slices

CAKE

¾ cup unsweetened applesauce

½ cup maple syrup

¼ cup water

2 tablespoons gelatin powder

¾ cup (84 grams) coconut flour

¾ cup (90 grams) tapioca flour

1 teaspoon baking soda

¼ teaspoon sea salt

1 teaspoon ground cinnamon

½ teaspoon ground ginger

½ cup avocado oil

1 tablespoon lemon juice

1 teaspoon vanilla extract

1. Preheat the oven to 325°F. Line an 8-inch cake pan with parchment paper (see the Lining Cake Pans tutorial on page 287). Set aside.

2. First, make the spiced maple topping and arrange the pears. In a small saucepan, stir the oil, maple syrup, maple sugar, cinnamon, ginger, allspice, cardamom, cloves, and salt to combine. Place on the stovetop, turn the heat to low, and cook for 5 minutes, or until the mixture has warmed and the sugar has dissolved. Pour into the prepared cake pan. Arrange the pear slices in a slightly overlapping pattern evenly along the bottom of the pan. Set aside.

3. Next, prepare the cake batter. In a small saucepan, whisk the applesauce, maple syrup, and water to combine. Sprinkle with the gelatin and set aside for at least 5 minutes, so the gelatin can bloom and absorb the liquid.

4. In a large bowl, combine the flours, baking soda, salt, cinnamon, and ginger. Stir to combine. In a medium bowl, whisk the oil, lemon juice, and vanilla to combine and set aside.

5. Place the saucepan with the gelatin mixture on the stovetop on the lowest heat setting. Whisk as it warms and take off the heat when the gelatin has dissolved (around 120°F—do not overheat). Add the warm gelatin mixture to the bowl with the oil and whisk or use an electric mixer on low speed to combine thoroughly, then add to the bowl with the flours and continue to mix until fully combined. Your mixture will be thicker than usual cake batter—this is normal.

6. Pour the mixture into the prepared cake pan and use a spatula to level the surface, as the mixture will be too thick to naturally even out. Bake for 1 hour 10 minutes, or until golden brown and just firm to the touch. Allow to cool completely in the cake pan placed on a wire rack, then turn out onto a plate or rack and let sit for another hour for the gelatin to set. It keeps for up to 5 days in the refrigerator.

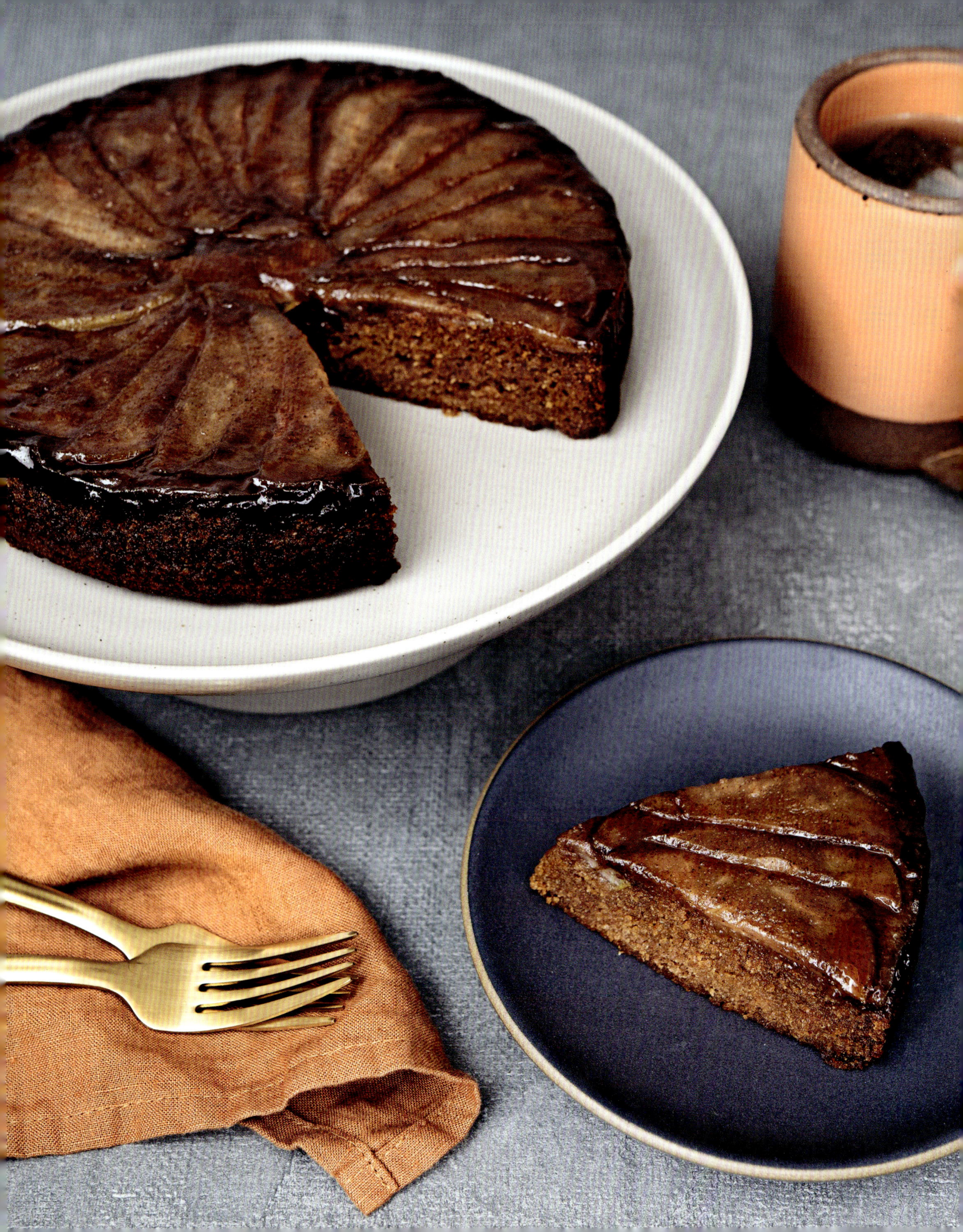

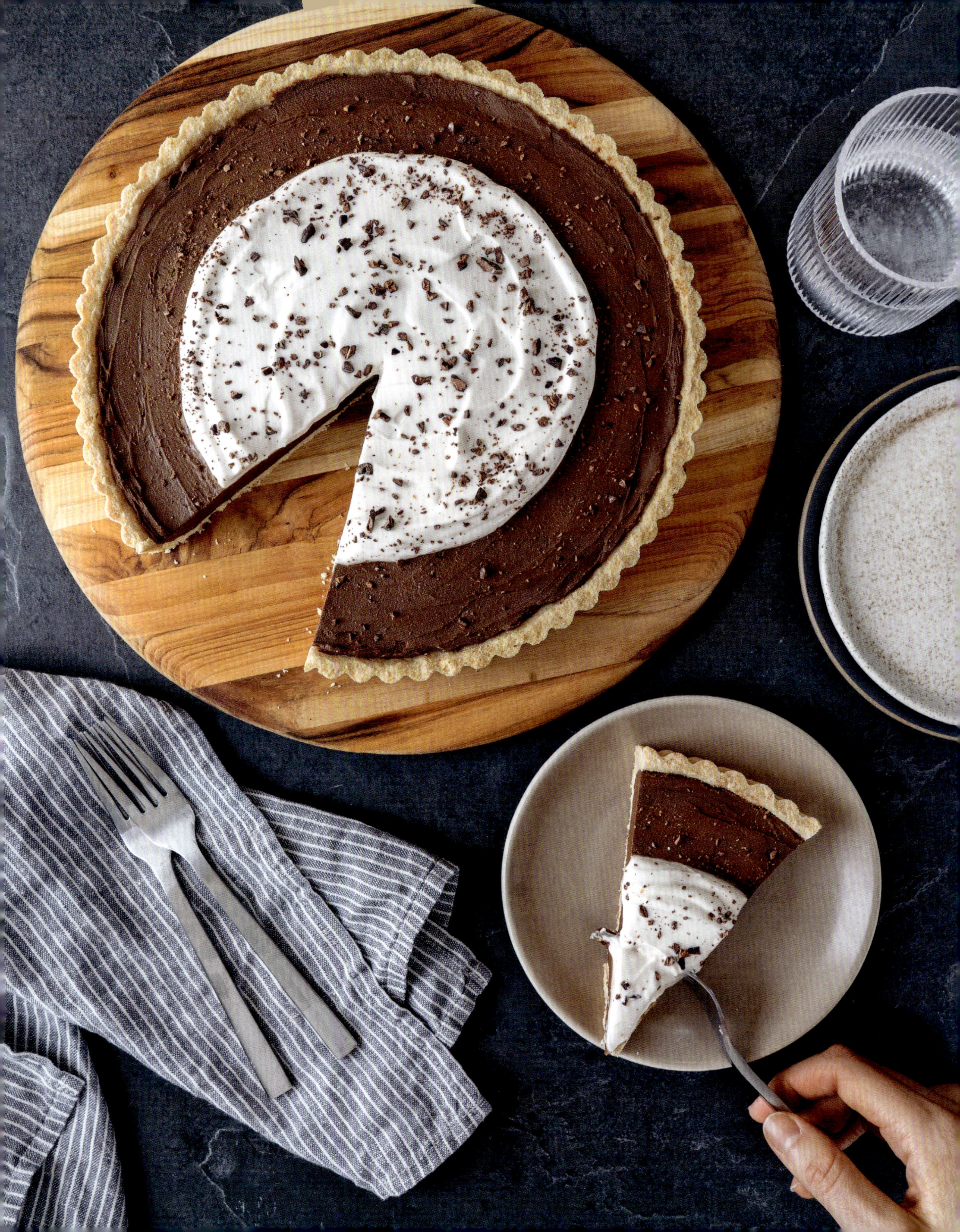

Chocolate Cream Pie

1 HOUR
30 MINUTES, PLUS
2 HOURS TO SET

MAKES
8 SERVINGS

1¼ cups (200 grams) sweet white rice flour

½ cup maple sugar

¼ cup (30 grams) tapioca flour

½ teaspoon sea salt, divided

½ cup palm shortening

1 tablespoon water, plus more if needed

9 ounces dark chocolate chips (check ingredients)

3 cups mashed avocado (3 to 4 avocados)

⅓ cup maple syrup

1 teaspoon vanilla extract

2 tablespoons cacao powder

1 recipe Maple-Yogurt Cream (page 192)

Cacao nibs, for garnish (optional)

1. Preheat the oven to 350°F.

2. First, make the crust. Place the rice flour, maple sugar, tapioca flour, and ¼ teaspoon of the salt in the bowl of a food processor and pulse once to combine. Add the shortening and process on low speed until a crumbly mixture forms; don't overmix. Add the water and pulse to combine until a crumbly dough comes together. If the mixture is too dry, add additional water 1 teaspoon at a time until the dough comes together, but it is best if the mixture is on the dry side.

3. Place the mixture in the bottom of a 9-inch tart pan. Use your hands to gently work the mixture across the bottom and up the sides, pressing it into an even form but taking care not to work the dough too much to preserve the crumbly texture. Prick with a fork and bake for 12 to 14 minutes, until just beginning to brown. Remove from the oven and set on a wire rack to cool for 20 minutes.

4. When the crust has cooled, make the filling. Place the chocolate chips in a small saucepan and heat over low heat, stirring occasionally, until they are just melted. Take off the heat and set aside.

5. In the bowl of the food processor or a high-powered blender, combine the avocado, maple syrup, vanilla, cacao powder, and remaining ¼ teaspoon of salt and process on low speed until the avocado is fully smooth and combined, 1 to 2 minutes. Pour in the melted chocolate and process until smooth. Immediately pour into the cooled tart crust, using a spatula to smooth into the sides of the crust. Place in the refrigerator to set for at least 2 hours.

6. When the tart is ready to serve, spoon the Maple-Yogurt Cream over the top and garnish with cacao nibs, if desired.

CHAPTER 18

Modified AIP 4-Week Meal Plan and Shopping Lists

In this chapter you'll find four complete weeks of done-for-you meal plans and corresponding shopping lists to help you get started right away. Some notes:

- **Servings:** Each week of the meal plans serve one person for generous servings of breakfasts, lunches, and dinners. If you find the quantities are too large, freeze any extra servings for later. (If you need a meal plan that serves two people, visit THEAUTOIMMUNEPROTOCOL.COM/PRINTABLES for a downloadable meal plan that serves two.)
- **Schedule:** Cooking from scratch is only required on nights and weekends; most meals simply need to be reheated or assembled quickly. Scratch-cooked meals are noted in color and bold type with the corresponding page number for the recipe. Meals to be eaten as leftovers are shown in regular font.
- **Prep day:** They day before the meal plan starts and every subsequent Sunday is designated as prep day—most weeks you'll do some extra batch-cooking on these days. Take note of which meals are to be prepped ahead on prep day.
- **Bone broth:** You can either purchase or make broth for cooking recipes called for in the plans (see page 119 for my recipe). Bones are on the shopping lists, but you can eliminate that if you purchase or have a stash of broth already.
- **Storage:** You will need to freeze and thaw portions of meals for use later in the meal plan; it is always handy to freeze in single-serving portions, but I've noted where you can freeze three or four servings together if you want. I've given you two days thawing time for single portions of meals that will need only a quick reheat when the time comes to enjoy them. You can reduce this if you use a microwave to quickly thaw your meals.

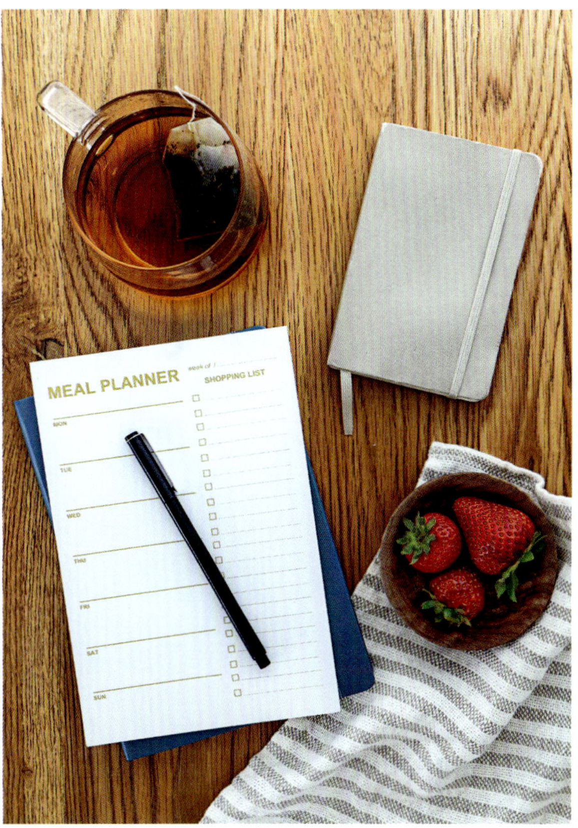

- **Shopping for fresh items:** You will need to shop before cooking dinner on Sundays and Wednesdays—if you want to shop on different days, adjust accordingly. Always cross-reference your shopping list with what you have left over from the previous shopping session to make sure you don't buy anything you may still have in stock (especially things like lemons or fresh herbs).
- **Shopping for pantry items:** Before each shopping session, compare the provided shopping list with items you have in your pantry and add as needed.

MODIFIED AIP MEAL PLAN: Week 1

	BREAKFAST	LUNCH	DINNER	NOTES
SUNDAY PREP	**NUTRIVORE BREAKFAST BATCH COOK,** page 144 **HERBED QUINOA BOWL WITH ROASTED SALMON,** page 231 **HEALING BONE BROTH,** page 119 (optional)			*Portion 5 cups of Healing Bone Broth to keep in the refrigerator to use next week; freeze 4 cups together for use in week 3 and freeze the remaining separately*
MONDAY	Nutrivore Breakfast	Herbed Quinoa Bowl with Roasted Salmon	**SAVORY BEEF AND BEAN CHILI,** page 235	*Freeze 4 portions of Savory Beef and Bean Chili (together or individually)*
TUESDAY	Nutrivore Breakfast	Herbed Quinoa Bowl with Roasted Salmon	Savory Beef and Bean Chili	
WEDNESDAY	Nutrivore Breakfast	Herbed Quinoa Bowl with Roasted Salmon	Savory Beef and Bean Chili	
THURSDAY	Nutrivore Breakfast	Herbed Quinoa Bowl with Roasted Salmon	**HEARTY PORK AND CABBAGE STEW,** page 158	*Freeze 3 portions of Hearty Pork and Cabbage Stew (together or individually)*
FRIDAY	Nutrivore Breakfast	Savory Beef and Bean Chili	Hearty Pork and Cabbage Stew	
SATURDAY	Nutrivore Breakfast	Hearty Pork and Cabbage Stew	**CURRIED BEEF VEGETABLE PIE,** page 171	*Freeze 4 portions of Curried Beef Vegetable Pie (together or individually)*
SUNDAY	**SPICED PORK SKILLET BREAKFAST,** page 225	Curried Beef Vegetable Pie	**BACON CHICKEN RANCH SALAD,** page 153	
SUNDAY PREP	**LEMONGRASS GINGER BREAKFAST SOUP,** page 143			*This meal can be batch-cooked anytime on Sunday for the following week; freeze 4 portions*

MODIFIED AIP MEAL PLAN: Week 2

	BREAKFAST	LUNCH	DINNER	NOTES
MONDAY	Spiced Pork Skillet Breakfast	Bacon Chicken Ranch Salad	Curried Beef Vegetable Pie	
TUESDAY	Spiced Pork Skillet Breakfast	Bacon Chicken Ranch Salad	Curried Beef Vegetable Pie	
WEDNESDAY	Lemongrass Ginger Breakfast Soup	Bacon Chicken Ranch Salad	**PORK TENDERLOIN WITH CABBAGE,** page 172	
THURSDAY	Lemongrass Ginger Breakfast Soup	Pork Tenderloin with Cabbage	**CHICKEN AND CHICKPEA CURRY,** page 247	
FRIDAY	Lemongrass Ginger Breakfast Soup	Pork Tenderloin with Cabbage	Chicken and Chickpea Curry	*Pull out 3 portions of Hearty Pork and Cabbage Stew to thaw for Sunday*
SATURDAY	**LEMON TARRAGON TURKEY SKILLET,** page 137	Pork Tenderloin with Cabbage	Chicken and Chickpea Curry	
SUNDAY	Lemon Tarragon Turkey Skillet	Chicken and Chickpea Curry	Hearty Pork and Cabbage Stew	
SUNDAY PREP	**NUTRIVORE BREAKFAST BATCH COOK,** page 144			*This meal can be batch-cooked anytime on Sunday for the following week*

MODIFIED AIP MEAL PLAN: Week 3

	BREAKFAST	LUNCH	DINNER	NOTES
MONDAY	Lemon Tarragon Turkey Skillet	Hearty Pork and Cabbage Stew	Chicken and Chickpea Curry	*Pull out 4 portions of Savory Beef and Bean Chili to thaw for Wednesday*
TUESDAY	Nutrivore Breakfast	Hearty Pork and Cabbage Stew	Chicken and Chickpea Curry	
WEDNESDAY	Nutrivore Breakfast	Savory Beef and Bean Chili	**THAI LIME CHICKEN LETTUCE CUPS,** page 229	
THURSDAY	Nutrivore Breakfast	Thai Lime Chicken Lettuce Cups	Savory Beef and Bean Chili	
FRIDAY	Nutrivore Breakfast	Thai Lime Chicken Lettuce Cups	Savory Beef and Bean Chili	*Pull out 4 portions of Curried Beef Vegetable Pie to thaw for Sunday* *Pull out 4 cups of Healing Bone Broth to thaw for making stew on Sunday*
SATURDAY	Nutrivore Breakfast	Thai Lime Chicken Lettuce Cups	Savory Beef and Bean Chili	*Pull out 4 portions of Lemongrass Ginger Breakfast Soup to thaw for Monday*
SUNDAY	Nutrivore Breakfast	Curried Beef and Vegetable Pie	**COZY WHITE BEAN STEW,** page 236	*Soak beans in the morning to make Cozy White Bean Stew in the evening*

MODIFIED AIP MEAL PLAN: Week 4

	BREAKFAST	LUNCH	DINNER	NOTES
MONDAY	Lemongrass Breakfast Soup	Curried Beef and Vegetable Pie	Cozy White Bean Stew	
TUESDAY	Lemongrass Breakfast Soup	Curried Beef and Vegetable Pie	Cozy White Bean Stew	
WEDNESDAY	Lemongrass Breakfast Soup	Curried Beef and Vegetable Pie	Cozy White Bean Stew	
THURSDAY	Lemongrass Breakfast Soup	Cozy White Bean Stew	**FALL VEGGIES AND BEEF WITH QUINOA AND TAHINI SAUCE,** page 252	*Soak the buckwheat groats in the evening to make Buckwheat Porridge on Friday*
FRIDAY	**BUCKWHEAT BREAKFAST PORRIDGE,** page 219	Cozy White Bean Stew	Fall Veggies and Beef with Quinoa and Tahini Sauce	
SATURDAY	Buckwheat Porridge	Fall Veggies and Beef with Quinoa and Tahini Sauce	**CAULI-SHRIMP STIR-FRY,** page 167	
SUNDAY	Buckwheat Porridge	Fall Veggies and Beef with Quinoa and Tahini Sauce	Cauli-Shrimp Stir-Fry	

MODIFIED AIP SHOPPING LIST: Week 1

PANTRY ITEMS

OILS/VINEGARS

- ☐ Apple cider vinegar
- ☐ Avocado oil
- ☐ Olive oil

SPICES

- ☐ Black pepper
- ☐ Cardamom (ground)
- ☐ Cinnamon (ground)
- ☐ Coriander (ground)
- ☐ Cumin (ground)
- ☐ Garlic powder
- ☐ Ginger powder
- ☐ Onion powder
- ☐ Sea salt
- ☐ Smoked sea salt
- ☐ Turmeric powder

OTHER

- ☐ Capers (check ingredients)
- ☐ Fish sauce
- ☐ Maple syrup
- ☐ Quinoa
- ☐ Tamarind paste
- ☐ Unsweetened dried tart cherries or raisins (check ingredients)

BROTH

- ☐ 5 cups bone broth, homemade (page 119) or store-bought

SUNDAY

MEAT

- ☐ 1½-pound salmon fillet, skin on
- ☐ 3 pounds ground beef
- ☐ 1 pound ground pork

PRODUCE

- ☐ 1 yellow onion
- ☐ 1 red onion
- ☐ 3 pounds sweet potatoes
- ☐ 1 large beet
- ☐ 2 bunches kale
- ☐ 1 cucumber
- ☐ 1 bunch radishes
- ☐ 1 lemon
- ☐ 5 avocados

HERBS

- ☐ 1 head garlic
- ☐ 2 large bunches parsley
- ☐ Fresh mint (½ cup)
- ☐ Fresh oregano, rosemary, or thyme
- ☐ Fresh cilantro, for garnish

OTHER

- ☐ 12 ounces sauerkraut or other fermented vegetables (check ingredients)
- ☐ 1 (14-ounce) can pumpkin puree
- ☐ 3 (14-ounce) cans mixed beans (black, pinto, and/or kidney beans)

WEDNESDAY

MEAT

- ☐ 3 pounds ground pork
- ☐ 2 pounds ground beef

PRODUCE

- ☐ 3 yellow onions
- ☐ 2 pounds light-fleshed sweet potatoes
- ☐ 1 regular sweet potato
- ☐ 3 large carrots
- ☐ 3 pounds parsnips
- ☐ ½ green cabbage
- ☐ 6 ounces brussels sprouts
- ☐ 1 bunch celery
- ☐ 8 ounces mushrooms
- ☐ 1 green apple

HERBS

- ☐ 1 head garlic
- ☐ 1-inch piece fresh ginger
- ☐ Fresh dill

OTHER

- ☐ 16 ounces sauerkraut, homemade (page 120) or store-bought (check ingredients)

MODIFIED AIP SHOPPING LIST: Week 2

PANTRY ITEMS

OILS/VINEGARS

- ☐ Apple cider vinegar
- ☐ Avocado oil
- ☐ Coconut oil
- ☐ Olive oil

SPICES

- ☐ Bay leaves
- ☐ Cinnamon (ground)
- ☐ Coriander (ground)
- ☐ Cumin (ground)
- ☐ Garlic powder
- ☐ Ginger powder
- ☐ Onion powder
- ☐ Sea salt
- ☐ Turmeric powder

OTHER

- ☐ Brown rice
- ☐ Honey
- ☐ Tamarind paste

BROTH

- ☐ ½ cup bone broth, homemade (page 119) or store-bought

SUNDAY

MEAT

- ☐ 3 pounds bone-in, skin-on chicken thighs
- ☐ 1½ pounds chicken breasts
- ☐ 4 slices thick-cut uncured bacon (check ingredients)

PRODUCE

- ☐ 1 yellow onion
- ☐ 1 red onion
- ☐ 2 large sweet potatoes
- ☐ 1 large head romaine lettuce
- ☐ 2 large zucchinis
- ☐ 5 ounces spinach
- ☐ 1 bunch green onions
- ☐ 1 bunch radishes
- ☐ 12 ounces button mushrooms
- ☐ 2 lemons
- ☐ 2 avocados

HERBS

- ☐ 1 head garlic
- ☐ 3 inches fresh ginger
- ☐ 3 lemongrass stalks
- ☐ Fresh dill
- ☐ Fresh thyme
- ☐ Fresh parsley

OTHER

- ☐ 4 ounces plain unsweetened coconut yogurt (check ingredients)

WEDNESDAY

MEAT

- ☐ 1½-pound pork tenderloin
- ☐ 2 pounds chicken breast
- ☐ 1 pound ground turkey

PRODUCE

- ☐ 1 yellow onion
- ☐ 4 shallots
- ☐ 1 small sweet potato
- ☐ 3 carrots
- ☐ 5 ounces baby spinach
- ☐ ½ red cabbage (about 1½ pounds)
- ☐ 1 large or 2 small zucchinis
- ☐ 1 bunch Tuscan kale
- ☐ 8 ounces mushrooms
- ☐ 1 lime
- ☐ 1 lemon
- ☐ 1 green apple

HERBS

- ☐ 1 head garlic
- ☐ 1 inch fresh ginger
- ☐ 1 lemongrass stalk
- ☐ Fresh tarragon (¼ cup)
- ☐ Fresh cilantro (garnish)

OTHER

- ☐ 1 (14-ounce) can coconut milk (check ingredients)
- ☐ 1 (14-ounce) can chickpeas

MODIFIED AIP SHOPPING LIST: Week 3

PANTRY ITEMS

OILS/VINEGARS

- ☐ Avocado oil
- ☐ Olive oil

SPICES

- ☐ Cinnamon
- ☐ Garlic powder
- ☐ Ginger powder
- ☐ Onion powder
- ☐ Sea salt

OTHER

- ☐ Coconut aminos
- ☐ Fish sauce
- ☐ Toasted rice powder (see note on page 229 on making your own)

SUNDAY

MEAT

- ☐ 1 pound ground beef
- ☐ 1 pound ground pork

PRODUCE

- ☐ 3 pounds sweet potatoes
- ☐ 2 bunches kale

HERBS

- ☐ Fresh oregano, rosemary, or thyme

OTHER

- ☐ 12 ounces sauerkraut or other fermented vegetables, homemade (page 120) or store-bought (check ingredients)

WEDNESDAY

MEAT

- ☐ 1½ pounds ground chicken

PRODUCE

- ☐ 2 shallots
- ☐ 1 head romaine lettuce
- ☐ 1 lime

HERBS

- ☐ 1 inch fresh ginger
- ☐ 1 lemongrass stalk
- ☐ 1 bunch cilantro or Thai basil
- ☐ Mint (2 cups)

MODIFIED AIP SHOPPING LIST: Week 4

PANTRY ITEMS

OILS/VINEGARS

- ☐ Apple cider vinegar
- ☐ Avocado oil
- ☐ Olive oil

SPICES

- ☐ Black pepper
- ☐ Cinnamon
- ☐ Coriander (ground)
- ☐ Cumin (ground)
- ☐ Garlic powder
- ☐ Onion powder
- ☐ Sea salt

OTHER

- ☐ Buckwheat groats
- ☐ Coconut aminos
- ☐ Coconut flakes (optional)
- ☐ Coconut sugar
- ☐ Ground flax seeds
- ☐ Hulled hemp seeds
- ☐ Quinoa
- ☐ Pea, hemp, or rice protein powder
- ☐ Tahini (sesame butter)

BROTH

- ☐ 1 quart bone broth, homemade (page 119) or store-bought

SUNDAY

PRODUCE

- ☐ 1 yellow onion
- ☐ 1 carrot
- ☐ 2 large parsnips
- ☐ 1 bunch celery
- ☐ 2 cups oyster mushrooms (or sub button mushrooms)
- ☐ 1 lemon

HERBS

- ☐ 1 head garlic
- ☐ 1 bunch cilantro

OTHER

- ☐ 1 pound dry Great Northern beans

WEDNESDAY

MEAT

- ☐ 1 pound ground beef
- ☐ 1 pound medium shrimp, peeled, deveined, and without tails

PRODUCE

- ☐ 1 red onion
- ☐ 1 white onion
- ☐ 1 pound butternut squash
- ☐ 1 pound brussels sprouts
- ☐ 14 ounces frozen riced cauliflower
- ☐ 6 ounces shiitake mushrooms (or sub button mushrooms)
- ☐ 1 bunch green onions
- ☐ Fresh fruit (for topping 4 servings of porridge)

HERBS

- ☐ Fresh cilantro (garnish)

OTHER

- ☐ 12 ounces plain unsweetened coconut yogurt (check ingredients)
- ☐ 1 (14-ounce) can coconut milk (check ingredients)

Appendixes

KITCHEN SETUP GUIDE

First: Gather Kitchen Essentials

Setting up your kitchen for AIP cooking shouldn't require a major shopping trip or unusual tools. In fact, you likely have most of what you need to start preparing the delicious, nutrient-dense recipes in this book at home already. While kitchen stores may tempt you with endless tools and appliances, the truth is that good cooking relies more on basic techniques and quality ingredients than on expensive or specialty equipment. This guide will help you assess what you already have, make the most of your current tools, and identify any essentials you might want to upgrade or add over time so that you can make the most of your resources.

Start by taking stock of your kitchen basics. A sharp knife, a sturdy cutting board, and a few reliable pots and pans will carry you through most recipes in this book with ease. If any of your essentials need maintenance—like sharpening a dull knife or replacing a worn-out spatula—prioritize those small improvements before considering new purchases. The goal is to create a functional and efficient kitchen space that supports your cooking, not to clutter it with unnecessary tools. With just a few well-chosen essentials, you'll be ready to tackle any recipe with confidence. If you are looking for specific brands and recommendations for any of the listed tools, visit THEAUTOIMMUNEPROTOCOL.COM/COOKINGTOOLS for more information and direct links.

BASIC TOOLS: These are basic kitchen items you'll need to make most of the recipes in this book and should be prioritized first in your assessment of what needs maintenance or what you need to purchase before beginning your healing diet.

- Baking sheets (having two can be handy)
- Blender
- Colander or mesh strainer
- Cooking utensils: mixing spoon, ladle, metal and silicone spatulas, whisk, tongs
- Cutting board (one large and one smaller, for different types of ingredients)
- Roasting dish (preferably large; having two can be handy)
- Stockpot (preferably large)
- Measuring spoons and cups
- Mixing bowls of various sizes
- Sharp knives (an 8-inch chef's knife and a paring knife)
- Skillet (preferably large)
- Storage containers (preferably glass)

AFFORDABLE, USEFUL TOOLS: These are tools that are not required to make the recipes in this book but can make certain tasks much easier. After you've got all your basic tools set up, you can consider adding these to your collection.

- Box grater and/or Microplane zester
- Handheld citrus juicer
- Mini prep or immersion blender
- Mandoline slicer Spiralizer
- Thermometer
- Garlic press
- Bench scraper
- Kitchen shears

ADVANCED TOOLS: Once you have all your basics and some of the smaller, more affordable tools in your set, you can consider some bigger, more expensive items and appliances. I like to consider counter space and/or storage space when adding a larger cooking tool to my collection, in addition to noting what functions it will serve to help me prepare meals.

- **FOOD PROCESSOR:** This appliance is handy for processing raw vegetables and creating other mixtures, purees, and doughs. Additionally, for those who have joint pain or limited hand mobility, a food processor can be used to minimize chopping and make scratch-cooking more achievable.
- **HIGH-POWERED BLENDER:** This tool is different from a regular blender because it has the capability of processing thicker foods, like soups and thick purees. I recommend either owning a food processor and an immersion blender, or a high-powered blender on its own, as both are not necessary.
- **DUTCH OVEN:** This large, somewhat shallow pot with a heavy lid can be used both on the stovetop and in the oven. A Dutch oven can double as a roasting dish, a stockpot, or even a sauté pan; it's one of the most flexible cooking vessels in the kitchen. There are many great brands out there at different price points; I recommend getting one that is at least 6 quarts, but having the extra space in an 8-quart is handy for batch-cooking.
- **MULTI-COOKER:** An electric, programmable, countertop cooker is a handy advanced tool. Most combine two functions: slow cooking and pressure cooking. While it isn't required that you have one to make any of the recipes in this book, they can be big time-savers for tasks like making bone broth or cooking dried beans from scratch.

There are several kitchen tools that I *don't* find necessary while on AIP. These include stand mixers, juicers, toasters, waffle irons, tortilla presses, ice cream makers, countertop fryers, air fryers, and dehydrators. While each of these appliances can certainly be useful and even enjoyable for specific recipes or occasional treats, they aren't necessary for everyday meal preparation. Many of their functions can be achieved with more versatile tools you likely already own, making them more of a luxury than a necessity in a well-equipped healing kitchen. If you already own some of these items, consider storing them away—you can always bring them out later once you've expanded your diet or when you want to make something specific that requires them.

Next: Organize Your Space

A well-organized kitchen makes cooking easier, more enjoyable, and far more efficient. Start by clearing out anything that doesn't serve your cooking needs—whether it's unnecessary gadgets, duplicate tools, or non-kitchen items that have found their way onto your counters. If you're hesitant to part with certain items, consider boxing them up and storing them elsewhere to free up valuable workspace. Creating designated spots for mail, keys, or other household clutter can also prevent distractions and keep your kitchen focused on what it's meant for—cooking.

Once you've cleared the clutter, arrange your appliances and tools in a way that supports your daily cooking habits. Keep frequently used items, like knives, cutting boards, and your go-to appliances, easily accessible, while storing occasional-use tools in cabinets or drawers. If you haven't already, take time to organize your pantry as well—having a well-stocked and tidy pantry makes meal preparation much smoother. With your kitchen set up for efficiency, you'll feel more inspired to cook AIP meals and enjoy the process from start to finish.

CORE AND MODIFIED AIP PANTRY GUIDES

Before beginning the elimination phase of AIP, it's helpful to stock your pantry with some foundational ingredients that you'll frequently use in meal prep. These lists aren't exhaustive guides to everything allowed on Core or Modified AIP (see pages 62 and 66 for the full lists), but rather the essential ingredients featured in recipes throughout this book. By keeping these pantry staples on hand, you'll only need to shop for fresh ingredients each week, making meal prep simpler and more efficient.

CORE AIP BASIC PANTRY ITEMS

FLOURS

- ☐ Arrowroot starch/flour
- ☐ Cassava flour
- ☐ Coconut flour
- ☐ Tapioca starch/flour

SWEETENERS

- ☐ Coconut sugar
- ☐ Honey
- ☐ Maple sugar
- ☐ Maple syrup

COOKING FATS

- ☐ Avocado oil
- ☐ Coconut oil
- ☐ Extra-virgin olive oil

VINEGARS

- ☐ Apple cider vinegar
- ☐ Champagne vinegar
- ☐ Red wine vinegar

ASSORTED FOODS AND FLAVORINGS

- ☐ Anchovies
- ☐ Canned fish (check ingredients)
- ☐ Coconut aminos
- ☐ Coconut milk (check ingredients)
- ☐ Fish sauce
- ☐ Gelatin
- ☐ Mackerel
- ☐ Salmon
- ☐ Sardines
- ☐ Tuna

GROUND SPICES

- ☐ Cinnamon
- ☐ Garlic powder
- ☐ Ginger powder
- ☐ Onion powder
- ☐ Sea salt
- ☐ Turmeric

MODIFIED AIP BASIC PANTRY ITEMS

FLOURS

- ☐ Arrowroot starch/flour
- ☐ Coconut flour
- ☐ Sweet white rice flour
- ☐ Tapioca starch/flour

GRAINS, PSEUDO-GRAINS, AND LEGUMES

- ☐ Buckwheat
- ☐ Dried or canned legumes, all varieties: black, navy, pinto, Great Northern, chickpeas, lentils
- ☐ Pea protein powder
- ☐ Quinoa (whole-grain)
- ☐ Rice (whole-grain), all varieties: basmati, brown, jasmine, wild
- ☐ Rice cakes or crackers (check ingredients)
- ☐ Rice noodles (pad Thai, udon, or pasta-style)
- ☐ Soba noodles (buckwheat only)

SEEDS

- ☐ Cacao powder
- ☐ Flax (whole or ground)
- ☐ Hemp seeds
- ☐ Pumpkin seeds
- ☐ Sesame seeds
- ☐ Sunflower seeds
- ☐ Sunflower seed butter
- ☐ Tahini (sesame butter)

SWEETENERS

- ☐ Coconut sugar
- ☐ Honey
- ☐ Maple sugar
- ☐ Maple syrup

COOKING FATS

- ☐ Avocado oil
- ☐ Coconut oil
- ☐ Extra-virgin olive oil
- ☐ Ghee

VINEGARS

- ☐ Apple cider vinegar
- ☐ Champagne vinegar
- ☐ Red wine vinegar

ASSORTED FOODS AND FLAVORINGS

- ☐ Anchovies
- ☐ Canned fish (check ingredients)
- ☐ Coconut aminos
- ☐ Coconut milk (check ingredients)
- ☐ Fish sauce
- ☐ Gelatin
- ☐ Mackerel
- ☐ Salmon
- ☐ Sardines
- ☐ Tuna

GROUND SPICES

- ☐ Black pepper
- ☐ Cardamom
- ☐ Cinnamon
- ☐ Coriander
- ☐ Cumin
- ☐ Garlic powder
- ☐ Ginger powder
- ☐ Onion powder
- ☐ Sea salt
- ☐ Turmeric

LINING CAKE PANS

If you are making the Citrus and Cherry Celebration Cake (page 190) or the Spiced Pear Upside-Down Cake (page 270), you'll need to know how to properly line both the bottoms and sides of your cake pans to prevent sticking. Make sure to use parchment paper, which is heat-resistant and suitable for baking, and not wax paper, which should only be used for storage.

First, set the bottom of your cake pan on a piece of parchment paper. Trace a circle the size of the bottom of your pan and cut it out about ⅛ inch inside the tracing line. You now have a round for the bottom.

Next, cut a couple of strips of parchment paper that are 5 inches wide and long enough to cover the length of the inside wall of the pan (if you need two strips, make sure they overlap at least 1 inch; more is fine). Fold the strips lengthwise at the 2-inch mark and then cut slits to the fold line every ½ inch or so of the short side. This will help the strips sit nicely in the round pan.

Place the wall strip in the pan before adding the round for the bottom on top. This will keep the slits underneath. Your pan is now fully lined and ready to use for the recipe!

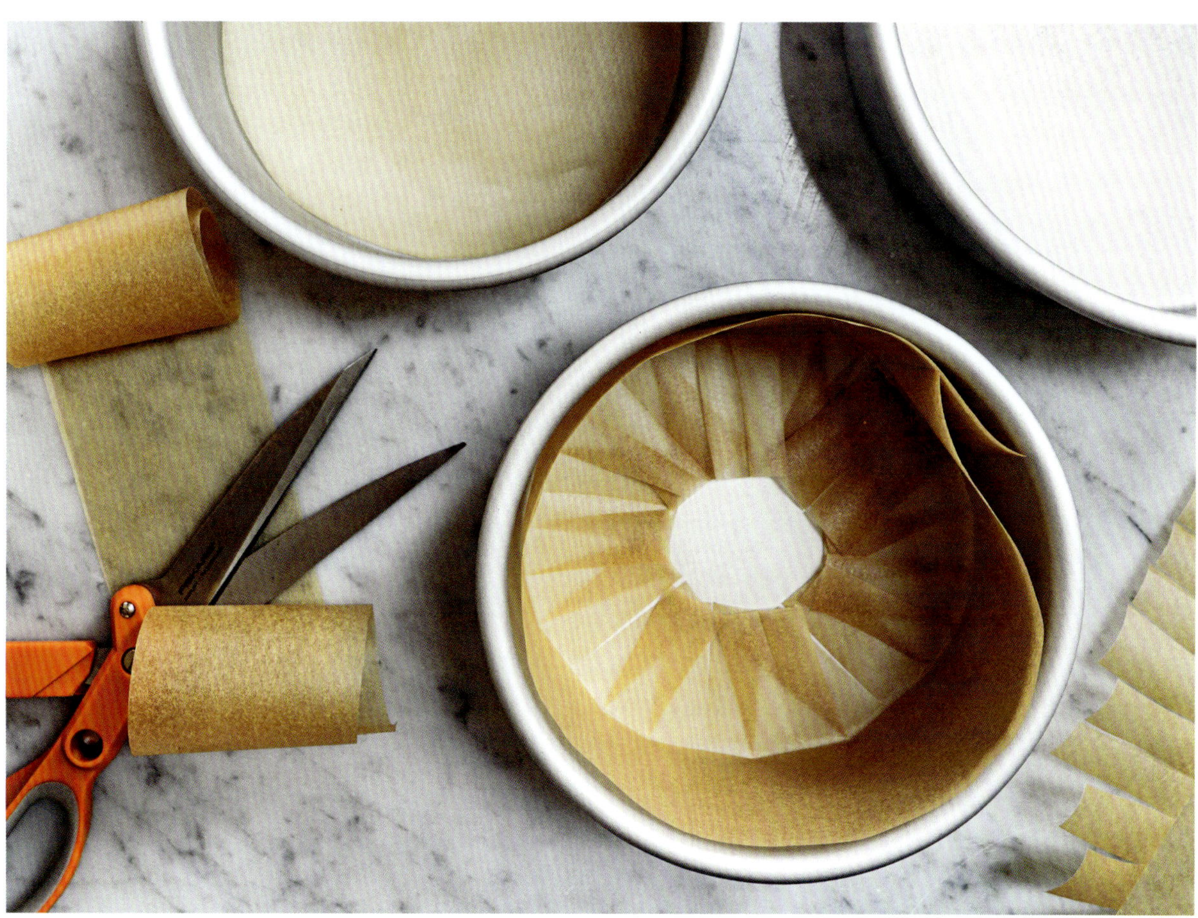

Resources

Food Sourcing

Azure Standard
WWW.AZURESTANDARD.COM

Butcher Box
WWW.BUTCHERBOX.COM

Crowd Cow
WWW.CROWDCOW.COM

Eat Wild
WWW.EATWILD.COM

Local Farm Markets.org
WWW.LOCALFARMMARKETS.ORG

Local Harvest
WWW.LOCALHARVEST.ORG

National Farmers Market Directory
NFMD.ORG

Natural Grocers
WWW.NATURALGROCERS.COM

Pick Your Own
WWW.PICKYOUROWN.ORG

Sprouts Farmers Market
WWW.SPROUTS.COM

Thrive Market
WWW.THRIVEMARKET.COM

Urban AIP Meal Delivery
WWW. URBANAIP.COM

US Wellness Meats
WWW.GRASSLANDBEEF.COM

Vital Choice Wild Seafood and Organics
WWW.VITALCHOICE.COM

Whole Foods Market
WWW.WHOLEFOODSMARKET.COM

Wild Fermentation
WWW.WILDFERMENTATION.COM

Ingredients/Snacks

Artisan Tropic
WWW.ARTISANTROPIC.COM

Bare Bones Broth
WWW.BAREBONESBROTH.COM

Bob's Red Mill
WWW.BOBSREDMILL.COM

Bonafide Provisions Broth
WWW.BONAFIDEPROVISIONS.COM

Coconut Secret
WWW.COCONUTSECRET.COM

Crown Maple Syrup and Sugar
WWW.CROWNMAPLE.COM

Culina Coconut Yogurt
WWW.CULINAYOGURT.COM

Edward & Sons
WWW.EDWARDANDSONS.COM

Great Lakes Gelatin
WWW.GREATLAKESWELLNESS.COM

GT's Kombucha and CocoYo
WWW.GTSLIVINGFOODS.COM

Healthy Traditions
WWW.HEALTHYTRADITIONS.COM

Jackson's
WWW.SNACKJACKSONS.COM

Kettle & Fire Broth
WWW.KETTLEANDFIRE.COM

Lotus Foods
WWW.LOTUSFOODS.COM

Lundberg
WWW.LUNDBERG.COM

McCormick Gourmet
WWW.MCCORMICK.COM/GOURMET

Natural Value
WWW.NATURALVALUE.COM

Nutiva
WWW.NUTIVA.COM

Once Again
WWW.ONCEAGAIN.COM

Otto's Naturals
WWW.OTTOSNATURALS.COM

Primal Kitchen
WWW.PRIMALKITCHEN.COM

Real Salt
WWW.REALSALT.COM

Red Boat Fish Sauce
WWW.REDBOATFISHSAUCE.COM

Seasnax
WWW.SEASNAX.COM

Sip Herbals
WWW.SIPHERBALS.COM

Sunfood Organics
WWW.SUNFOOD.COM

Sweet Apricity
WWW.SWEETAPRICITY.COM

Kitchen Tools

Bamboo Spoons
WWW.AUTOIMMUNEWELLNESS.COM/BAMBOOSPOONS

Berkey Filters
WWW.USABERKEYFILTERS.COM

Cuisinart
WWW.CUISINART.COM

GIR Spatula
WWW.GIR.CO

Instant Pot
WWW.INSTANTPOT.COM

Kitchen Aid
WWW.KITCHENAID.COM

Lodge Cast Iron
WWW.LODGECASTIRON.COM

Made In
WWW.MADEIN.COM

Mickey Recommends
WWW.AUTOIMMUNEWELLNESS.COM/SETTING-UP-YOUR-AIP-KITCHEN

Nordic Ware Bundt
WWW.NORDICWARE.COM

Spiralizer
WWW.AUTOIMMUNEWELLNESS.COM/SPIRALIZER

Sur la Table
WWW.SURLATABLE.COM

ThermoWorks
WWW.THERMOWORKS.COM

Vitamix
WWW.VITAMIX.COM

Autoimmune Protocol Online Resources

The AIP BIPOC Network
WWW.AIPBIPOC.ORG

The AIP Certified Coach Practitioner Directory
WWW.AIPCERTIFIED.COM

The AIP Summit and Monthly Webinars
WWW.AIPSUMMIT.COM

The Autoimmune Protocol Website and Resources
WWW.THEAUTOIMMUNEPROTOCOL.COM

The Autoimmune Wellness Blog and AIP Recipe Archive
WWW.AUTOIMMUNEWELLNESS.COM

The Autoimmune Wellness Podcast
WWW.AUTOIMMUNEWELLNESS.COM/AWP

Finding a Doctor

Academy of Integrative Health and Medicine
WWW.AIHM.ORG

The AIP Certified Coach Practitioner Directory
WWW.AIPCERTIFIED.COM

The American Association of Naturopathic Physicians
WWW.NATUROPATHIC.ORG

American College for Advancement in Medicine
WWW.ACAM.ORG

Canadian Association of Naturopathic Doctors
WWW.CAND.CA

The Institute for Functional Medicine
WWW.IFM.ORG

International College of Integrative Medicine
WWW.ICIMED.COM

Autoimmune Disease Organizations

The AIP BIPOC Network
WWW.AIPBIPOC.ORG

Autoimmune Association
AUTOIMMUNE.ORG

Arthritis Foundation
WWW.ARTHRITIS.ORG

Celiac Disease Foundation
WWW.CELIAC.ORG

Crohn's and Colitis Foundation of America
WWW.CCFA.ORG

Endometriosis.org
WWW.ENDOMETRIOSIS.ORG

Graves' Disease and Thyroid Foundation
WWW.GDATF.ORG

International Foundation for Autoimmune Arthritis
WWW.AIARTHRITIS.ORG

Lupus and Allied Diseases Association
WWW.NOLUPUS.ORG

Lupus Foundation of America
WWW.LUPUS.ORG

Myasthenia Gravis Foundation of America, Inc.
WWW.MYASTHENIA.ORG

The Myasthenia Gravis Holistic Society
WWW.MGHOLISTICSOCIETY.ORG

The Myositis Association
WWW.MYOSITIS.ORG

National Alopecia Areata Foundation
WWW.NAAF.ORG

National Multiple Sclerosis Society
WWW.NATIONALMSSOCIETY.ORG

National Psoriasis Foundation
WWW.PSORIASIS.ORG

National Scleroderma Foundation

Platelet Disorder Support Association
WWW.PDSA.ORG
WWW.SCLERODERMA.ORG

Sjögren's Foundation
WWW.SJOGRENS.ORG

References

Chapter 1: Autoimmune and AIP Basics

1. Fairweather, DeLisa, and Noel R. Rose. 2004. "Women and Autoimmune Diseases." *Emerging Infectious Diseases* 10 (11): 2005–11. doi: 10.3201/eid1011.040367.
2. Tucker, Miriam E. "Closing the Care Gap in Autoimmune Disease," last modified October 4, 2018, https://autoimmune.org/closing-care-gap-autoimmune-disease/.
3. Scott, I. C., et al. 2016. "Impact of Intensive Treatment and Remission on Health-Related Quality of Life in Early and Established Rheumatoid Arthritis." *RMD Open* 2 (2): e–e000270. doi: 10.1136/rmdopen-2016-000270.
4. Li, Jiaomei, et al. 2024. "Thyroid Antibodies in Hashimoto's Thyroiditis Patients Are Positively Associated with Inflammation and Multiple Symptoms." *Scientific Reports* 14 (1): 27902–12. doi: 10.1038/s41598-024-78938-7.
5. Autoimmune Wellness. "Stories of Recovery Index," last modified January 2022, accessed January 9, 2025, https://autoimmunewellness.com/stories-recovery-index/.
6. Konijeti, Gauree G., et al. 2017. "Efficacy of the Autoimmune Protocol Diet for Inflammatory Bowel Disease." *Inflammatory Bowel Diseases* 23 (11): 2054–60. doi: 10.1097/MIB.0000000000001221.
7. Lee, Joy, et al. 2019. "Clinical Course and Dietary Patterns among Patients Incorporating the Autoimmune Protocol for Management of Inflammatory Bowel Disease (P12-010-19)." *Current Developments in Nutrition* 3 (Suppl 1): nzz035.P12–19. doi: 10.1093/cdn/nzz035.P12-010-19.
8. Abbott, Robert D., et al. 2019. "Efficacy of the Autoimmune Protocol Diet as Part of a Multi-Disciplinary, Supported Lifestyle Intervention for Hashimoto's Thyroiditis." *Cureus* 11 (4): e4556. doi: 10.7759/cureus.4556.
9. Ihnatowicz, Paulina, et al. 2023. "Effects of Autoimmune Protocol (AIP) Diet on Changes in Thyroid Parameters in Hashimoto's Disease." *AAEM. Annals of Agricultural and Environmental Medicine/Annals of Agricultural and Environmental Medicine* 30 (3): 513–21. doi: 10.26444/aaem/166263.
10. Konijeti et al., "Efficacy of the Autoimmune Protocol Diet."
11. Chandrasekaran, Anita, et al. 2019. "An Autoimmune Protocol Diet Improves Patient-Reported Quality of Life in Inflammatory Bowel Disease." *Crohn's and Colitis 360* 1 (3): otz019. doi: 10.1093/crocol/otz019.
12. Chandrasekaran, Anita, et al. 2019. "The Autoimmune Protocol Diet Modifies Intestinal RNA Expression in Inflammatory Bowel Disease." *Crohn's and Colitis 360* 1 (3): otz016. doi: 10.1093/crocol/otz016.
13. Lee et al., "Clinical Course and Dietary Patterns."
14. Abbott et al., "Efficacy of the Autoimmune Protocol Diet."
15. Ihnatowicz et al., "Effects of Autoimmune Protocol (AIP) Diet."
16. Taylor, Julianne. "Rheumatoid Arthritis and the Paleo Diet—a Qualitative Study," last modified August 17, 2020, accessed November 27, 2024, https://autoimmunewellness.com/rheumatoid-arthritis-and-the-paleo-diet-a-qualitative-study/.
17. McNeill, Julianne, et al. 2023. "What Is the Efficacy of the Autoimmune Protocol (AIP) Diet in People with Rheumatoid Arthritis? A Mixed-Methods Pilot Intervention Study." *Medical Sciences Forum* 18 (1): 10. doi: 10.3390/msf2023018010.
18. Philpott, H., et al. 2016. "Allergy Tests Do Not Predict Food Triggers in Adult Patients with Eosinophilic Oesophagitis. A Comprehensive Prospective Study Using Five Modalities." *Alimentary Pharmacology & Therapeutics* 44 (3): 223–33. doi: 10.1111/apt.13676.
19. Pitsios, Constantinos, et al. 2022. "Allergy-Test-Based Elimination Diets for the Treatment of Eosinophilic Esophagitis: A Systematic Review of Their Efficacy." *Journal of Clinical Medicine* 11 (19): 5631. doi: 10.3390/jcm11195631.
20. Capobianco, Ivan, et al. 2024. "Adverse Food Reactions in Inflammatory Bowel Disease: State of the Art and Future Perspectives." *Nutrients* 16 (3): 351. doi: 10.3390/nu16030351.
21. Yan, Manli, et al. 2024. "Analysis of the Correlation between Hashimoto's Thyroiditis and Food Intolerance." *Frontiers in Nutrition (Lausanne)* 11: 1452371. doi: 10.3389/fnut.2024.1452371.
22. Kuang, Rebecca, et al. 2023. "Nightshade Vegetables: A Dietary Trigger for Worsening Inflammatory Bowel Disease and Irritable Bowel Syndrome?" *Digestive Diseases and Sciences* 68 (7): 2853–60. doi: 10.1007/s10620-023-07955-9.
23. Gombart, Adrian F., et al. 2020. "A Review of Micronutrients and the Immune System—Working in Harmony to Reduce the Risk of Infection." *Nutrients* 12 (1): 236. doi: 10.3390/nu12010236.
24. Reider, Carroll A., et al. 2020. "Inadequacy of Immune Health Nutrients: Intakes in US Adults, the 2005–2016 NHANES." *Nutrients* 12 (6): 1735. doi: 10.3390/nu12061735.
25. Ihnatowicz et al., "Effects of Autoimmune Protocol (AIP) Diet."
26. Abbott et al., "Efficacy of the Autoimmune Protocol Diet."
27. Konijeti et al., "Efficacy of the Autoimmune Protocol Diet."
28. Chandrasekaran et al., "The Autoimmune Protocol Diet Modifies Intestinal RNA Expression."

Chapter 3: Elimination Phase

1. Bryce, Paul J. 2016. "Balancing Tolerance or Allergy to Food Proteins." *Trends in Immunology* 37 (10): 659–67. doi: 10.1016/j.it.2016.08.008.
2. Philpott, et al., "Allergy Tests Do Not Predict Food Triggers."
3. Pitsios, et al., "Allergy-Test-Based Elimination Diets."
4. Konijeti et al., "Efficacy of the Autoimmune Protocol Diet."
5. Turnbull, J. L., et al. 2015. "Review Article: The Diagnosis and Management of Food Allergy and Food Intolerances." *Alimentary Pharmacology & Therapeutics* 41 (1): 3–25. doi: 10.1111/apt.12984.

Chapter 4: Reintroduction Phase

1. Turnbull et al., "The Diagnosis and Management of Food Allergy."
2. Philpott et al., "Allergy Tests Do Not Predict Food Triggers."
3. Lee et al., "Clinical Course and Dietary Patterns."
4. Taylor, "Rheumatoid Arthritis and the Paleo Diet."
5. Fritscher-Ravens, A., et al. 2019. "Many Patients with Irritable Bowel Syndrome Have Atypical Food Allergies Not Associated with Immunoglobulin E." *Gastroenterology (New York, NY, 1943)* 157 (1): 109–118.e5. doi: 10.1053/j.gastro.2019.03.046.
6. Wahls, Terry L., et al. 2021. "Impact of the Swank and Wahls Elimination Dietary Interventions on Fatigue and Quality of Life in Relapsing-Remitting Multiple Sclerosis: The WAVES Randomized Parallel-Arm Clinical Trial." *Multiple Sclerosis Journal—Experimental, Translational and Clinical* 7 (3): 20552173211035399. doi: 10.1177/20552173211035399.

Chapter 5: Nutrient Density and Lifestyle

1. Konijeti et al., "Efficacy of the Autoimmune Protocol Diet."
2. Abbott et al., "Efficacy of the Autoimmune Protocol Diet."
3. Ihnatowicz et al., "Effects of Autoimmune Protocol (AIP) Diet."
4. Konijeti et al., "Efficacy of the Autoimmune Protocol Diet."
5. Abbott et al., "Efficacy of the Autoimmune Protocol Diet."
6. Haas, Elson, and Buck Levin. 2012. *Staying Healthy with Nutrition: The Complete Guide to Diet and Nutritional Medicine*. 21st-century ed. Celestial Arts.
7. Reider, Carroll A., et al. 2020. "Inadequacy of Immune Health Nutrients: Intakes in US Adults, the 2005–2016 NHANES." *Nutrients* 12 (6): 1735. doi: 10.3390/nu12061735.
8. Gombart, Adrian F., et al. 2020. "A Review of Micronutrients and the Immune System–Working in Harmony to Reduce the Risk of Infection." *Nutrients* 12 (1): 236. doi: 10.3390/nu12010236.
9. Newsholme, Philip. 2001. "Why Is L-Glutamine Metabolism Important to Cells of the Immune System in Health, Postinjury, Surgery or Infection?" *The Journal of Nutrition* 131 (9): 2515S—22S. doi: 10.1093/jn/131.9.2515s.
10. Mar-Solís, Laura M., et al. 2021. "Analysis of the Anti-Inflammatory Capacity of Bone Broth in a Murine Model of Ulcerative Colitis." *Medicina (Kaunas, Lithuania)* 57 (11): 1138. doi: 10.3390/medicina57111138.
11. Monjotin, Nicolas, et al. 2022. "Clinical Evidence of the Benefits of Phytonutrients in Human Healthcare." *Nutrients* 14 (9): 1712–54. doi: 10.3390/nu14091712.
12. Leeuwendaal, Natasha K., et al. 2022. "Fermented Foods, Health and the Gut Microbiome." *Nutrients* 14 (7): 1527. doi: 10.3390/nu14071527.
13. Latoch, Agnieszka, et al. 2024. "Edible Offal as a Valuable Source of Nutrients in the Diet—A Review." *Nutrients* 16 (11): 1609. doi: 10.3390/nu16111609.
14. Mendivil, Carlos O. 2021. *Fish Consumption: A Review of Its Effects on Metabolic and Hormonal Health*. Vol. 14. London, England: SAGE Publications.
15. Zielinski, Mark R., et al. 2019. "Fatigue, Sleep, and Autoimmune and Related Disorders." *Frontiers in Immunology* 10: 1827. doi: 10.3389/fimmu.2019.01827.
16. Grabovac, Igor, et al. 2018. "Sleep Quality in Patients with Rheumatoid Arthritis and Associations with Pain, Disability, Disease Duration, and Activity." *Journal of Clinical Medicine* 7 (10): 336. doi: 10.3390/jcm7100336.
17. Ananthakrishnan, Ashwin N., et al. 2013. "Sleep Disturbance and Risk of Active Disease in Patients with Crohn's Disease and Ulcerative Colitis." *Clinical Gastroenterology and Hepatology* 11 (8): 965–71. doi: 10.1016/j.cgh.2013.01.021.
18. Song, Huan, et al. 2018. "Association of Stress-Related Disorders with Subsequent Autoimmune Disease." *JAMA: The Journal of the American Medical Association* 319 (23): 2388–400. doi: 10.1001/jama.2018.7028.
19. Sun, Yue, et al. 2019. "Stress Triggers Flare of Inflammatory Bowel Disease in Children and Adults." *Frontiers in Pediatrics* 7: 432. doi: 10.3389/fped.2019.00432.
20. Yılmaz, Volkan, et al. 2017. "Rheumatoid Arthritis: Are Psychological Factors Effective in Disease Flare?" *European Journal of Rheumatology* 4 (2): 127–32. doi: 10.5152/eurjrheum.2017.16100.
21. Markomanolaki, Zoe S., et al. 2019. "Stress Management in Women with Hashimoto's Thyroiditis: A Randomized Controlled Trial." *Journal of Molecular Biochemistry* 8 (1): 3–12. https://www.ncbi.nlm.nih.gov/pubmed/31404454.
22. Alishiri, Gholamhossein, et al. 2017. "Effect of Stress Management on Quality of Life in Females with Rheumatoid Arthritis." *Iranian Journal of Psychiatry and Behavioral Sciences* 11 (3). doi: 10.5812/ijpbs.9605.
23. Sharif, Kassem, et al. 2018. "Physical Activity and Autoimmune Diseases: Get Moving and Manage the Disease." *Autoimmunity Reviews* 17 (1): 53–72. doi: 10.1016/j.autrev.2017.11.010.

Index

C

D

E

F

Q

R

S

T

U

V

W

Y

Z

Gratitude

No book is made alone—especially one full of research and recipes. I'm endlessly thankful to the people who helped shape this book from start to finish. To Donna Loffredo, my editor, and her team at Rodale, for not only seeing the potential in AIP but wanting to craft a beautiful and useful book that would serve the autoimmune community for years to come. To Leda Scheintaub, for bringing clarity and accuracy to these pages. To Jaidree Braddix, my agent, for honing my vision and advocating for me every step of the way. I am lucky to have you in my corner!

I am grateful to many for helping shape the recipes and photography in this book. To Jenny Davis, Lynne Yeamans, and the Rodale art and design teams—this book is a work of art due to your craft. To Felix Madrid, Hannah Jones, and Grace Hoober, my photoshoot A-team—thank you for the hours of cooking, endless loads of dishes, and great ideas. To James Sullivan and Spencer Norris, who provided technical advice and production sourcing. To Kyle Johnson, for photographing me in my studio kitchen. Our collaboration on the original AIP cookbook more than a decade ago eventually led to this project—it feels right to have your images in this book, too. To Wendy Sullivan and Leila Cearley, who lent some gorgeous pieces from their pottery collections.

I also want to thank those who kept nurturing the AIP community while I was engaged in research and writing. To Jaime Hartman, my partner at AIP Certified Coach and fellow AIP community leader, I am endlessly proud of the work we do together and grateful to you for managing most of our shared ventures while I was busy with this project. To Jaime Nicole Martin, for continuing to show up for the AIP community through your work with the AIP BIPOC Network. And to the AIP Certified Coaches, for your work with AIP research and serving individuals seeking health; this work is both necessary and important to the growth of the AIP movement.

This book is also the product of endless support from my family and friends. To Noah, your steadiness and encouragement were the backbone of this project. Your belief in me never wavered, and that made all the difference. I adore you. My family—Rose, Brian, James, Kyle, and Katie—thank you all for supporting me as I navigated the process of creating yet another book, and for doing the "hard" job of being my primary taste-testers. To Alaina Moore, for being the friend who could completely understand the demands of creation under the strain of a new health crisis. And to Stacy Pulice, Susan McCauley, and Mary Cloos, for being the friends who listened when things got hard and I needed a boost of encouragement.

Last, I'd like to thank the AIP community—your collective wisdom, curiosity, and resilience has shaped this movement in powerful ways. This book stands on the foundation you helped build, and I am deeply inspired by you.

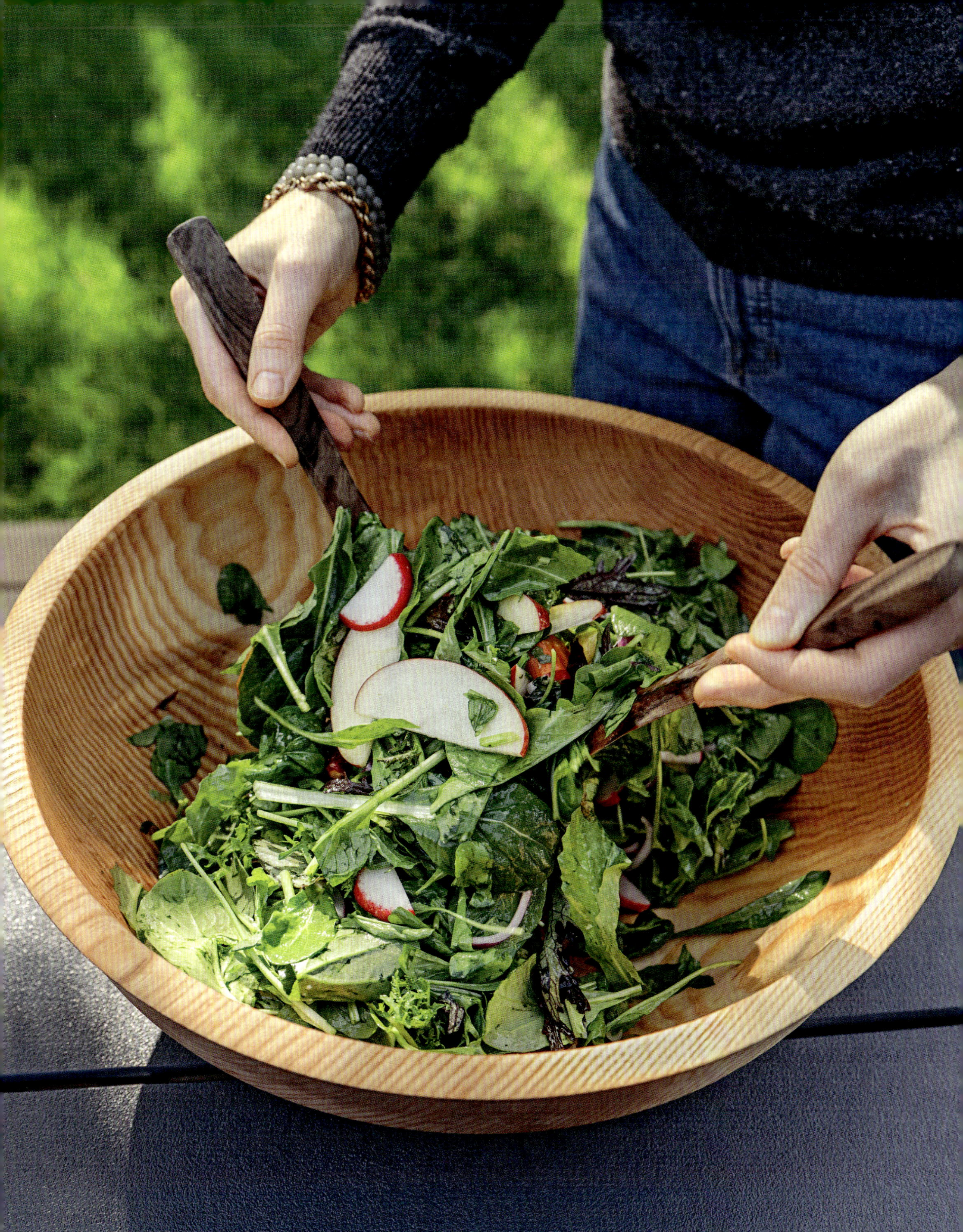

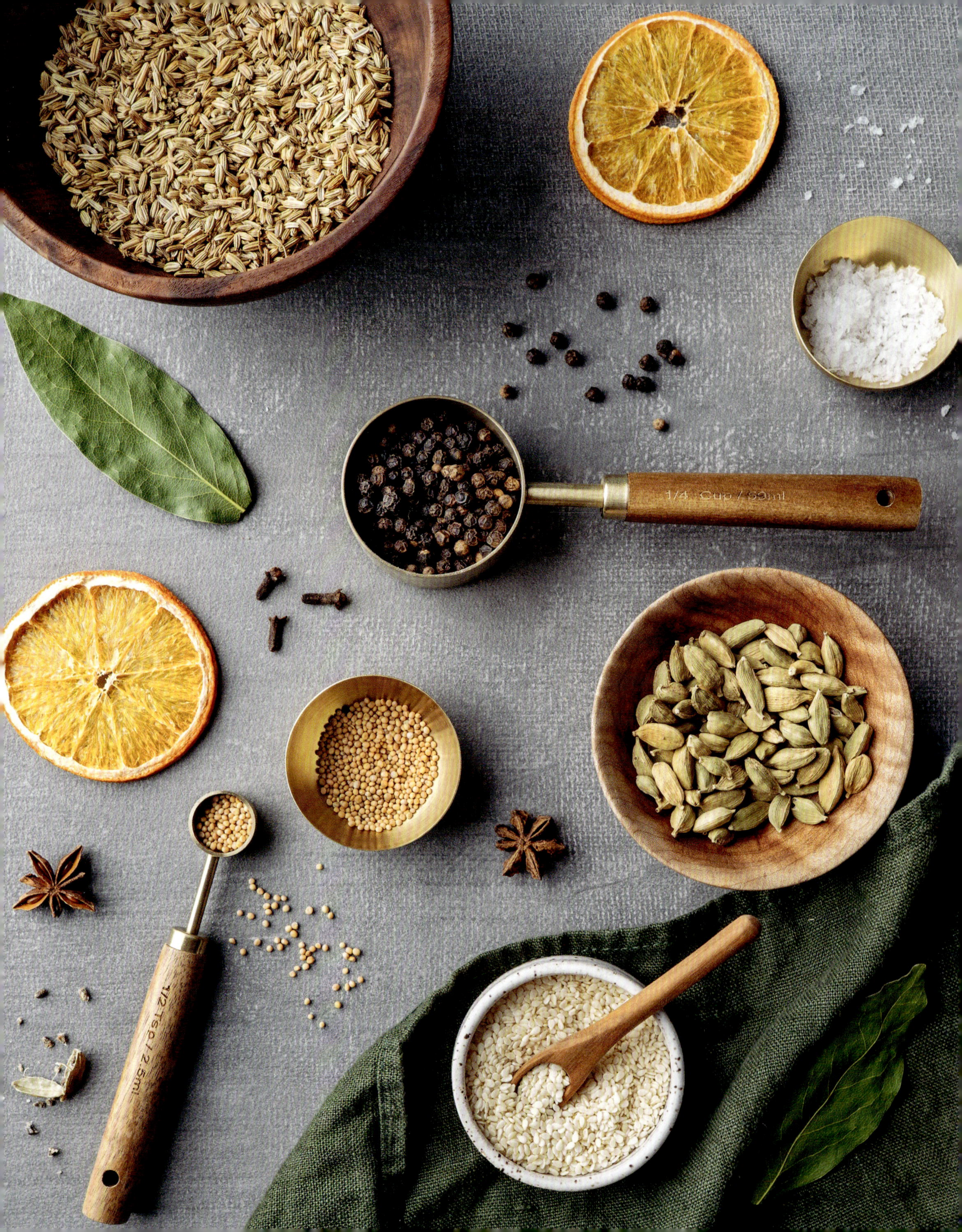
1/4 Cup / 59ml
1/2 Tsp / 2.5ml

Rodale Books
An imprint of Random House
A division of Penguin Random House LLC
1745 Broadway, New York, NY 10019
RODALEBOOKS.COM | RANDOMHOUSEBOOKS.COM
PENGUINRANDOMHOUSE.COM

"Healing Bone Broth" and "Fermented Vegetables" were originally published in *The Autoimmune Wellness Handbook* by Mickey Trescott, NTP, and Angie Alt (New York: Rodale Wellness, 2016).

Photographs by the author except for photos on pages 2, 3, 13, 19, 48, 301, and 304 which are by Kyle Johnson.

Library of Congress Cataloging-in-Publication Data

ISBN 9780593980835
Ebook ISBN 9780593980842

Printed in China

2 4 6 8 9 7 5 3 1

First Edition

BOOK TEAM:
Editor: Donna Loffredo | Editorial Assistant: Mia Pulido
Creative Director: Jenny Davis
Art Director: Lynne Yeamans
Designer: Zaiah Antwi
Managing Editor: Allison Fox
Production Editor: Cassie Gitkin
Production Manager: Kevin Garcia
Photographer: Mickey Trescott
Food and Prop Stylist: Mickey Trescott
Compositor: Merri Ann Morrell
Copy Editor: Leda Scheintaub
Proofreaders: Marisa Crumb, Mindy Fichter, Ella Maoz, Jinah Yoon
Indexer: Thérèse Shere
Publicist: Hannah Dirgins
Marketer: Elizabeth Groening

The authorized representative in the EU for product safety and compliance is Penguin Random House Ireland, Morrison Chambers, 32 Nassau Street, Dublin D02 YH68, Ireland.
HTTPS://EU-CONTACT.PENGUIN.IE

About the Author

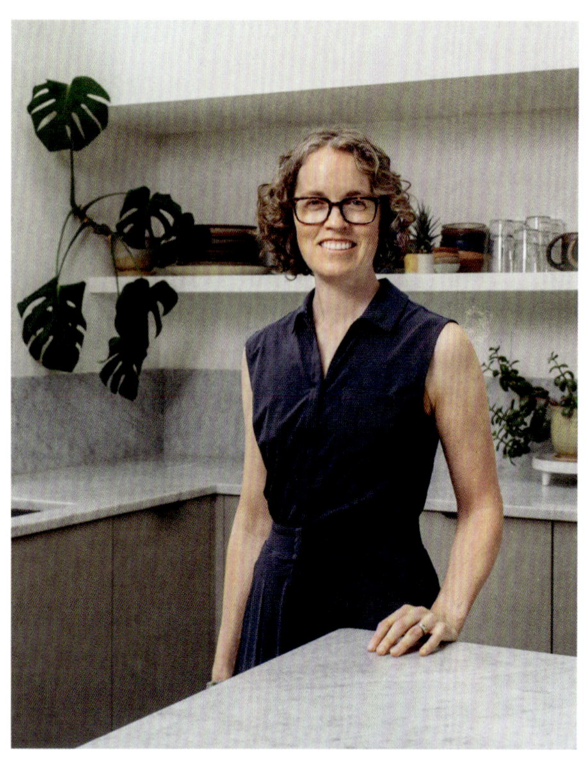

MICKEY TRESCOTT, M.SC., is an author, recipe creator, and holistic nutritionist, widely recognized for her expertise in living well with autoimmune disease and implementing the Autoimmune Protocol. She is the author of three best-selling and award-winning books: *The Autoimmune Paleo Cookbook, The Autoimmune Wellness Handbook,* and *The Nutrient-Dense Kitchen*. Beyond her authorship, Mickey is the leading voice in the autoimmune community through her influential website, Autoimmune Wellness (autoimmunewellness.com), her podcast *The Autoimmune Wellness Podcast*, and associated social media channels, which have collectively served millions of wellness-seekers since 2012. Mickey lives in Portland, Oregon, where she is perpetually working on a sustainable home renovation, playing pickleball, and developing an edible suburban yard with her husband, Noah.

MICKEYTRESCOTT.COM

INSTAGRAM.COM/MICKEYTRESCOTT

YOUTUBE.COM/MICKEYTRESCOTT

THEAUTOIMMUNEPROTOCOL.COM